GCSE
Health and Social Care
FOR EDEXCEL

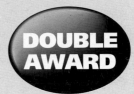

DOUBLE AWARD

Elizabeth Haworth
Carol Forshaw
Neil Moonie

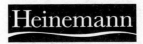

Heinemann

Heinemann Educational Publishers,
Halley Court, Jordan Hill, Oxford OX2 8EJ
A division of Harcourt Education Limited

Heinemann is a registered trademark of Harcourt Education Limited

OXFORD MELBOURNE AUCKLAND JOHANNESBURG BLANTYRE
GABORONE IBADAN PORTSMOUTH NH (USA) CHICAGO

© Elizabeth Haworth and Carol Forshaw, 2002

First published 2002
2006 2005 2004 2003 2002
10 9 8 7 6 5 4 3 2 1

A catalogue record for this book is available from the British Library
on request.

ISBN 0 435 47141 4

Pages designed by Artistix, Thame, Oxon
Typeset and illustrated by ⚐ Tek-Art, Croydon, Surrey
Printed and bound in Italy by Printer Trento S.r.l.

Acknowledgements
Every effort has been made to contact copyright holders of material
reproduced in this book. Any omissions will be rectified in subsequent
printings if notice is given to the publishers.

Tel: 01865 888058 www.heinemann.co.uk

Contents

Acknowledgements

Elizabeth Haworth would like to thank her family, Mike, Emma and Ben, for their patience and unquestioning support throughout the writing process. She would also like to thank her parents for having faith in her and for providing encouragement; her stepdaughter Sarah Haworth, BA, for factual input from the International Labour Organisation in Geneva on AIDS and HIV; her stepdaughter Rachel Johnson, BA, MSc, and husband Mike, BA, MSc, for their suggestions; Sally Forshaw, RGN, RM, BA, Nursing Development Manager of the Ashton, Leigh and Wigan Primary Care Trust, for providing factual backup and help with some of the text; and Ann Amsbro, BA, CSS, for factual support.

Carol Forshaw would like to thank her partner Ellis and her friend Pat for their unwavering support during the time it took to write this book, her sisters Christine Rigby, BSc, MSc, SRN, and Gillian Moss, RGN, RSCN, Dip. Nursing, for their professional help and advice, and her parents for their support.

The authors would both like to thank their colleagues in the Science Department at Lowton High School for putting up with their endless discussions about the book and their Headteacher for her support.

Photo acknowledgements

Robert Harding p. 223
Trevor Hill p. 11
Format/Brenda Prince p.23, p.213
Format/Jacky Chapman p.170 (top right)
Format/Joanne O'Brien p.52, p.197
Format/Judy Harrison p. 202, p.232
Format/Melanie Friend p.62
Format/Miriam Reik p.158
Format/Pam Isherwood p.226
Format/Paula Solloway p.39, p.101
Format/Roshini Kempadoo p.189
Foundation for the Study of Infant Death p.98
Photodisc p.170 (top left and bottom), p.187
S&R Greenhill p.22, p.48, p.120, p.170 (middle), p.171, p.203, p.213, p.224, p.237
Science Photo Library p.63

The authors and publisher would also like to thank the following organisations for allowing us to reproduce material in this book:

The Centre for Policy on Ageing for permission to reproduce an extract from 'Home Life: A Code of Practice for Residential Care' (1984) on p.77.

The Department of Health for permission to reproduce 'National surveys of NHS patients, General Practice 1998: Summary of key findings (Oct 1999, NHS Executive) on p.40 and Table 17 from 'Health and Personal Social Services Statistics' on p.45.

The Nursing and Midwifery Council for permission to reproduce an extract from 'Code of Professional Conduct' (2002) on p. 78.

The Royal College of Nursing for permission to reproduce an extract from 'Guidance on Employing Nurses in General Practice' (2002) on p.81.

Introduction

How to use this book

This book has been written for students who are working to the 2002 National Standards for the GCSE in Health and Social Care (Double Award). It covers the three compulsory units:

1 Health, social care and early years provision
2 Promoting health and well-being
3 Understanding personal development and relationships

By working through the units, you will find all the knowledge and ideas you need to successfully complete both your portfolio coursework for Units 1 and 2, and the external assessment for Unit 3.

Special features

Throughout this book, there are a number of features which are designed to encourage discussion and group work, and to help you to see how theory is put into practice in Health and Social Care. These activities will not only help you achieve your GCSE in Health and Social Care, but will also enable you to build up a portfolio of key skills.

The features of this book are:

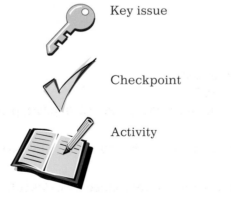

Key issue		The key issue covered in each chapter.
Checkpoint		Definitions of key terms.
Activity		Activities that encourage you to apply theory in a practical way.

 Red arrows indicate core level activities to be attempted by everyone.

 Green arrows indicate extension activities to be attempted by students aiming to gain a higher grade pass. There are also more in-depth practice activities at the end of some chapters.

Case study

Case studies of real (or simulated) issues in health and social care. Questions on the case studies will enable you to explore the key issues and broaden your understanding of the subject.

Check your knowledge

Questions to check your knowledge at the end of each section.

Did you know?

Interesting facts and snippets of information about health and social care

Snapshot

Close-ups of people either working in or affected by health and social care services, and the problems and challenges they face.

How you will be assessed

Assessment is by means of portfolio work for Units 1 and 2 and an externally set test for Unit 3. Your portfolio is marked by your teacher and is moderated by the exam board. The Unit 3 test is set and marked by the exam board. Sample assessment material can be found at the end of each unit.

Finally, good luck with your studies and your chosen career.

Unit 1

Health, social care and early years provision

Introduction to Unit 1

Learning about the areas of care that are provided, the way in which the services are organised and the different jobs available will help to prepare you to make your own decisions about a career in health, social care and early years work.

What you will learn

In this unit you will learn about:

- the range of care needs of major client groups;
- the types of services that exist to meet client group needs and how these are organised;
- the ways people can obtain care services and the barriers that can prevent people from gaining access to services;
- the major work roles and skills of the people who provide health, social care and early years services; and
- the values that underpin all care work with clients.

You will understand more about the work of health, social care and early years service providers by:

- understanding how services are developed in response to social policy goals and to meet the needs of individuals; and
- knowing about the different services and job roles.

Assessment

This unit is assessed through portfolio work. Your overall result for the unit will be a grade from G to A*.

By the end of this chapter you will have learnt how care services are designed to meet the health, development and social care needs of major client groups. You should understand that services are shaped to meet the needs of individual users. The major client groups are:

- babies and children
- adolescents
- adults
- older people
- disabled people.

You will learn how services are developed and provided to meet social policy goals, such as reducing child poverty, homelessness and drug misuse in the population as a whole. You will also learn that health authorities and local authorities assess the care needs of local populations in order to identify likely service demand in a local area. You should also be able to identify and describe the reasons why individuals may require and seek to use health, social care and early years services.

Client groups

Different groups of people, because of their age or physical abilities, have different health needs. These different groups of people are called *client groups*. The ones you need to know about are shown in Figure 1.1. These are the client groups who need to use care services – you need to learn them.

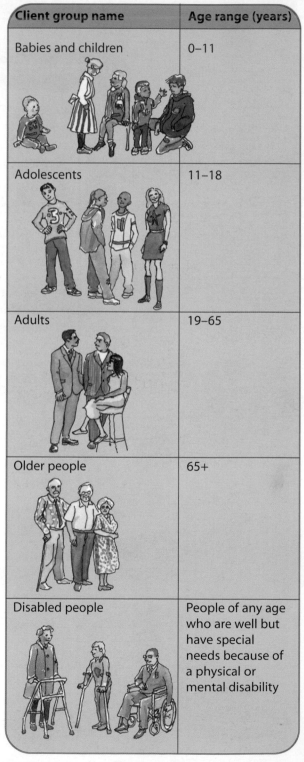

Client group name	Age range (years)
Babies and children	0–11
Adolescents	11–18
Adults	19–65
Older people	65+
Disabled people	People of any age who are well but have special needs because of a physical or mental disability

Figure 1.1 The major client groups

Health, developmental and social care needs

In order to understand who needs to use care services and why, you need to know the general needs of each of the client groups. These can be divided into the following categories:

- **Health needs:** Those things we need in order to stay *physically* healthy (see Figure 1.2).

- **Developmental needs:** Those things we need in order to develop *intellectually*. For example, as a baby develops into a child the baby needs more advanced toys to stimulate her or his brain (see Figure 1.3).

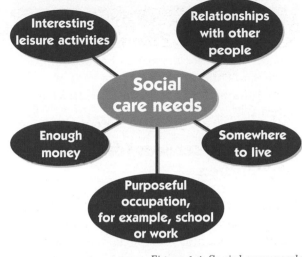

Figure 1.4 Social care needs

- **Social care needs:** Those things we need throughout our lives to support us *socially and emotionally* and to keep us *settled* in our community (see Figure 1.4).

However, other needs vary from client group to client group. We will look at the extra needs of each group so that you can understand how care services are designed and shaped to meet the health, development and social care needs of these groups and individual members of these groups.

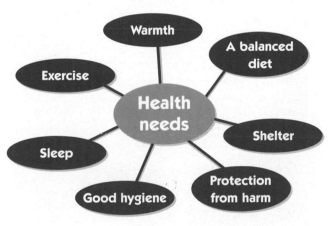

Figure 1.2 Health needs

Babies and children (aged 0–11 years)

Care services for babies and children are designed to help their carers to meet all their needs.

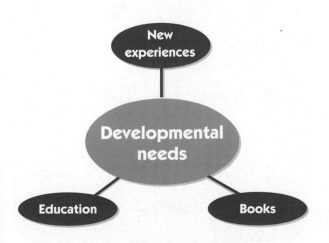

Figure 1.3 Developmental needs

Activity

- Work with a partner and write down the needs of a newborn baby.
- Discuss why the needs of a baby change as the baby grows older.
- Try to write down as many ways as you can think of how someone caring for a child can make sure all the child's needs are met.

Early years services

The early years services are those services that provide health, social care and education services to children between the ages of 0 and 8 years. Some examples are shown in Figure 1.5.

Health care services for babies and children

In addition to the health care offered to all people, there are special services for children:

- **Maternity services:** Before a baby is born and up to 10 weeks after the birth, the mother and child are looked after by a midwife.
- **Health screening:** From the age of 10 weeks all children are seen in their own homes by health visitors, who give children regular developmental tests. These tests are for growth and development, sight and hearing.
- **Vaccination and immunisations:** Children are given a programme of injections (starting at the age of 8 weeks) to protect

Setting	Provider	Description
Childminders	Private; registered with local authority	A childminder looks after other people's children in the childminder's own home. This might include looking after other children after school as well as looking after children under 5 years of age during the day
Nannies	Private; no registration required	A nanny looks after children in the children's own home
Day nurseries	Statutory or private; inspected by OFSTED	A day nursery is open all year round and children under 5 years of age can stay all day
Workplace nurseries	Statutory or private; inspected by OFSTED	A workplace nursery is organised by an employer and the places are often subsidised. This means the employee does not pay the full cost
Crèches	Private or local authority run	Crèches look after children under 8 years of age for short periods of time. For example, they are found in new shopping centres, allowing parents to shop for a few hours
Playgroups	Voluntary or private	Playgroups are non-profit-making groups designed to give children under 5 years of age an opportunity to play. Sessions are often two to three hours long
Nurseries or kindergartens	Statutory or private; inspected by OFSTED	Nurseries and kindergartens offer sessions in mornings and afternoons that allow children under 5 years of age to learn and play
Nurseries within schools	Run by local education authority	Some infant or primary schools have a nursery attached. The nurseries take children from 3 to 4 years of age. No charge is made to the parents
Infant and primary schools	Run by local education authority; inspected by OFSTED	Infant and primary schools take children from the age of 5 years. The normal school day is about six hours long
After-school clubs	Voluntary or private	After-school clubs look after children over the age of 5 years after school has finished during term time. They are often used by working parents
Holiday play schemes	Run by local authorities and private and voluntary groups	Holiday play schemes look after children over the age of 5 years during school holidays. They are often used by working parents

Figure 1.5 Child care settings

them from whooping cough, polio, tetanus, measles and other infectious diseases. These immunisations are given by the doctor or at the local baby clinic.

- **School health services:** Once they start school, children are seen by a school nurse and given health education. If any health problems are detected, the nurse can refer the children to their own doctor who may send them to a specialist.
- **Dental services:** Dental check-ups and orthodontic treatment (straightening the teeth) are free to children up to the age of 16 years.
- **Community and hospital services:** If children need referral to specialist treatment, they may see a *paediatrician*, *audiologist*, *speech therapist*, *optician* or *dietician*.

All these services are free to children under the age of 16 years.

Checkpoint

- A **paediatrician** is a doctor who treats sick children.
- An **audiologist** is someone who specialises in hearing problems.

Find out what a **dietician** does.

Education for babies and children

Local education authorities (LEAs for short) are responsible for delivering nursery, primary and secondary education in their areas. Every 4-year-old is entitled by law to receive some nursery education, either in a school, a private day nursery or a playgroup. Any nursery wanting to be funded by the government has to be inspected by OFSTED, the school inspection service.

Checkpoint

- Entitled means having a right to something.
- The **curriculum** is what schools or government-funded nurseries are told they have to teach children by the Department for Education and Skills (DfES).
- **OFSTED** is the school inspection service.

In 1996 the government identified six desirable learning outcomes for children aged under 5 years. Each of the early years services should be working towards these outcomes to help the child grow fully in all parts of his or her development. The areas the government identified for action are:

1. language and literacy;
2. maths and numeracy;
3. creativity;
4. knowledge of the world;
5. personal and social development;
6. physical development.

These outcomes are now known as the Early Learning Goals and nurseries must follow them as they form the basis for the curriculum for 3 – 5-year-old children. Children are expected to be in full-time education in the school term following their fifth birthday but many children start in reception a year earlier.

Activity

Sophie is 18 months old. Every morning, Monday to Friday, she is taken to the Sticky Fingers nursery owned by Mrs Bancroft. She arrives at 7.30 am so that her parents can leave and get to work on time. Sophie has her breakfast in the nursery and her lunch and evening meal because her parents cannot collect her until 6.00 pm. Sophie's parents pay £80.00 per week for her nursery care but don't mind the cost because they know that qualified nursery nurses are caring for Sophie.

Sophie is learning so much by being with other children. She is beginning to play with the other children as well as joining in with the painting activities organised by the nursery nurses.

Discuss with another person the following:

1. Is the nursery privately owned or not?
2. What kind of service is being offered to Sophie and her parents?
3. What are the benefits to Sophie and her parents of using the nursery provision?

1. How are the activities organised by the nursery contributing to the Early Learning Goals?

Social care services for babies and children

The Department of Social Security (now the Department for Work and Pensions) is responsible for providing benefits for children and families, and it also runs the Child Support Agency. A number of benefits are available for children and families, and the main ones are as follows:

- **Child Benefit:** A fixed payment to all parents who have a child or children.
- **Maternity Benefit:** Money paid to working mothers while they are on leave from work to have a baby.
- **Family Credit:** Payments for families with a child or children where the family's income is low.

The benefits system is complex and changes frequently.

Local authorities are responsible for a range of services, particularly for registering people who work with children in early years settings. These settings may be statutory, private or voluntary (see Figure 1.5). Look at page 16 to find out what private, statutory and voluntary mean.

One such service is foster care and adoption. Fostering can be divided into three kinds:

1 short term
2 long term
3 teenage.

A child or teenager is fostered in someone else's home because the social services and, sometimes, the parents or carers believe there is a need for help. This can be because:

- the child's parents or carers are ill or unable to look after the child and there is no-one else to care for him or her;
- the child has been abused in some way (either physically or mentally); or
- the child has been neglected.

Foster parents are paid for looking after a child or teenager. The money is used to support the child with clothes and other expenses. The foster parents take only a small amount to cover the cost of their caring work. Very often a child is able to return home after a period of time. Occasionally, a child will never return home, for .

a variety of reasons. Instead, the child may be adopted (this means living with someone else permanently), sometimes by the foster family.

The National Childcare Strategy

The government has made a decision to focus attention on the early years to ensure that preschool children are provided with good-quality care and education. There have been a number of key developments in this area, some of which have already been mentioned:

- A national framework of qualifications for people who work with children to ensure everyone understands the levels and achievements attained through the various training courses currently on offer.
- The pre-school curriculum entitled Early Learning Goals.
- Inspection by OFSTED of all pre-school settings to ensure they are following a balanced programme of learning and play.
- Early Years Development Partnerships, where all local authorities have to produce a plan to show how the local health, social care and education services are working together for children.

Early Years Development Partnerships and Plans

These partnerships and plans are seen as the key to ensuring there is good quality local provision for all children. Some of the key aims of the plans are to:

- make sure every 4-year-old has three terms of good quality pre-school education;
- include children with specials needs within the same care and education settings as other children;
- show how the provisions of the Children Act 1989 and other laws relating to children are fulfilled;
- promote training for all early years workers (for example, NVQs in early years care); and
- provide grants for training.

For example, a childminder might decide she would like to be NVQ trained so that she is better equipped to help the children she looks after. She could apply for a grant from her local authority to help her with training to achieve this.

Adolescents (aged 11–18 years)

Many of the services already described for children, such as vaccinations and immunisations, school health services, dental services and community and hospital services, continue to apply in adolescence, although after the age of 16 years adolescents have to pay for the services if they are not in full-time education. However, adolescents also have their own unique health needs: they are at an age when they are no longer really children but are not yet adults. Health promotion (that is, providing information about things like contraception or the dangers of smoking, alcohol, drugs and unprotected sex, becomes important in adolescence.

Services for adolescents are not provided because the government is trying to be nice to them but because certain groups of people (who were asked by the government to look into some of the problems facing our society) have identified several problems that either continue into, or start in, adolescence such as poverty and drug misuse. These groups of people have made their findings known to the government and, as a result, targets are set to try to start to ease some of these problems. These are known as social policy goals (which are covered in more detail later in this chapter).

One way of trying to meet some of these social policy goals is to provide services designed to help adolescents with these problems. Providing health promotion services that highlight the dangers of habits as smoking, it is hoped, stops some adolescents either starting or continuing with these habits. This cuts the cost of health treatment for problems arising as a result of these habits, both in adolescence and later in life.

Activity

The government is very concerned about the fact that the average weekly consumption of alcohol among pupils aged 11–15 years has increased steadily from 5.3 units in 1990 (equivalent to almost 3 pints of normal-strength beer) to 10.4 units in 2000.

▶ Discuss in a group what services you think need to be provided to try to reduce the consumption of alcohol by adolescents.

▶ Discuss what else can be done to address the problem of adolescent drinking. Think about role models such as family members, teachers and friends, and advertising, both in the media and in shops. Write down what is the biggest influence on you as an adolescent to encourage you to:
- drink
- not to drink.

The school nurse, medical centres, doctors' surgeries, libraries and various support agencies provide a lot of health promotion in the form of advice or free leaflets. Schools also provide much of this in certain areas of the curriculum, such as personal and social health education (PSHE), religious studies, health and social care, drama and citizenship. Services such as the youth service, child protection and youth offending also offer advice and help.

You will probably be an adolescent yourself and will be aware that, although your physical needs have not changed much, your emotional, social and intellectual needs have. Figure 1.6 shows some of these developing needs.

Checkpoint

If you are **assertive** you can argue a point or stand up for yourself without being aggressive, and you can say no to people about things you don't want to do.

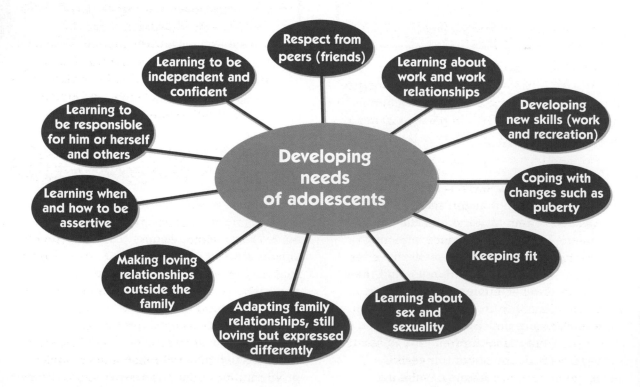

Figure 1.6 The developing needs of adolescents

Case study

Julie

Julie is a 15-year-old school girl who is very bright and hard working. She has an active life outside school, caring for and riding her horse and training at the local athletics club twice a week. However, she is now in Year 11 and is beginning to feel the strain of trying to balance her hobbies with the increasing demands of her schoolwork. She has not told her family about her worries. She is becoming withdrawn and depressed and is liable to flare up at the slightest criticism made by her family. Her parents are very worried about her as she is reluctant to discuss any of her worries with them.

1 What services can her parents call upon to help Julie cope with her problems?

2 What services can Julie call upon without her parents' knowledge?

3 Is there a service you think is, or should be, provided in school to help students like Julie? Describe such a service and say why you think it could help adolescents.

Social services for adolescents

The social services already described for children (such as foster care) can also apply to adolescents. Other social services that apply to children (and adolescents in particular) include the following:

- **Residential care** (see below).

- **Child protection:** Social services have a child protection register that lists children and young people whose welfare and safety are felt to be at risk. Social workers monitor their welfare and, if the situation becomes worse, the child or young person is moved to foster care or a residential home while help is offered to the family and child to try to solve the problem. Anyone who comes to the notice of social services from the police, concerned neighbours, other family members or schools as suspected of being abused or neglected in any way, or in danger because of problems in the family, is visited. His or her needs are assessed and his or her name is put on the register until such time as the situation is thought to be resolved. Such children and young people are assigned a social worker for them to contact if the need arises. All schools have a child protection officer to whom any suspicions of abuse are reported; this information is then passed on to social services who visit the family and monitor the situation closely.

- **Youth offending services:** These services are used mainly by adolescents but sometimes by children as well. They give support to young people who have committed an offence and provide them with legal advice (as well as help) to get them back into school or employment or to get benefits when they have been in a youth custody centre. They also support the families of the youth offenders.

- **Youth work:** Social services employ special workers who work with young people. These workers might come into school on certain days of the week to talk to teenagers about their problems or to ask them what facilities they would like providing to occupy them in the evenings. Alternatively, these workers might be available in local community centres. They might also run youth clubs and activities aimed at different age groups.

Adults (aged 19–65 years)

Adults are served by the health services in much the same way as children and adolescents, although adults will develop more serious medical conditions as they grow older, and they may require a wider range of specialist care. Health care for adults includes general hospital services (for example, operations such as hysterectomies, physiotherapy after accidents, strokes, etc.), and recuperation and rehabilitation advice after conditions such as a heart attack. Some adults may also need mental health care (as do children and adolescents but less commonly than adults), which is provided either by community nursing or in residential care. Complementary therapies, such as osteopathy, aromatherapy and chiropractic, are now used alongside more conventional medical treatments, and doctors often refer adults to these services although most are run privately outside the National Health Service. Family planning clinics and hospices are other health care services used by adults.

Adults' educational (developmental) needs are provided by further education establishments (such as universities), local colleges on day release, correspondence courses or night classes at local schools or colleges.

Social services that are provided for adults include refuges for adults at risk of violence, homelessness services, support services such as the Samaritans and advice services such as the Citizen's Advice Bureau. Many of these have to be provided because adults are having problems with relationships.

Older people (65+ years)

As people become older, they may need more help with daily living. Local authorities have the *duty* to assess the needs of older people and the power to provide services in order to meet those needs. They offer a range of services to meet the needs of older people.

Checkpoint

Duty in this example means being required by law to assess the needs of older people.

The help that may be offered includes the following:

- Nursing care at home.
- Personal care (e.g. help with bathing, getting up, getting dressed).
- Domestic help (e.g. shopping, housework, laundry and pension collecting).
- Equipment (e.g. bath seats, commodes, wheelchairs, bed rails and hoists).

- Aids for dressing, eating and carrying out everyday tasks.
- Help with continence problems, including pants and other aids.
- Help with speech and swallowing problems after an illness such as a stroke.
- Foot care and chiropody (podiatry).
- Residential care.
- Day care facilities.

Residential care services

In social care services, the term 'residential' often means a client living in a care home with other people. This could be a residential home where care workers are on duty at all times.

The social services and the independent sector (private business) provide residential services. Residential care is also provided by charitable groups. The following are some examples of people who live in residential care homes:

- Older people who can no longer care for themselves.
- People with physical disabilities who need practical help with moving, eating and dressing.
- Children with no carers – e.g. children whose parents have died or who cannot care for them.
- People with learning disabilities who need support managing their own lives.

Residential care is included here because older people are the main users of residential care services, but it is important to realise (from the bullet points you have just read) that these services are also for those with disabilities and for children with no carer.

Sheltered accommodation

Another kind of residential care is called sheltered housing. Clients live independently in their own homes (rented or purchased) and help is immediately available if they need it. A warden is on duty at all times. Their job is to make sure the clients are safe and well. The clients are also encouraged to join in with a range of social activities that are planned and ...ided for them, usually by the residents and

Case study

A residential home for older people

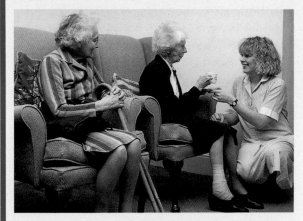

Hello, my name is Cath and I am a care worker at a residential home for older people. I only work 15 hours a week because I am also a student at my local college. When I go into work first thing in the morning, the night duty staff tell me about our residents and what sort of night they have had. They tell me if Mrs Hall has not been able to sleep or if Mr Bancroft had a good night out with his daughter. They make sure all the clients' records are up to date before they leave duty.

The first thing I do is awaken the clients I work with. Sometimes I find Mary already up and dressed (usually waiting for her breakfast!). I always have to help George. He can't get out of bed easily, so with the help of other staff I use the hoist to get him up and on to his favourite chair. Some of my clients eat their breakfast in bed if they are not feeling too well. If this is the case then I take them their breakfast.

1. Identify three ways in which Cath helps her clients.
2. Identify the differences for the clients living in residential care compared with those living in their own homes.
3. Why do you think somebody might need to go into residential care? Give reasons under the headings 'Health needs' and 'Social needs'.

1. Identify three different needs Cath's clients have.
2. How can Cath help her clients with these needs?

---

warden of the accommodation. Clients do not have to join in unless they want to. They are still completely independent and make their own choices about their lives.

Day care services

Day care centres are provided by both the health and social services. Those provided by health services are discussed on page 23 in Chapter 2. In the case of social services, the main purpose is to provide social support activities for the clients, not medical treatment and health care. The types of activities provided are shown in Figure 1.7.

Day care centres are very important in the lives of many older clients or those with special support needs. Often clients are collected from their own homes or residential homes and

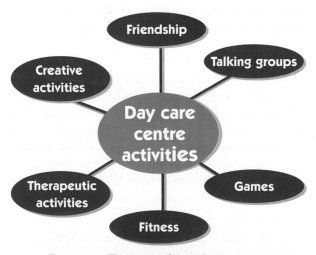

Figure 1.7 The types of social support activities provided in day care centres

taken to the day care centre in minibuses run by social services or voluntary groups.

Disabled people

Irrespective of the particular disability a person may have, he or she is likely to have additional needs to those without a disability (for example, appropriate, suitably adapted facilities and resources, and access to services that allow that person to lead an independent life). In addition to the services already mentioned for other client groups, some disabled people need additional specialist nursing and medical services, including physiotherapy, psychology, occupational therapy and rehabilitation services.

Checkpoint

Access means the route that enables a person to take advantage of a particular service.

Health services for people with a disability

People who have physical or learning disabilities require the kind of care that enables them to live as full a life as possible. We need a wide range of services for those people. Primary health care teams and community services, as well as hospitals, often provide these services. The kinds of service you might come across are as follows:

- **Supported community living:** People with special needs sharing a house in the local community and being supported by a health care worker.
- **Day care centres:** Often based in local hospitals providing, for example assessment, treatment and occupational therapy.
- **Hospital care:** To treat a specific illness or disability.
- **Home care:** Medical care provided in the home to allow the client the opportunity to stay within his or her own community.

Day centres for people with learning disabilities

There is a range of services for people with learning disabilities, as in the case of Stephen in the following activity.

Case study

Stephen is 17 years of age and has Down's syndrome. He lives at home with his parents. Every day he takes the bus to the Woodlands Centre, five kilometres from where he lives. At Woodlands he is able to take part in a range of sporting and recreational activities, which he thoroughly enjoys. These include horse riding at the local riding centre. Stephen is also part of the horticulture group, which raises plants for sale at a garden fair twice a year. The money they raise helps to pay for the extra facilities the centre needs.

Each day a group of the clients at the centre works out a menu for lunch and then walks to the supermarket to buy the ingredients. Then with the support of one of their carers they cook lunch for everyone. Stephen is also learning computer skills. This is very useful as he has his own computer at home.

▶ Discuss with a partner the services that are available to Stephen at the centre. How does each service help Stephen achieve a better standard of life? Make notes of your discussion.

Domiciliary care

Domiciliary care is care that is provided in the client's own home. This can include:

- help with personal hygiene (e.g. bathing, dressing and using the toilet);
- household care and cleaning;
- transport; and
- shopping.

The availability of these services usually varies from one place to another. It often depends on the amount of money the social care services has to spend on client care. In some places clients are asked to contribute a small amount to the cost of the service provided.

Social policy goals

When the government commissions a group of people to look into one of the problems facing our society (such as homelessness, child poverty and drug misuse), that group of people will report back on the particular area they have been asked to investigate. Based on their report a policy will be written to help tackle the problem and *targets* will be set to implement the policy – that is, to put it into action. These targets are known as *social policy goals*.

Checkpoint

- **Commission** means to instruct or give authority to a group of people to do a particular task.
- **Implement** means to put into action.
- A **policy** is a general plan of action.

An example of such a group of people is the Policy Action Team (PAT) on Young People. The team was made up of experts from the voluntary sector and business and people with a research background, as well as senior Whitehall officials. PAT was put together in 1998 to look at how the government can improve the way policies and services work for young people following a report published in September 1998 about social exclusion.

Checkpoint

- **Whitehall** is a street in London where there are many government offices. We use the phrase 'Whitehall officials' to mean people who work for the government.
- **Social exclusion** refers to people who are excluded from opportunities to have a healthy and economically comfortable life. Some factors that create social exclusion are poverty, family conflict, poor educational opportunities and poor services.
- **Initiatives** are new ideas for, or first steps taken towards, solving a problem.

Exclusion among young people emerged as a particular issue in the September 1998 report. The Policy Action Team therefore investigated and, in their report (published in March 2000), said that the most important task facing society is to ensure that every young person, no matter who he or she is, has the best possible start in life and the opportunity to develop and achieve his or her full potential. However for a minority of young people, achieving this ambition will not be easy, with too many of them appearing to be destined for a life of underachievement and social exclusion.

The PAT used a case study about a young man called Matthew to illustrate the problems facing young people. Matthew was abused by his stepfather and older half-brother at home and was bullied at school. He began taking drugs and getting involved in crime and, at the age of 16, he was kicked out of home. When he was 17 he spent six months in jail.

The PAT suggested that the government should support young people such as Matthew more effectively through their adolescence and should act earlier to stop them developing problems in the first place. This means developing and providing services to do this.

The report states that a large minority of young people experience a range of acute problems, including homelessness, poverty, drug addiction, illiteracy (an inability to read or write), mental illness and serial offending. It highlighted facts such as the following:

- One in five children are growing up in households where no-one has a job, which means these children are experiencing poverty.
- The UK has more 15 – 16-year-old drug users than any other European Union country.
- In England and Wales half of all 16 – 19-year-olds have tried drugs.
- There are approximately 32,000 homeless 16 – 21-year-olds in Britain.
- There are more homeless 16 – 17-year-olds, in the UK than in other European Union countries.

Checkpoint

Acute in this context means serious. **Serial** means at regular intervals.

Some of these problems are partly due to the following:

- Not enough work has been done to prevent them.
- The services designed to meet the needs of the poorest young people have been badly designed and have been provided haphazardly rather than where they are needed.
- The services are restricted rather than being available to all who need them.
- The services have not been adapted to new problems experienced by young people, such as poor mental health, drug abuse and family conflict.
- The money has not always gone to the right places, which has meant that some of the most deprived areas have had less money spent on them.
- When the policies and services were designed, the young people they were supposed to help were not consulted about their needs.
- The services often work in isolation from each other.

The Policy Action Team therefore made the following recommendations:

- Shifting the balance of effort and resources into preventing young people experiencing problems, rather than coping with young people when they have encountered the problems and are in serious trouble.
- Improving individual services for young people.
- Designing policies around the needs and priorities of young people, by involving them in the policy-making process.

A report such as that produced by the Policy Action Team for Young People therefore provides facts and examples and it makes recommendations to which service providers can respond in order to develop and provide services that contribute towards meeting social policy goals, such as reducing child poverty, homelessness and drug misuse in the population as a whole.

Health needs assessment

In addition to policy decisions made centrally by the government, there are also regional groups.

Strategic health authorities and primary care trusts (explained in more detail in Chapter 2), along with the local authority, need to assess the care needs of the local population so they can plan and develop the health and care services that are needed in their local area. Each area develops its own Health Improvement Programme, and this, along with the Primary Care Investment Plan, is an important local document that helps in this process. Public and service users, local authorities and health service providers pool their ideas, efforts and resources to improve health and to reduce the gap between those who are disadvantaged and those who are not. They outline the current position of many of the important health areas within their districts which allows them to identify any likely service demand in the area. These documents are the basis on which all the organisations involved develop plans to make significant health improvements within the local population by:

- promoting healthy living;
- preventing ill-health;
- providing health and social care when needed; and
- reducing the problems of the poor and disabled.

Checkpoint

- **Primary care trusts** are regional organisations that involve all the health care services in the area. They identify which services are needed in their area and then arrange for various organisations to deliver those services.
- **Strategic health authorities** are bodies that monitor (watch over) the primary care trusts and the National Health Service trust (hospitals).
- **Local authorities** provide such services as social services and schools in a particular area.

The government publishes its national health priorities in reports, and these priorities are incorporated into local documents. One such report is the NHS Plan, which was published in July 2000. This report set targets for the NHS on such issues as:

- heart disease and stroke;
- cancer;

- accidents;
- mental health;
- children's health; and
- improving waiting times.

It also set targets for the NHS to work with social services on the rehabilitation of older people to help them live independently and on increasing the participation of drug users in drug treatment programmes (as well as targets for social services on education and adoption).

The reasons why individuals use health, social care and early years services

Individuals use health, social care and early years services because they may need the following:

- **Care:** To be looked after in some way.
- **Support:** To be given help of some kind (e.g. encouragement or money).
- **Advice:** To be given an opinion or information as to what to do.
- **Medical treatment:** To have a medical problem dealt with.

At various stages in an individual's life, he or she may require help to meet his or her health, development and social care needs. Care services are designed to meet these needs and are shaped to meet the needs of individual users – so an individual will seek to use those services as and when it becomes necessary.

Check your knowledge

Read through the whole chapter and then try to answer the following questions:

1 Name the five major client groups.
2 What age range is covered by each of the client groups?
3 What do we mean by development needs?
4 Give three reasons why an individual might seek the help of the early years services.
5 Name three health needs an adult has.
6 Name three social needs an older person has.
7 Name one social policy goal.
8 How can health and social care services help to reduce drug misuse?
9 Why do health authorities and local authorities assess the care needs of local populations?
10 What are the four general reasons why individuals need to seek the use of health, social care and early years services? Describe these reasons.

Case study

Gertrude

Gertrude Evans is 76 years old and a widow. She has recently been finding it harder to get about because her arthritis has been getting worse and she is distressed because she can no longer keep her house as spotlessly clean as she always has done. Her son, Charles, and daughter, Mary, are married, have children of their own and have moved to other parts of the country. Although they visit her regularly she is quite lonely because she cannot get out and about as much as she used to. To make matters worse, she has recently suffered a slight heart attack and has lost a lot of confidence because she is worried that any exertion will bring on another attack.

Charles and Mary are becoming increasingly worried about her but neither of them has the room to invite her to live with them. They decide they need to talk to someone about whether their mother's situation might be improved by having some help in her own home or by moving into some sort of residential care. Gertrude agrees she cannot go on as she is but is reluctant to leave the home where she brought up her family. She is happy for Charles and Mary to talk to someone on her behalf.

1 Identify the health and social care services Charles and Mary might contact to help with Gertrude's needs (for example, the local authority about home care help).

2 List the reasons why they would seek to use those particular services.

Chapter 2

Types of care services

What types of care services are provided to meet client group needs?

By the end of this chapter you will have found out about organisations and private sector practitioners that deliver health care, social care and early years services. You will be able to identify the main types of care services that are offered to different client groups.

You will learn who provides the services and where they are made available. You should understand that there may be national and regional variations. You should be able to identify local and national examples of service providers who operate in the following care sectors:

- **Statutory** (including NHS trusts and local authority services).
- **Private** (including private companies and self-employed practitioners).
- **Voluntary** (including charities, local support groups who use volunteers and not-for-profit organisations with paid employees).

You will learn how the different service providers work together to meet client group needs. You will also understand how informal carers (family, friends and neighbours) provide a large amount of care in the community.

Be prepared

Although this chapter describes in general who provides services and where these are made available, there may be national and regional variations. You need to be able to identify local examples of service providers in the three sectors named above, so a number of the activities in this chapter require you to find out details of such services in your own area. Be on the lookout for leaflets about services when you go to see the doctor, dentist or any other health and social care services.

The organisation of health, social care and early years services

Care services may be provided in one of three ways (see Figure 2.1):

- Statutory services have been set up because Parliament has passed a law that requires the services to be provided (e.g. accident and emergency departments in hospitals).
- Private organisations are run on a profit-making basis and are businesses (e.g. private residential homes).
- Voluntary organisations are run on a non-profit making basis (e.g. Barnardo's, an organisation that provides care for children and young people).

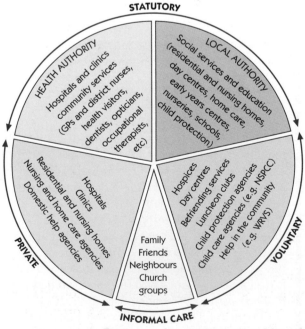

Figure 2.1 An overview of health and social care provision

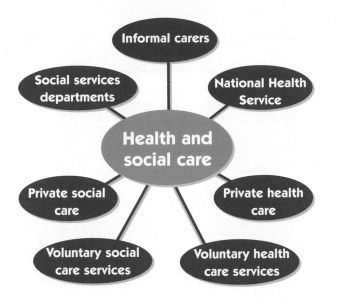

Figure 2.2 *The providers of health and social care*

People outside these formal agencies and organisations also provide health and social care. Informal care may be provided by family members, friends and neighbours (see Figure 2.2).

Statutory sector organisations

The two main providers of statutory services are the National Health Service (NHS) and local authority services. Statutory services are organised at government (national), regional and local levels (see Figure 2.3):

- **National** levels of the organisation include key government departments. The government is divided into various departments that have a responsibility for specific areas (e.g. the Department of Health deals with national issues concerning the NHS).
- **Regional** levels include regional services in the NHS, social services boards and the strategic health authorities.
- **Local** levels include local authority social services departments, hospital and primary care trusts and GPs.

The Secretary of State for Health in England and the Secretaries of State in Northern Ireland, Scotland and Wales are responsible for all aspects of health and social care provision. The Department of Health (DOH) in England has responsibility for:

- making policies in relation to health and social care and issuing guidelines;
- monitoring the performance of health authorities and social service departments, ensuring the quality of care; and
- allocating resources for the provision of health and social care.

National

Parliament
Secretary of State for Health
Department of Health
National voluntary organisations' headquarters

Regional

NHS strategic health authorities
Voluntary organisations' regional offices
Regional offices of private health and social care agencies

Local

NHS trusts
Local voluntary organisations
Local authorities social services departments
Primary care trusts
Voluntary organisations' local offices
Private health and social care agencies
Informal carers

Figure 2.3 *National, regional and local levels of health and social care provision*

Checkpoint

The **DOH** is responsible for:
- deciding what needs to be done and how it will be put into practice;
- providing safe, quality services; and
- deciding which part of the service gets what amount of money.

In Northern Ireland, health services and social services are organised as a single agency. This is called a *unified structure* and is provided outside political control. Although the organisation of health services in Scotland, Wales and Northern Ireland may be different from that in England, the range and provision of services are much the same (see Figure 2.4).

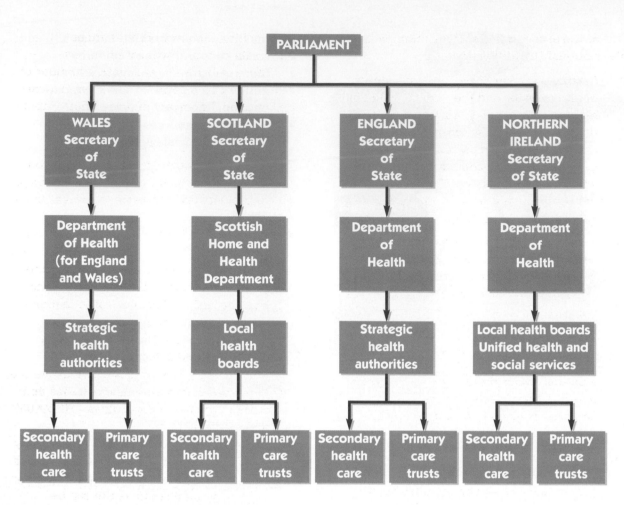

Figure 2.4 *The health care structures of England, Wales, Scotland and Northern Ireland*

The structure of health services

Before 1948, health services were provided in various ways: some by voluntary organisations, some by local authorities, some by employers, some by private care. There was no co-ordination of services. Generally people had to pay for their health care. Many poor people could not afford health care if they needed it.

The National Health Service (NHS)

In July 1948, Nye Bevan, a government minister, founded the National Health Service (NHS). He wanted *free* health care for all at the time of use.

Did you know?

Before 1948, if people needed to see a doctor for coughs, colds or more serious illnesses, they often were not able to because they didn't have enough money. Many more people became very ill and sometimes died because they couldn't afford the medical care they needed.

Activity

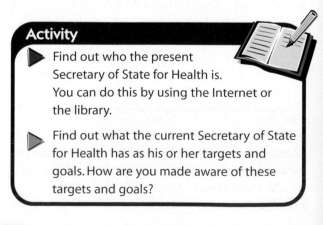

► Find out who the present Secretary of State for Health is. You can do this by using the Internet or the library.

► Find out what the current Secretary of State for Health has as his or her targets and goals. How are you made aware of these targets and goals?

There were, and still are, three main parts to the National Health Service.

1 **Primary care services:** These are family health services and they are provided by family doctors (GPs), practice nurses, district nurses, health visitors, dentists, opticians and pharmacists and are generally the first contact a person has with the health service. There is also a lot of preventative work in primary care (e.g. routine dental check-ups and eye tests).

2 **Secondary and tertiary care services:** Secondary care services include general hospitals; tertiary care services include such things as specialist hospital centres (e.g. specialist cancer care hospitals). The care is often provided following referral from a primary care or community health professional. For example, a GP may refer a patient to hospital for tests and special investigations. Secondary care is about the care that is given in hospitals, day case surgeries and outpatient clinics.

3 **Public health services:** This area is mainly concerned with health promotion and preventative work and includes health education programmes aimed at preventing illness and disease. Childhood immunisation programmes against illnesses such as smallpox and whooping cough and dental health care education programmes are good examples of public health services. Both the health services and local authorities have various roles in the promotion of better health.

Checkpoint

Opticians look at people's eyes and are able to prescribe glasses and contact lenses to correct vision problems.

Pharmacists (or chemists) dispense medicines that are prescribed by doctors or other health professionals.

Until recently there were only comparatively minor changes in the way the NHS was structured and, indeed, provided health care. However the NHS has now undergone major reforms that have been more far-reaching than any other changes undertaken since it was set up in 1948.

These reforms are set out in a number of government *White Papers*. The most radical and, indeed, important of these White Papers are as follows:

- **The New NHS: Modern Dependable (December 1997):** This document set out the ways in which the NHS would change to provide new and better services for the public.
- **A First Class Service: Quality in the New NHS (June 1998):** This document describes the quality, standards and efficiency the public should expect from the NHS and how the NHS will be monitored to make sure it is performing well.
- **The Health of the Nation (June 1991):** This document sets health targets for health care practitioners to achieve in the key areas of coronary heart disease and stroke, cancers, mental illness, HIV/AIDS and accidents.
- **Saving Lives – Our Healthier Nation (July 1999):** This document is about saving lives by promoting healthier living and looking at how inequalities in health can be reduced. Its main aims are to improve the health of:
  - the nation as a whole by increasing the length of people's lives and the number of years people spend free from illness; and
  - the worst-off in society and to narrow the health gap that exists between different groups in society.

It sets national targets for improving health by the year 2010:

- *Heart disease and stroke:* To reduce the death rate from heart disease and stroke and related illnesses amongst people of 65 years by at least a further third than in the *The Health of the Nation* document.
- *Cancers:* To reduce the death rate from cancer amongst people aged under 65 years by at least a further fifth.
- *Mental health:* To reduce the death rate from suicide and undetermined injury by at least a further sixth.
- *Accidents:* To reduce accidents by at least a further fifth.

As a result of this document, health promotion is being aimed at healthy schools (children), healthy workplaces (adults) and healthy neighbourhoods (older people).

NHS trusts to ensure they are providing good-quality and efficient services that meet the needs of the populations they serve.

Activity

Read the main aims of *Our Healthier Nation* and then answer the following questions:

1 List at least five factors that affect health but that people have little control over personally (for example, pollution).
2 Write down your ideas as to how each of these factors could be tackled by the government.
3 Why do you think the government picked the four areas it did for its national targets?
4 Produce a health promotion leaflet to encourage healthy schools. You need to identify the main factors involved, such as what children eat at school, the sort of accidents children could have at school, etc., before you start to design it.

Poorer people and those living in deprived areas are more likely to suffer from cancer, heart diseases and other related illnesses. People from better-off areas are more likely to recover from cancer.

1 Why do you think there is a health gap between different groups in society? Think of at least five different factors that are likely to affect poorer people and those who live in deprived areas more than those in better-off areas.
2 Based on the factors you identified in question 1, produce a health promotion leaflet as part of the healthy neighbourhoods campaign.

Strategic health authorities

It is proposed that there will be around 30 strategic health authorities in England by 2002. The primary function of these authorities will be to monitor the primary care trusts and the

Checkpoint

Monitoring providers of services means watching over the providers of those services to check that standards are as high as they should be and that everything which should be done is done so in the way it is meant to be.

Primary care trusts (PCTs)

Primary care trusts have replaced the primary care groups that first came into being in 1999. Primary care trusts are larger organisations, serving a population of (usually) 100,000–300,000 people. These are free-standing bodies that commission services and that provide a wide range of health services within the local community. Their work involves many of the duties the old health authorities previously carried out, including the following:

- Planning services within the PCT's area.
- Assessing primary health care needs in order to contribute to and to implement the government's Health Improvement Programme.
- Developing services within the area.
- Commissioning.
- Arranging service contracts (e.g. with hospitals).
- Managing services provided by GPs, dentists, opticians and pharmacists and monitoring the quality of services.
- Providing public information about services.
- Registering and dealing with complaints about the provision of services.

They are also able to:
- employ staff under their own terms and conditions; and
- buy, own and sell assets, such as land or buildings.

Most of a PCT's income is money directly from central government, which is, of course, public money (money that is paid in taxes by everyone to the government).

NHS trusts

National Health Service trusts are self-governing units within the health service. Trusts are managed by a board of directors and are accountable to central government. A trust can be either a hospital or a group of hospitals, or an ambulance service for a particular area.

A trust is able to:

- decide its own management structure;
- employ staff under its own terms and conditions of employment;
- buy, own and sell assets, such as land or buildings;
- carry out research; and
- provide facilities for medical, nursing and other forms of education/training.

Self-governing trusts receive most of their income from NHS contracts for providing commissioned services to PCTs.

All trusts, both primary care and NHS, must produce annual reports and maintain annual accounts, which must be published. This means the public can see how its money is being spent!

National Care Standards Commission (NCSC)

This is a new national organisation that commenced work in April 2002. Its responsibilities are to inspect, regulate and enforce standards where necessary in a range of caring environments. These include:

- private nursing homes;
- residential care homes;
- home care provider agencies;
- nurse agencies;
- private hospitals;
- adoption agencies;
- children's homes; and
- boarding schools.

The National Care Standards Commission is directly responsible to government and is divided into eight regions across England. These areas are again broken down into smaller area groups.

NHS Direct

NHS Direct is a telephone helpline that can provide information about health, illness and health services. Specially trained nurses can advise whether you should treat yourself at home, speak to a pharmacist, visit a GP practice, dentist, optician or walk-in-centre or go to hospital.

NHS walk-in centres

NHS walk-in centres are available in a number of towns and cities across England. They complement general practice by providing treatments for minor illnesses and injuries (e.g. strains and sprains), health promotion and self-care advice. They are run by nurses and an appointment isn't necessary. Most walk-in centres are open from 7.00 am to 10.00 pm, seven days a week.

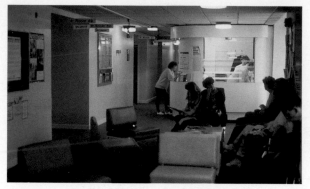
A walk-in centre

Activity

▶ Find out if there is a walk-in centre near you and the types of services it provides. You can find this out from the Internet, the library or by contacting your local medical centre.

▶ Find out what services are *not* provided by the walk-in-centre and why they are *not* provided.

Doctors' surgeries

A surgery provides a wide range of services (see Figure 2.5).

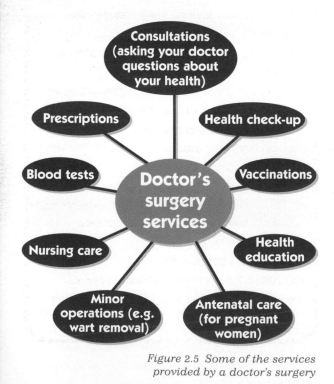

Figure 2.5 *Some of the services provided by a doctor's surgery*

Health centres

A health centre provides medical and health care as well as support and personal welfare services. The range of services provided depends on the kind of care required in your local area, how many people live there, how old they are and the amount of money available to spend. By building health centres, health service planners can organise most of the required services under one roof. The first health centres were started in the 1930s.

Dentists

Dentists are part of primary care services because they are usually the first people anyone with a mouth problem goes to. They are based in either a health centre or a dental surgery and offer a wide range of services, such as:

- treatments;
- check-ups;
- oral health education;
- hygienist treatment;
- orthodontics (making teeth straight); and
- minor oral surgery.

Hospitals

As you will know from earlier in this section, a hospital is an example of a trust – that is, it is managed by a board of directors and is accountable to the government. Hospitals provide secondary care: clients usually go to a hospital because a health professional has referred them there. Clients use hospitals for:

- operations and consultations;
- treatment for infections, accidents or illness;
- health education; and
- rehabilitation after an operation or illness.

Sometimes a client who needs special treatment or help will have to go to a specialist hospital, which are often called 'centres of excellence'. These specialise in such care as:

- heart transplants;
- terminal illness (care of people who are dying);
- paediatric care (children's specialists);
- mental health care; and
- maternity and women's health.

Community health care

Clients can have health care in their own homes as well as in hospitals, health centres and doctors' surgeries. The services provided in the community are often based at a health centre or a surgery and are carried out by primary health care teams. Services can also be provided by a community health care trust attached to a hospital. Examples of community health care services are shown in Figure 2.6.

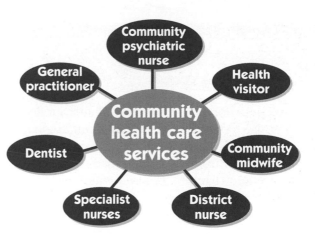

Figure 2.6 Community health care services

Case study

Nell

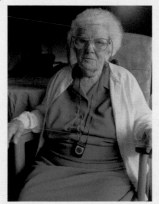

Nell is 79 years old. She lives by herself with her two cats. She has very bad arthritis and leg ulcers that will not heal up. She cannot get around much by herself. Once a day she is visited by a district nurse who treats her leg ulcers and gives her a weekly vitamin injection.

Every evening a care worker comes at about 7 o'clock to help her wash and get changed for bed. She also makes sure that Nell has remembered to take her tablets. On Wednesdays Nell is taken by hospital transport to the day care centre at the local hospital. A physio-therapist helps her with exercises to keep her joints mobile. She has lunch with her friends and really looks forward to the day.

The nurse at the day hospital always has a chat with Nell to make sure everything is going well at home.

1   List the various services Nell receives.
2   What are the benefits to Nell of receiving the services mentioned?
3   What would happen to Nell if these services were not available to her?

Check your knowledge

1   What is meant by the term 'statutory services'?
2   What is the difference between a private organisation and a voluntary organisation?
3   Which are the main two providers of statutory services?
4   What do we mean by a 'unified structure'?
5   What is the difference between primary and secondary care?
6   Write down one example of a tertiary service.
7   Name two examples of public health services.
8   Which government White Paper aims to reduce inequalities in health care?
9   How many strategic health authorities were set up in England during 2002?
10 Name three areas of work covered by primary care trusts.
11 What is an NHS trust?
12 What is the name of the new national organisation set up to inspect, regulate and enforce standards in a range of care establishments?
13 What is NHS Direct?
14 What is the purpose of walk-in centres?
15 Why are some hospitals called centres of excellence?

The structure of the social services

The introduction of the National Health Service in 1948 also meant a range of health and social care services came under the direct control of the Minister of Health. It was hoped this direct control would result in a more unified and co-ordinated range of services. The responsibility for providing for old and disabled people, and children by the local authorities was extended further. Also, services for people with mental health problems were strengthened through the setting up of the Provisional Council for Mental Health. However, until the 1960s these three areas of care were operated quite separately from one another. The publication of the *Seebohm Report* in 1968 resulted in the merging of the children's departments and the welfare services. Then, in 1970, the Local Authority Social Services Act set out a new framework for social care provision, which requires the local authorities in England to set up Social Services Committees (see Figure 2.7).

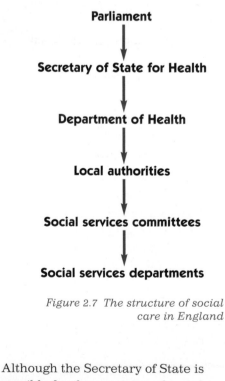

Parliament

↓

Secretary of State for Health

↓

Department of Health

↓

Local authorities

↓

Social services committees

↓

Social services departments

Figure 2.7 The structure of social care in England

Although the Secretary of State is responsible for the provision of social care, it is the local authorities who administer those services. In England and Wales, county councils, metropolitan councils and the London boroughs run the local authorities. In Northern Ireland, there are four boards that administer the combined health and social services. In Scotland, regional local authorities control social services departments. However, the powers and responsibilities of local authorities are defined by Parliament, which passes legislation outlining the local authorities' duties.

Local authorities have the responsibility for the co-ordination of many aspects of social care in their communities, including services for children, for people with learning disabilities and for people with mental health problems, as well as responsibilities for housing, education, leisure facilities, refuse collection and highways.

Each local authority must appoint a Director of Social Services and must have a Social Services Committee. Some local authorities have separate directorates for each of their responsibilities (e.g. social services, housing, education, etc.). Others combine these departments at senior management level; for example, one director might oversee housing and community care services which could include services for older people and services for adults with disabilities (see Figure 2.8).

The organised structures of social services departments have changed considerably in the last few years. This has happened so they can carry out their new roles and responsibilities as required by new legislation, particularly the NHS and Community Care Act 1990. As mentioned earlier, this Act made local authorities the *purchasers* of care, rather than the *providers* of care. Many social services departments reorganised their staffing structures to reflect these changes in responsibilities (see Figure 2.9).

Activity

1   Why do you think the government wanted to change the role of local authorities from providers to purchasers?
2   What might be the advantages and disadvantages?

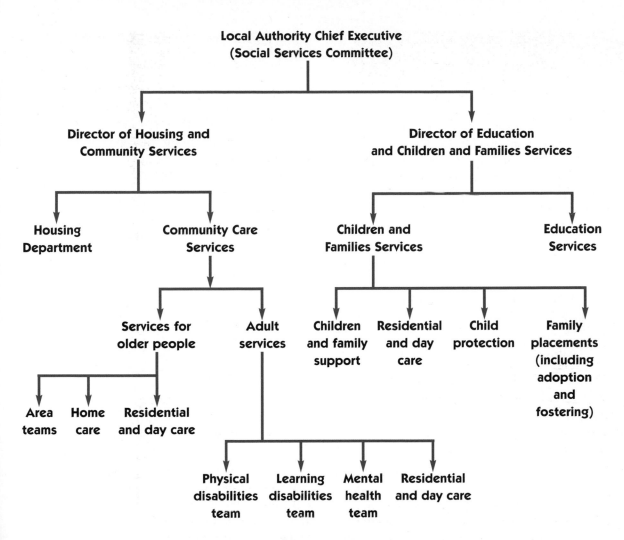

Figure 2.8 Combining different social care functions: an example

Before 1990 Local authorities were providers of care. This meant they had to:	Since 1990 Local authorities are providers of care. This means they have to:
Own and run care homes and residential homes	Pay private care homes to look after clients
Employ all the staff	Provide money to the owners to pay their staff
Train all their staff	Provide money to the owners to train their staff
Provide services such as cleaning	Find private cleaning companies to come in and clean the institutions
Run a catering department	Bring in 'contract caterers' to provide food

Figure 2.9 Changes in local authority responsibilities since the NHS and
Community Care Act 1990

The role of social services departments

The role of the social services departments has changed as their function as direct providers of services has decreased and their role as assessors of need and purchasers of services has increased. Their main role now is to offer advice and to provide access to services – such as residential care – for all client groups (e.g. children, people with physical or learning disabilities, people with mental health problems or older people). Previously, local authorities owned and managed a number of residential homes themselves. Today they are more likely to purchase residential care for individuals in private or non-profit-making residential homes.

Social workers are employed within the social services departments and their role is to assess the needs of people requiring social care services. Social workers are often organised into teams that deal with a specific client group (e.g. children and family teams). Teams consist of health and social care workers (e.g. teams dealing with people with mental health problems may work side by side with social workers and community psychiatric nurses).

With their increased role in the purchasing of services, many social services departments have created special commissioning and **contracting** sections. These new sections operate alongside the divisions created as a result of the 1990 Act (e.g. complaints, inspection and registration units, quality monitoring and planning and development). Planning and development has become even more important as social services departments are required to work closely with health service colleagues as well as with the private and voluntary sectors.

Checkpoint

Contracting means employing someone who does not regularly work for your organisation to do a specific job for you – for example, employing cleaners through an agency.

Joint work and planning

Health and social services must now work together to modernise the front-line care they provide for people. In September 1998, the targets set for achieving this were outlined in *Modernising Health and Social Services: National Priorities Guidance 1999–2002*. The priorities contained in this document included the following:

- Cutting waiting lists and waiting times.
- Modernising mental health and primary care services.
- Reducing deaths from cancer and coronary heart disease and improving the health of the most disadvantaged in society.
- Improving the quality and safety of children's services and providing better rehabilitation services for older people.

Previous governments tried to encourage joint planning between the health and local authorities. However, this was difficult to achieve because of the different ways the authorities were structured. For example, in terms of health, the care of older people who were mentally ill was the responsibility of the mental health services whereas, in terms of social care, the same people came under the remit of services for older people.

Other problems have arisen because health authorities (now primary care trusts) and local authorities do not share the same geographical boundaries. For example, one primary care trust may cover all or part of a local authority's area (see Figure 2.10), or one local authority's area may come under the responsibility of a number of primary care trusts.

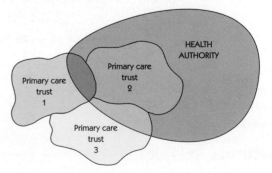

Figure 2.10 A primary care trust that covers more than one local authority area

Check your knowledge

1 How has the role of the social services changed over the years?
2 Name three services offered by social services.
3 What does the word 'residential' mean?
4 Why are social workers often organised into teams?
5 What does contracting mean?
6 What is the function of a general Social Care Council?
7 What were the targets set in September 1998 for the modernisation of care?
8 Why do you think it is important to cut waiting lists and waiting times? What effect will achieving this have on health and well-being?
9 Why was it hard to modernise mental health services for older people when older people come under the responsibility of both mental health services for health care and services for older people for social care? List some difficulties you could imagine arising.
10 Suggest a way these difficulties could be overcome.
11 Give some examples of when an older person might need a rehabilitation service.

Early years services

Structure

The early years services are those services that provide health, care and education services to children between the ages of 0 and 8 years when not at school. As with the health and social services, the early years services involve both the statutory sector and private groups.

Statutory services

The government's role is to provide statutory services directly, or to supervise services through government departments. The four main government departments concerned with children are shown in Figure 2.11. Funding from these central government departments is passed on to local authorities in the form of grants. The authorities then use these grants to provide services for children and families in their areas. The three main services are health, education and social services.

Department	Responsible for
1 Department of Health (DOH)	Health services, including hospitals and local health care
2 Department for Education and Skills (DfES)	All aspects of education and skills, including standards in schools and day nurseries
3 Department for Work and Pensions	Providing benefits for children and families
4 Office of the Deputy Prime Minister (ODPM)	Local government, housing, planning and the countryside

Figure 2.11 Government departments concerned with children

Other services for children

As we saw in Chapter 1, there are special services for children (in addition to the health care for all), such as health screening, vaccinations and immunisations. These are all free to children under the age of 16 years. The local education authorities are responsible for providing nursery, primary and secondary education, while the Department for Work and Pensions is responsible for providing benefits for children and families. Details of these, plus notes on the National Childcare Strategy and the Early Years Development Partnership and Plans, can be found in Chapter 1. It would be a good idea to read those sections of Chapter 1 again to make sure you are fully aware of what is delivered by the early years services.

Voluntary organisations

The UK has a long tradition of voluntary services and this sector has always been involved in the provision of health and social care. Today, the National Council for Voluntary Organisations (NCVO) is the central co-ordinating agency in England. Its main function is to provide links between voluntary organisations, official bodies and the private sector. Councils in Scotland, Wales and Northern Ireland have similar roles. There are over 20,000 voluntary organisations in the UK and more than 170,000 of these are registered as charities. Throughout the UK, the Home Office is the government department responsible for co-ordinating government interests in the voluntary sector (see Figure 2.12).

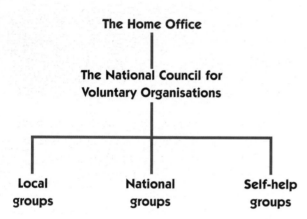

Figure 2.12 *The structure of voluntary organisations in England*

There are thousands of voluntary organisations involved in health and social care, ranging from national agencies such as Age Concern to small local groups. In recent years *self-help groups* have greatly increased in number. These are usually set up by people who share a particular concern and who want to help other people in similar situations.

Funding for voluntary organisations comes from various sources, such as contracts with health authorities or local authorities, fund-raising events, charitable donations from individuals, groups of people or businesses and through grants from grant-awarding bodies. Voluntary organisations tend to focus on specific issues (see Figures 2.13 and 2.14).

Area of concern	Organisation
Personal and family problems	Family Welfare Association; Child Poverty Action Group; Relate (formerly Marriage Guidance); Barnardo's; ChildLine; National Council for One-Parent Families; National Society for the Prevention of Cruelty to Children; Claimants' Union (advice on social security benefits); Samaritans (for lonely, depressed and suicidal people); Women's Aid
Health and disability	WRVS (Women's Royal Voluntary Service); MIND (National Association for Mental Health); Gamanon (for people with gambling problems); Help the Aged; Brook Advisory Centres; Royal Institute for the Blind; Royal National Institute for Deaf People; Alcoholics Anonymous; British Red Cross Society; Haemophilia Society
National organisations whose work is religious in inspiration	Salvation Army; Church Army; TocH; Church's religious Urban Fund; Church of England Children's Society; Young Men's Christian Association (YMCA); Catholic Marriage Advisory Council; Jewish Welfare Board

Figure 2.13 *Voluntary organisations and their principal areas of concern*

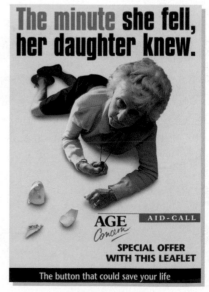

Figure 2.14 *Age Concern*

The range and extent of services available from private organisations have increased considerably in recent years. In particular, there was a rapid growth in private health care in the 1970s and 1980s when central government introduced the idea of a *mixed economy of care*. It is now government policy that NHS and private and voluntary health care provision should co-operate in meeting the nation's health needs. Private health care may be provided by NHS hospital trusts or in totally separate health care facilities. Similarly, the government expects local authorities to use private and voluntary agencies to provide them with social care rather than own and manage those services themselves. Consequently, a number of small businesses have emerged in recent years, such as home-help services.

Private health and social care organisations

The work of private organisations in the provision of health and social care has always been important. These organisations charge for their services with the intention of making a profit. Some of the services provided by the private sector are shown in Figure 2.15.

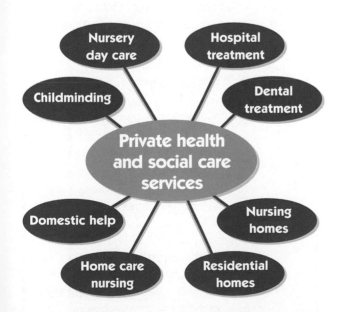

Figure 2.15 Health and social care services provided by the private sector

Different service providers working together to meet client group needs

Primary care trusts and local authorities have, as a result of government reforms, agreed to work together more in areas of care that overlap. Examples have already been mentioned in this chapter.

Good examples of this are often seen in the care of older people. Instead of a number of different professionals assessing the needs of an older person, one professional will assess and pass on the relevant information to the relevant person in the other organisation. For example, an older person may need assistance in getting up and washed each morning but this 'home care' service may be provided either by people employed directly by the authority or by people employed by a private agency. In the latter case, the local authority may have a contract with the agency to provide home care for such people.

Informal carers

In recent years the term **carer** has been used to describe anyone (other than a paid worker) who is looking after someone who cannot manage without help because of age, illness or disability. The carer may be a family member, friend or neighbour. Many carers are children or young people, or are elderly themselves and in poor health (e.g. a wife looking after a disabled partner, a parent looking after a child with learning difficulties, an adult looking after a parent who has dementia – memory loss usually associated with old age – or a child who is looking after a sick or disabled parent).

The work of a carer can be very difficult and demanding and typically involves:

- helping people to get into and out of bed;
- helping with washing and dressing, and eating and drinking;
- helping people with bathing or showering;
- housework and shopping; and
- helping people take medication.

Informal carers often belong to a local group, such as a church, or a group set up to advise and help others.

Young carers

The Carers Recognition and Services Act 1995 says that: 'A Young Carer is a child or young person under the age of eighteen who is carrying out significant tasks and assuming a level of responsibility for another person, which would normally be taken by an adult.' Across the UK there are about 32,000 young carers who are caring for someone in the family who is ill, disabled, elderly or with a drug or alcohol problem. Caring tasks range from general household chores (such as doing the housework, getting the shopping and doing the washing) to full personal care (such as helping them to wash and dress, keeping them company and stopping them having an accident).

Associations exist to support these young carers (such as the National Carers Association), which give advice on how to get help from the social services. These associations can arrange for someone to sit with the family member or can organise Meals on Wheels, or they can arrange for help around the house to give the young carer some time off. Other associations provide someone to talk to who will listen to and believe what the carer says, information about the relative's problem and help with school work.

Case study

Jenny

Jenny is 15 years old and very bright. Her mother is single and an alcoholic. She has made Jenny promise not to tell anyone else about her drink problem, which was brought on by the trauma of getting divorced and of which she is very ashamed. Jenny often comes home from school and finds her mother lying on the sofa drunk. This means that, before Jenny can settle to her homework (she is in her final GCSE year), she has first of all to tidy the house, make something to eat for herself and her mother, persuade her mother to eat and do any other jobs that need doing, such as ironing a school shirt for the next day. She often has to help her mother clean herself up after she has been sick while semi-conscious and get her into fresh clothes.

When she eventually gets to do her schoolwork she is often interrupted by her mother singing or shouting or, if her mother is feeling guilty (which she often does), apologising repeatedly for being a nuisance. At the weekend Jenny does tasks such as washing but won't go out much other than to get some shopping because she is worried her mother might drink even more and hurt herself.

1 What effect is Jenny's situation likely to have on her health, development and social needs?
2 What can she do to get some help?
3 What sort of help would be of benefit to Jenny?
4 What kind of help would be of benefit to her mother?

1 Write down all the ways each of your suggestions in question 3 above will help Jenny's health, development and social needs and explain why you think this.
2 Write down all the ways each of your suggestions in question 4 above will help her mother's health, development and social needs.
3 What do you think will happen to Jenny if she doesn't get any help soon?
4 What do you think will happen to Jenny's mother if she doesn't get some help soon?

Care services offered to different client groups

Many different care services have already been mentioned in this chapter. Figure 2.16 lists some examples.

Client group	Health care services	Social care services	Early years services
Children	(Including maternity services, health visitors), general hospital services, mental health care, speech therapy, dentistry	Residential care, child education, family centres, support group services	Playgroups and nursery health crèches, after-school care, toy libraries, child guidance, parent and toddler support groups
Adolescents	School medical services, primary health care, general hospital services, dental services, mental health care, health promotion (smoking, sexual health, drugs, alcohol)	Foster care, residential care, youth offending services, child protection, youth work, support group services	
Adults	Primary health care (including community provision of district and community mental health nursing), general hospital services, mental health care, family planning clinics, health promotion (smoking, sexual health, drugs, alcohol), complementary therapies, hospices	Housing/homelessness services, residential care, refuges, day centres, counselling support (e.g. Samaritans), information and advice services, social work, support groups, service user organisations	
Older people	Primary health care (including district and community mental health nursing), occupational therapy, complementary therapies, dentistry, chiropody/podiatry, specialist hospital services (general and mental health), nursing homes, hospices	Sheltered/supported housing residential care, home helps, day centres, lunch clubs, information and advice services, social work, support group services, service user organisations	
Disabled people (additional services)	Any of the above according to individual and local needs. Additionally, specialist medical and nursing services, physiotherapy, psychology, occupational therapy, complementary therapies, specialist education and training services (work-related and rehabilitative training schemes, for example)	Any of the above according to individual and local needs. Additionally specialist support and provision through service user organisations, direct payment personal assistance, social education (life skills education and supported work schemes, for example)	Any of the above according to individual and local needs. Separate specialist education provision and support services are provided in addition to integration within mainstream provision

Figure 2.16 Some examples of care services offered to different client groups

Sheltered accommodation is housing (usually ground-floor flats or small bungalows) where people live independently, (either rented or bought) that is available for people over the age of 55 years and that is warden controlled. Warden controlled means a person is on site 24 hours a day in case an older person needs help.

Residential care usually means that a person lives in a 'care home' with other people. This could be a residential home where care workers are on duty at all times. The social services and the independent sector (private business) provide residential services. Charitable groups also provide residential care. Different types of people may live in residential care homes. For example:

- Older people who can no longer care for themselves.
- People with physical or mental disabilities.
- Children with no carers (e.g. children whose parents have died or who cannot care for their children).

Case study

Mrs Stringer

Mrs Stringer is an 80-year-old woman. She was widowed seven years ago and lives alone in a two-bedroomed house. None of her family lives nearby and Mrs Stringer is very isolated. Two months ago Mrs Stringer fell and broke her left hip. She has now been discharged from hospital but her mobility is greatly reduced and she is unable to manage the stairs properly. She also has angina and problems with arthritis in many of her joints. Following an assessment by the social worker, the following services were provided and recommendations made.

Local authority

1. A recommendation was made for Mrs Stringer to be moved into sheltered accommodation as soon as possible.
2. A home carer has been provided (the local authority has a contract with a private agency for home care services) to help her with washing and dressing. In the evening she can still manage to get herself into bed.
3. Once a week the local authority provides her with help for her shopping, for collecting her pension and for general household tasks (also provided through the private home care agency).
4. Meals on Wheels are provided five days a week as she has difficulty preparing substantial meals (the WRVS prepare and deliver meals on behalf of the local authority).

5. Day care is provided at a local centre one day a week (Age Concern run the centre and arrange the transport for Mrs Stringer).

The primary care trust

1. A district nurse attends to dress Mrs Stringer's surgical wound and to monitor her medication.
2. The podiatrist attends to cut Mrs Stringer's toenails as she can no longer manage to do this herself.
3. The occupational therapist has arranged for Mrs Stringer to have a Zimmer frame to help her walk and to have a bath seat, grab rails and raised toilet seat fitted.

Informal carer

Mrs Stringer's niece visits each Sunday and provides a meal that day. She also does all her aunt's laundry for her.

▷ 1. List all the tasks Mrs Stringer gets help with.
2. Does Mrs Stringer receive a 'mixed economy of care' package?
3. What is meant by a 'mixed economy of care'?
4. Is Mrs Stringer receiving primary care, secondary care or both? Give examples to illustrate your answers.

▷ 1. What other care needs might Mrs Stringer have in the future and who might provide these?

Chapter 3

Ways of obtaining care services and barriers to access

Key issue

How can people gain access to care services and what can prevent people from being able to use the services they need?

In this chapter you will learn that the ways people gain access to care services are known as 'methods of referral'. You will learn that the three different methods of referral are as follows:

1   **Self-referral:** A person chooses to ask for or go to the services him or herself.
2   **Professional referral:** A person is put in contact with a service by a care practitioner, such as a doctor, nurse or social worker.
3   **Third-party referral:** A person is put in contact with a service by a friend, neighbour, relative or other person who is not employed as a care practitioner (e.g. the person's employer or a teacher).

You will also be able to identify barriers that might prevent people from making use of the services they need, including the following:

- **Physical barriers** – for example, stairs, a lack of lifts and a lack of adapted toilet facilities can prevent access by people with mobility problems.
- **Psychological barriers** – for example, fear of losing independence, the stigma associated with some services and not wanting to be looked after can deter people from making use of care services. Mental health problems can also prevent those in need from accessing services.
- **Financial barriers** – for example, charges and fees can deter and exclude people who have not got the money to pay for the services they need.
- **Geographical barriers** – for example, in rural areas the location of an organisation or practitioner may be a barrier to use if

there is also a lack of public transport or a long bus or car journey is required to get there.

- **Cultural and language barriers** – for example, cultural beliefs about who should provide care and how illness and social problems should be dealt with, as well as difficulties in using English, may deter members of some communities from using care services.
- **Resource barriers** – for example, lack of staff, lack of information about services, lack of money to fund services or a large demand for services can prevent people from gaining access to services when they need or want them.

You should be able to identify ways in which services and the individuals they serve might overcome these barriers. You should also understand that poor integration of services, rationing and the 'postcode lottery' might affect availability of services in your local area.

Be prepared

You will need a copy of the booklet *Your Guide to the NHS*, available from your local medical centre, hospital, walk-in centre or doctor's surgery, for an activity later in this chapter. You will also need the address and/or phone number of your local social services and early years services.

Try to read newspapers and cut out any articles about shortages of nurses or social service workers, about lack of hospital beds, unfair allocation of money to services in different parts of the country, long waiting lists or about any other crisis in the care services. Keep the cuttings inside your book or folder. They will be a useful source of reference for discussions in class when you are learning about resource barriers later in this chapter. Also, try to watch the news and, again, watch out for any item about a crisis in the care services.

Referral

A client can gain access to the health and social care services in different ways. For example, he or she could arrange to see a doctor him or herself or someone else could make an appointment for the client. Whichever way the client manages to make use of the service, it is called a *referral*.

There are three different forms of referral:

1. The client chooses to ask for or go to the services by him or herself (e.g. rings to makes an appointment with the doctor). This is called **self-referral**.

2. The client is put in contact with the service by a professional (e.g. the doctor sends the client to the hospital for an X-ray). This is called a **professional referral**.

3. The client is put in contact with a service by someone who is not a professional (e.g. an employer sends the person to the doctor for a medical check-up). This is called **third-party referral**.

Self-referral

Self-referral is the main way most people receive health and social care. Examples for health services include a person going to a walk-in centre for treatment for a sprained ankle or making an appointment at the doctor's because he or she is feeling unwell. For social care, an elderly person might go to a day care centre.

Professional referral

A person can only receive hospital treatment if he or she is either admitted to hospital as an emergency case or is referred there by another professional, usually his or her doctor. If a doctor thinks there is something wrong with a patient that requires specialist help, the doctor refers the patient to an outpatient clinic or arranges admission straight on to a hospital ward if the care is more urgently needed.

For social care, a health visitor might contact social services to arrange Meals on Wheels for an elderly patient.

Third-party referral

Third-party referral is the way many of those who cannot look after themselves are referred to services. A person might ring to call the doctor out to visit an elderly neighbour or might make a dental appointment for a relative.

In the area of social care, a person might ring a nursery to enquire about a place for his or her child or a teacher might contact social services if he or she is concerned about a pupil, perhaps suspecting child abuse. All schools have a named person who is responsible for making this kind of referral.

Activity

Read the following case studies.

Jim

Jim lives alone in his two-bedroomed bungalow. Since his wife died last year he has not been able to cook and clean very well for himself. He has a very good neighbour, Mrs Parker, who often calls in and gives him a meal she has made for him whilst cooking for her own family. The last time Mrs Parker visited Jim she noticed he was looking poorly and he said he thought he had a chill coming on. When she visited yesterday he was in bed coughing – his breathing was very noisy and laboured. She went home and called the doctor.

Mrs Shah

Mrs Shah was worried about her legs. She had noticed that by the end of a working day they were really aching. She knew they had never done this before. She decided she needed to visit the doctor. She telephoned the surgery and made an appointment. Dr Smith examined her legs and said she thought Mrs Shah needed to see a specialist. Dr Smith said she would write to the hospital and ask for an appointment for Mrs Shah.

▶ Working in pairs, decide which kinds of referral are being used in each case. It might be more than one method in any one case.

▶ When you see the school nurse, for example for a medical or injection, what kind of referral is being used? Think about who makes the appointment. Give reasons for your answer.

Barriers to referral

Most of us find it easy to use the health and social care services that are provided for us. However, for a variety of reasons some people find it difficult to get access to such services and these reasons are known as *barriers to referral*. The main ones are shown in Figure 3.1.

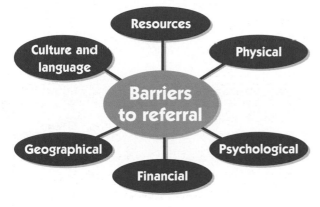

Figure 3.1 The barriers to referral

Physical barriers

Think about the problems that might arise because the building or environment a service is located in is not suitable for some clients. Older buildings often have steps up to the entrance. Clients with mobility problems will find it hard to get into such buildings. This does not mean only those with physical disabilities – parents with babies or children will also have problems. Parents are not happy to leave expensive prams and buggies outside buildings because of the risk of theft. Many new buildings are now being built with ramps as well as steps. Once inside the building, a lack of lifts and a lack of adapted toilet facilities can prevent further movement around the building.

Problems with communication caused by a person who has slurred speech is another physical barrier. If someone cannot make him or herself understood, he or she will avoid using the service. Similarly, a blind person will have difficulty moving around an unfamiliar building. It is therefore important that interpreters or guides are provided.

Activity

Mike is a wheelchair user. He has just started attending his local college to study for a degree. He goes to the education authority to organise his financial benefits and to make arrangements for his home care service to change times as he will now be out of the house at different times of the day. When he gets to the building he wheels himself to the front door, only to find ten steps leading up to the entrance. There is no other way in. Mike asks a passer-by to go in to ask someone to come out and speak to him. The security man comes out and carries Mike and his wheelchair up the stairs. Mike is very embarrassed and feels everyone is staring at him.

▶ Discuss with a partner ways in which the service can be improved to help people with problems such as Mike's.

▷ Write a letter to the education authority putting the case for the changes you feel are necessary to help people like Mike. Try to make the changes as simple as possible because any alteration that is very costly is unlikely to be done quickly. Give reasons why you think the changes are necessary.

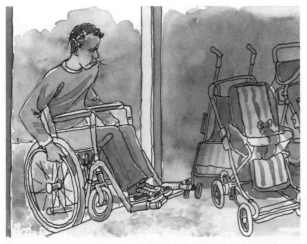

A physical barrier to referral

Accommodation	Visual disability	Hearing disability	Intellectual disabilities
Build ramps	Use conversation rather than written instructions or pictures	Do not shout – make sure sure face is visible for lip reading	Use pictures and signs
Install lifts	Explain details	Use pictures or write messages	Use clear, simple speech
Wide doorways	Check what client *can* see	Learn to sign	Be calm and patient
Adapt toilets	Check spectacles are being worn and are clean	Use a professional communicator	Set up small-group meetings
Handles at wheelchair level	Help client to touch things	Check hearing aids, etc., are being used and are in working order	Make sure client is not isolated
Check areas are clear of clutter, are well it and quiet		Sit close to the client	
Places to leave equipment (e.g. prams, etc.) safely			

Figure 3.2 *Ways of overcoming physical barriers*

Overcoming physical barriers between client and care worker

Figure 3.2 lists some ways physical barriers may be overcome.

Psychological barriers

Psychological barriers arise because of the feelings and attitudes of a client towards a service.

Fear is a very powerful barrier to people using the health and social care services. Some older people may be scared of hospitals because their parents told them about workhouses when they were young. Poor people were sent to live in these before the NHS started. Others are frightened to know what is wrong with them and others may fear having their homes taken away from them or losing their independence. Sometimes people are too proud to use the services. For many older people, not having to ask for help is part of the pride they have in themselves.

Those with mental health problems might not access services because they either do not

realise they need help or they might feel there is a stigma attached to getting help with such problems. They would prefer to try to cope with their own problems than to go and ask for help with something they see as shameful. The same might happen with problems such as alcoholism or being overweight, or with sexually transmitted diseases.

Checkpoint

In this context, a **stigma** is a mark of social disgrace, or something to feel ashamed of.

Overcoming psychological barriers

If someone is reluctant to contact a care service, that person might be encouraged to do so by one of the following means:

- Reading and reacting to the information given in the many leaflets and posters which are freely available in places that people go to regularly, such as supermarkets, health food shops, libraries, pharmacies and health centres.

- Seeing leaflets, cards, posters or other sources advertising telephone helplines. The potential but reluctant client does not even have to leave home to get the details of the helpline or to ring it. The BT phone book contains details about a wide variety of telephone helplines, as does *Yellow Pages*. Health lines include NHS Direct, a confidential 24-hour telephone helpline staffed by nurses who will give advice at any time of the day or night. There are also helplines for social welfare, alcohol, drugs, bereavement, disability, emotional support, family and parents, older people and children. A child with a problem might be scared to tell anyone about their problem because they are frightened someone will take them away from home or will split them from a friend. A child might see a poster or a card in a phone box advertising one of the telephone helplines (such as Childline or NSPCC) and might ring the number because they have no one else to turn to, and someone on the telephone seems safe and anonymous.

- Using the Internet. NHS Direct Online is a website that provides information about health services and a variety of conditions and treatment choices, as well as details about self-help groups. The information given is clear and helpful and might encourage someone to consult a care service.

- Using NHS Direct information points if the person does not have access to the Internet at home. These are touch-screen terminals that can be found in public places (such as supermarkets and pharmacies) and the service is free.

- Asking for advice at a pharmacist, which might seem less threatening than going to see a doctor or to the hospital.

- Finding someone to go with him or her to the care service (e.g. taking a friend along as a 'birth partner').

- Using walk-in centres. Nurses staff these and there is usually a card you can pick up to show if you don't want to say what your problem is at the reception desk.

- Asking someone to make contact for him or her. Family or friends might ring a health, social care or early years service and ask them to contact the person who needs help. Care workers (such as social workers or community nurses) will go to a client's home to talk to him or her to reassure the client and so encourage him or her to see an appropriate carer if necessary.

In all these examples, once contact has been made, the care worker – be it at the end of a telephone line or face to face – will use his or her training to explain carefully, clearly and kindly the options available and, hopefully, persuade someone who is afraid of using a care service to overcome his or her fears. The care worker will make appointments for the client and sometimes collect and escort the client to the appointment.

Activity

Emily is 42 years of age. She has just found a lump in her breast and is terrified it is cancer. She will not make an appointment with the doctor and she has not told her partner. What would she do if they told her it was cancer? She thinks that if she ignores it, it might go away.

▶ Discuss with a partner how fear is making Emily react. What should she be doing?

▶ Think of three reasons that might make it easier for Emily to go to the doctor.

Financial barriers

Lack of money can be a major barrier to people using care services, many of which have to be paid for. Some clients might not be able to afford the bus or train fares to reach the service they need. Also, the services clients need might not be available in their area because there is not enough money. Charges and fees can therefore discourage and exclude those people who do not have the money to pay for the services they need.

Overcoming financial barriers

The NHS plan, which the Prime Minister launched in July 2000, describes how increased funding will improve the NHS. The NHS list of core principles (that is, the things the NHS believes are important and is committed to) states that the NHS will provide a universal service for all based on clinical need, not ability to pay. What this means is that anyone who is examined and found to be in need of treatment will receive that treatment, even if they cannot afford to pay for it.

Another core principle is that public funds for health care will be devoted solely to NHS patients. From April 2001, the NHS will not take into account the value of a person's home for the means-testing rules for the first three months of residential or nursing home care. From October 2001, nursing care was made free in any setting, including nursing homes. By 2004 a new level of service has been promised that will provide high-quality care closer to home so, hopefully, this will alleviate (help) the problem of paying fares to reach the required services.

These improvements to the NHS should help to overcome some of the financial barriers some people face for health care. All essential services (such as health screening, vaccinations and immunisations, school health services, dental services, maternity, community and hospital services and education provision) are free for children under the age of 16, so early years services should not present a financial barrier.

Checkpoint

Means-testing is when the value of all your assets, such as your house and your savings, is worked out to see how much you can afford to pay towards something yourself.

Activity

Allocate two people from the class to contact your local social services to find out what services have to be paid for and how they help people who cannot afford them. They can then present the information to the rest of the class. After this presentation, decide if you think lack of money is a barrier to people wanting to use social services in your area.

Geographical barriers

These problems are caused as a result of where the service is located in relation to where the client lives. Having too far to travel can be a major barrier to using the services, and so can having no public transport system. Some clients live in rural areas where public transport systems are limited.

Overcoming geographical barriers

In some areas hospitals will send an ambulance to collect a client who has no transport. The commitment of the NHS to provide a universal service, to respond to the different needs of different populations and to provide high-quality care closer to home will, it is hoped, help some clients to overcome geographical barriers. By 2004, the NHS says clients may be treated in a GP practice instead of having to travel to hospital for treatment. These improvements (along with the advice on treatment that is available on the Internet, over the telephone and on touch-screens) should help reduce geographical barriers to health care.

Bus services are timed and routed so that children can get to school on time (even for those children who live in rural areas), and day centres often lay on transport to get clients to day care centres. Again, advice is available on telephone helplines if someone has a problem and needs to contact social services. Thus some geographical barriers have been overcome.

Cultural and language barriers

These are problems people have because they are of a different culture, speak a different language or because they do not understand the way in which things are said.

Culture means the history, customs and ways people learn as they grow up. The expressions people use and the meanings non-verbal signs can have vary from one culture to another. People use different terms, such as jargon (technical language), slang and dialect, which might prevent others understanding them.

White middle-class people often expect other people to look them in the eye while talking, interpreting someone who looks away a lot as being dishonest. In other cultures (for example, among some black communities), looking down or away when talking is a sign of respect.

Cultural beliefs about who should provide care and how illness and social problems should be dealt with may deter members of some communities from using care services. Even in a medical setting, many Muslim women will react strongly against any physical contact with men (for example, in an examination by a male doctor or nurse). Such contact with men is considered to be humiliating and dirty, leaving the woman feeling sinful and spiritually unclean. Muslim women should be examined by women doctors if possible and Muslim men by male doctors.

Older male Muslim patients are often unaccustomed to dealing with women of professional status or in positions of authority and may sometimes be embarrassed and difficult with female health and social care workers. This is particularly likely with nurses, who traditionally have a low status in Muslim and Asian societies because they have physical contact with men in the course of their work.

Conservative Muslim women are traditionally clothed from head to foot, except for their hands and faces. For a Muslim woman to be asked to wear a backless hospital gown or a garment with a low neckline, therefore, is not only immoral but also humiliating, especially in the presence of strangers and particularly men. Most Muslim women do not undress fully except when they are alone. If Muslim women are allowed to uncover only parts of themselves at a time for physical examination in hospitals and clinics, this may avoid distress and encourage Muslim women to use care services.

Every adult Muslim is expected to say certain prayers at set times every day. If they are in hospital they may require a private place (or at least curtains drawn around the bed) for this, and they will need to wash certain parts of the body before praying. Bed-bound Muslims who have used a bedpan may wish to be given a proper wash with water before they can pray.

In Asian traditions, the head is regarded as the most sacred part of the body and most devout Sikh men and women never cut their hair (men do not shave their beards). Conservative Sikhs may become very distressed if hair on any part of the body is shaved or cut except for good medical reasons or in an emergency. It is therefore important that the need for such hair removal is explained to the patient or his or her family beforehand. Where it is essential to remove body hair it may be more acceptable to use a depilatory cream rather than a razor or scissors.

These are just a few examples of situations in which health and social care services need to respond in a supportive way to different cultural beliefs so as not to deter clients from using the services. The national survey of NHS patients, *General Practice*, published in October 1999, showed that nearly one in three clients said it was important to be able to see a GP from their

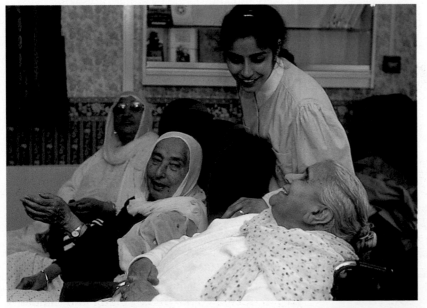

Health and social care services should respond positively to clients' cultural beliefs

own ethnic group (see Figure 3.3). Women were more likely to consider this important than men. The older patients of both sexes considered this to be more important (see Figure 3.4).

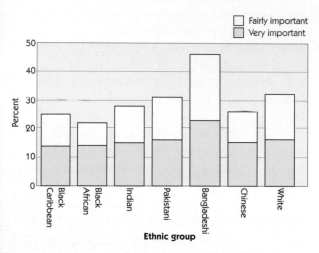

Figure 3.3 *The importance of seeing a GP of your own ethnic group, by age and sex of respondent*

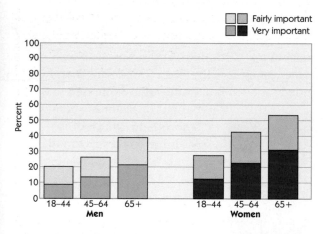

Figure 3.4 *The importance of seeing a GP of your own ethnic group, by ethnic group of respondent*

Figures 3.3, 3.4, 3.5 and 3.6 reproduced with permission from the Department of Health

Activity

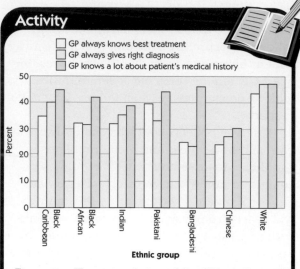

Figure 3.5 *The general view of the GP's skills and knowledge, by ethnic group of respondent*

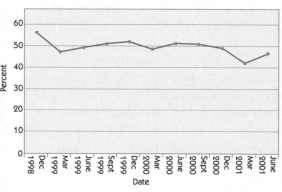

Figure 3.6 *Views of patient–GP communication, by ethnic group of respondent*

Look at the graph showing views of the GP's skills and knowledge by ethnic group of respondent (Figure 3.5).

▶ **1**   Are patients from ethnic minorities more or less critical of the doctor's skills than white patients?

2   How do you know this from the graph?

Look at the graph showing views of patient–GP communication by ethnic group of respondent (Figure 3.6).

▶ **1**   Are white respondents more or less likely to say their GP always gives enough information, listens and takes their opinions seriously?

2   What can you say about the number of respondents of Bangladeshi or Chinese origin who gave critical responses as compared with the number of white respondents?

Give reasons for all your answers.

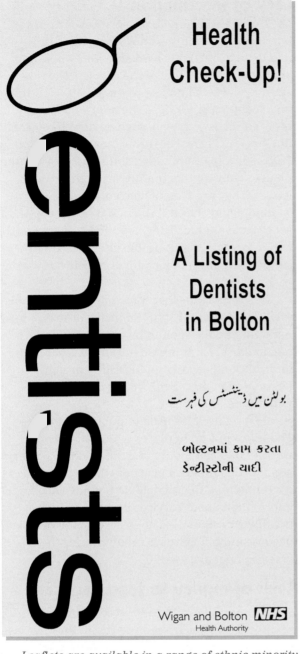

Health Check-Up!

A Listing of Dentists in Bolton

بولٹن میں ڈینٹسٹس کی فہرست

બોલ્ટનમાં કામ કરતા ડેન્ટીસ્ટોની યાદી

Wigan and Bolton **NHS**
Health Authority

Leaflets are available in a range of ethnic minority languages

The care services provide leaflets and posters in a wide range of ethnic minority languages so that information is readily available to all.

Similarly, arrangements have to be made for those who have difficulty using English. If people cannot make themselves understood because they speak a different language, including sign language, they will not use the service. It is therefore important that interpreters are provided.

Activity

Various cultural and language barriers were described above, and ways of overcoming these were suggested for some of them. Read through this section again and then copy and complete the table below. You will have to suggest ways of your own to overcome some of these barriers.

Barrier to services	Cultural or language?	How to overcome them?

▶ Work in groups. Identify the tasks you will need to do to complete this activity and divide them up fairly between the members of your group.

Contact your local health authority, social services and early years services. Ask them how they help people to overcome cultural and language barriers. Also ask them to send you leaflets in several different languages. The NHS, for example, has a form on which medical centres, hospitals, etc., can order free leaflets in a range of languages on specific health issues and details of how to access these services.

Put all the information gathered together and present it in such a way that it is clear and easily understood by the rest of the class.

Resource barriers

These are problems caused by a lack of resources (such as staff, information or funding), or because there is too much demand on certain services.

Lack of staff

Lack of staff can prevent people from gaining access to services when they want them. Nurses are currently being recruited from abroad to try to cope with the national shortage of nurses.

DEATHS OF SICK BABIES CAUSED BY LACK OF NURSES

A report published today warned that if an intensive care unit is busy a sick baby could be 50 per cent more likely to die. It states that there needs to be a rise in the number of neonatal intensive care nurses so that each sick baby has a specialist nurse looking after it.

Expert and patient groups welcomed the new report, saying that it 'reinforces the many concerns we have had about the state of neonatal care in this country'. One source said that 'These statistics show that the shortage of nurses is having a significant effect on the ability of such units to look after sick babies properly, leading to the death of babies, and this situation should not be tolerated by the government'. However, the report also said that although the number of deaths fell as the number of nurses grew, the risk of hospital infection grew as the number of doctors grew.

▶ **1** Why are there not enough one-to-one nurses? Give at least three answers.

2 Make suggestions as to what should be done to try to solve each of these three reasons.

3 What effect do you think it will have on the nurses who currently work in neonatal intensive care units if babies keep dying when they are busy?

▶ **1** Write down what personal qualities you think a nurse working on a neonatal intensive care unit needs to have and why.

2 Discuss in a small group whether you think more money should be raised by increasing taxes to pay for extra nurses.

Lack of information

Lack of information about services is another barrier. If a client does not know what is available, where it is available and when it is available, or how to use the service, that service will be of no use to the client. Health and social care services therefore publicise their services in places such as health centres, doctors' surgeries, libraries, hospitals, *Yellow Pages*, newspapers, television and other similar places. They do this mainly through printed leaflets that are free of charge, readily available and that tell the client about the services available. They need to be as attractive and informative as possible, and written in simple language so a client is encouraged to read them.

It is important that information is available in languages other than English – at least in the main languages spoken by the people in a particular area. It is also important that information is available in Braille or sign language for those with visual or hearing difficulties.

Posters are also used to publicise services. These are put up in places where the people who need to see them hang out, such as posters about drug helplines in areas where drug users go. It might be that people do not have access to information about services because they are travellers or homeless; therefore advertising via posters and billboards is important for these groups of people.

Lack of money to fund services

The amount of money allocated to health and social care varies from one area to another, as does the efficiency of the way in which that money is managed. If a client is unfortunate enough to live in an area where services are poorly integrated and funding is scarce, he or she is more likely to wait longer for treatment and, in some cases, be denied treatment because the local area cannot afford an expensive drug. It might be that the person living next door has a different postcode, which places them under the responsibility of a different health authority so that if he or she had the same medical condition needing the same expensive drug and that authority could afford it, he or she would get the treatment whilst the neighbour would not. This is known as a *postcode lottery* and can mean the difference between life and death for some people.

Figures released by the Department of Health show that spending per head of population varied considerably in 2000–2001, from £1,346 in Morecambe Bay, Cumbria, to £732 in Wigan and Bolton. Other places where expenditure was high were Camden and Islington in North London, with £1,067, and Sefton, Merseyside, with £1,040. This means that some health authorities are spending twice as much per head of population as others.

When the NHS was set up, it was assumed that because health would improve the costs of the services would eventually drop. This did not happen and costs have continued to go up. There are also more and more elderly people in the UK because people are generally living for longer so the money generated by national insurance and tax is not sufficient. This means there are always problems about deciding who takes priority when there is only a limited supply of money for treatment and equipment each month. Inevitably, some people will not get the treatment they need as quickly as they need it.

Large demand for services

A large demand for services can also prevent people from gaining access to services. If a person happens to have an appointment for a particular treatment that requires a hospital bed and there is a flu epidemic, the chances

Activity

Guide to hospitals highlights the postcode lottery of maternity care

Some mothers face a much harder labour than others due to the huge variation in care they receive in maternity hospitals. Decisions such as whether they get an epidural or how quickly they get hurried out of the delivery suite are decided by where they live. A report published today points out that the recommended safety limit for the number of babies delivered each year per midwife is 35, yet at more than 50 hospitals midwives are helping to deliver more babies than this. In the worst case the limit was exceeded by half as much again. At the 26 busiest maternity units more than one baby was being born in each bed per day, suggesting that women are being sent home too soon.

▶ 1 What effect might the amount of time spent in the delivery room have on (a) the mother and (b) the baby?

2 Why do you think there is a recommended safety limit on the number of babies a midwife helps to deliver each year?

3 What might be the possible consequences of sending a mother home too early on (a) the mother and (b) the baby?

▶ 1 In the worst case mentioned above, work out how many babies the midwife was delivering a year.

2 Other variations identified further on in the newspaper article are the number of Caesareans performed, the number of babies delivered by forceps, the number of babies born at home and the number of staff available at each birth. Discuss in a small group why each of these might happen and what effect, if any, each of these might have on the mothers, their partners and the babies.

3 Why does the headline refer to a 'postcode lottery'?

are the treatment will be postponed because there will be a huge demand for beds. Similarly, the chances of getting an appointment with a doctor are greatly reduced when there is an outbreak of measles or some other illness.

Summary of barriers to the use of services

Figure 3.8 summarises some of the barriers clients might experience when trying to gain access to services.

Activity

Resource barriers can cause distress to people and articles about them appear regularly in newspapers. The stories reported on pages 42 and 43 appeared in the newspapers within two days of each other.

▶ Read the NHS core principles shown in Figure 3. 7, which were written on the basis that increased funding will be used to improve the NHS. Pick out those that will help overcome some of the resource barriers mentioned in this section.

OUR COMMITMENT TO YOU – we want the NHS to be a high-quality health service. These are our aims as set out in the NHS Plan.

The NHS will provide a universal service for all based on clinical need, not ability to pay.

The NHS will provide a comprehensive range of services.

The NHS will shape its services around the needs and preferences of individual patients, their families and their carers.

The NHS will respond to different needs of different populations.

The NHS will work continuously to improve quality services and to minimise errors.

The NHS will support and value its staff.

Public funds for health care will be devoted solely to NHS patients.

The NHS will work together with others to ensure a seamless service for patients.

The NHS will help keep people healthy and work to reduce health inequalities.

The NHS will respect the confidentiality of individual patients and provide open access to information about services, treatment and performance.

Figure 3.7 The NHS core principles

▶ Read a copy of the booklet *Your Guide to the NHS*. Identify and then write down the targets (including the dates) that will help overcome each of the resource barriers described above. Explain clearly *how* they will help.

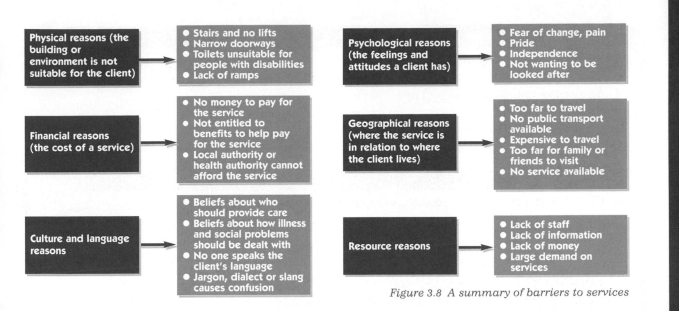

| Physical reasons (the building or environment is not suitable for the client) | • Stairs and no lifts
• Narrow doorways
• Toilets unsuitable for people with disabilities
• Lack of ramps | Psychological reasons (the feelings and attitudes a client has) | • Fear of change, pain
• Pride
• Independence
• Not wanting to be looked after |

| Financial reasons (the cost of a service) | • No money to pay for the service
• Not entitled to benefits to help pay for the service
• Local authority or health authority cannot afford the service | Geographical reasons (where the service is in relation to where the client lives) | • Too far to travel
• No public transport available
• Expensive to travel
• Too far for family or friends to visit
• No service available |

| Culture and language reasons | • Beliefs about who should provide care
• Beliefs about how illness and social problems should be dealt with
• No one speaks the client's language
• Jargon, dialect or slang causes confusion | Resource reasons | • Lack of staff
• Lack of information
• Lack of money
• Large demand on services |

Figure 3.8 A summary of barriers to services

Activity

Look at Figure 3.9, which shows (in the table) inpatient waiting lists and (in the graph) the number of patients waiting over 13 months carried over every 3 months from December 1998 to June 2001. Answer the following questions:

▶ 1 What type of referral will have been used for the waiting patients to be included on the waiting list?

2 What is meant by orthopaedics? (Look it up in a dictionary if you don't know.)

3 Which type of treatment had the largest percentage of patients waiting over 12 months?

4 Which type of treatment had the smallest percentage of patients waiting over 12 months?

5 Did the number of patients waiting go down, stay the same or go up over the time period shown in the graph?

▷ 1 Which type of treatment had the largest percentage increase in waiting time from up to 5 months to over 12 months?

2 Which type of treatment had the largest percentage increase in waiting time from up to 5 months to over 5 months?

3 What fraction of patients has been waiting less than 6 months for all treatment?

4 Between June 2000 and June 2001 the number of patients waiting over one year decreased by 4,700. Write a list of possible explanations for this decrease.

5 Find out what ophthalmology, gynaecology and urology involve.

In patient waiting lists: patients waiting for elective admission, June 2001, variation by specialty (ordinary admissions and day cases combined) England				
Specialty	**Total number waiting (thousands)**	**Months waiting (percent)**		
		0-5	**6-11**	**12+**
All specialties	1037.9	74.3	21.2	4.5
Trauma and orthopaedics	249.1	65.9	27.1	6.9
General surgery	187.0	75.5	20.4	4.2
Opthalmology	151.2	74.3	22.9	2.8
Ear, nose and throat	112.8	70.0	24.2	5.8
Obstetrics and gynaecology	83.8	84.6	13.3	2.1
Urology	73.0	79.5	16.8	3.7
Plastic surgery	42.2	70.8	22.9	6.3
Oral surgery	32.7	85.8	12.2	2.0
Others	106.1	82.1	15.0	2.9

Percentages may not sum due to rounding

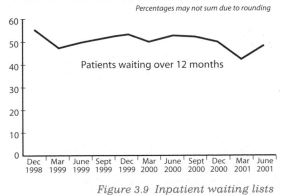

Figure 3.9 Inpatient waiting lists

Figure 3.9 reproduced with permission from the Department of Health

Check your knowledge

1. What is meant by referral?
2. Name the three different types of referral.
3. Give an example of each, but not one given in this chapter!
4. What does the phrase 'barrier to referral' mean?
5. Give an example of a physical barrier to referral.
6. How could this barrier be overcome?
7. Give an example of a psychological barrier to referral.
8. How might this barrier be overcome?
9. Who might experience a financial barrier to referral?
10. How could this person be helped to overcome this barrier?
11. Give an example of a geographical barrier.
12. Suggest how this barrier could be overcome.
13. Hospitals need to cater for the different needs of their patients. What dietary factors need to be considered when providing meals for Jewish patients?
14. Give an example of a religious barrier to health care.
15. Stick any newspaper articles you have collected in your book or folder. Highlight the parts that show what sort of barrier to referral has caused this crisis.

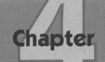

Chapter 4

The main jobs in health, social care and early years services

Key issue

What does care work involve and what skills do care practitioners need to perform their work roles?

By the end of this chapter, you should be able to compare the main work roles of care workers. You should understand the similarities and differences in the work roles of health, social care and early years workers, and know about the roles of practitioners who deliver care directly and those whose work is more indirectly involved with care. Examples are as follows:

- **Direct care:** Nurse, doctor, social worker, care assistant, nursery nurse.
- **Indirect care:** Medical receptionist, cleaner, porter.

You should understand why care workers need good interpersonal skills, and how care workers use communication skills to develop care relationships, to provide and receive information and to report on the work they do with clients.

You will need to know how effective communication can help support relationships with colleagues and with clients and their families, and how poor skills can reduce the effectiveness of care work or damage care relationships. You should also be able to recognise the differing communication needs of client groups using care services.

Groups of care workers

There are two main groups of care workers in health and social care services:

1 **Direct** carers: people who provide care directly to the client.
2 **Indirect** carers: people who provide a service to the direct carers that will ultimately benefit the client.

There are many different jobs in health and social care settings. In the following pages only a small proportion of these will be described. You will be able to find out about those jobs that are not described from career guides, in your careers library if you have one, at the library, on the Internet or from the health and social care services themselves.

Activity

In a group, write a list of as many different jobs as you can think of that are related to health, social and early years services. Do not turn the pages of this book or there will be no point in doing this! Then look through the tables and headings of this chapter to see if there are any areas you have not thought of.

Jobs in the direct provision of health care

The NHS is the biggest employer of staff in Europe but not everyone who is involved in the provision of health care is employed by the NHS (see Figure 4.1). Some health care professionals are employed by voluntary organisations, private companies or government departments or are self-employed. Many health care jobs require specialist training (for example, nurses or physiotherapists).

Nurses

From the beginning of their training, nurses may choose to specialise in one form of nursing. Alternatively, nurses undertaking the adult general nurse training may (on completion) continue to train in a very specific branch of nursing. For example:
- nurse practitioner;
- midwifery;
- health visiting;
- general practice nursing;
- school nursing; or
- district nursing.

Doctors	Nurses	Therapists	Others	Support staff
Gynaecologist	District nurse	Physiotherapist	Chemist	Environmental health officer
Psychiatrist	Community psychiatric nurse	Aromatherapist*	Pharmacist	Administrator
Cardiologist	Ward co-ordinator or manager (sister)	Speech therapist	Chiropodist	Health service manager
Dermatologist	Health visitor	Art therapist*	Radiographer	Ambulance crew
Physician	Hospital nurse	Hypnotherapist*	Dietician	Catering officer
General practitioner	Midwife	Counsellor	Optician	Domestic supervisor
Surgeon	Nursing auxiliary	Drama therapist*	Pathologist	Laboratory technician
Geriatrician	Nurse for people with learning disabilities	Acupuncturist*	Anaesthetist	Medical records officer
Neurologist	Occupational health nurse	Homoeopath*	Dentist	Medical secretary
Paediatrician	Paediatric nurse	Osteopath*		Radiotherapist
Rheumatologist		Psychologist		Receptionist

Note: *Complementary therapies.

Figure 4.1 A few of the main jobs in health care

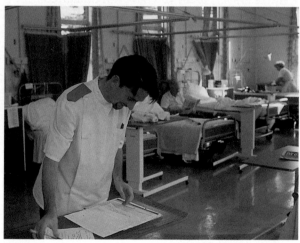

A hospital nurse at work

Nursing is physically, intellectually and emotionally demanding work. Being faced with illness and injury is always traumatic for patients and their relatives. Nurses have to have very good *communication* and *interpersonal* skills as they often need to be able to deal with very difficult situations, distressed patients and relatives. Nurses often have to work unsociable hours, late nights, early mornings, weekends and bank holidays and may be required to work all night. This demands *adaptability* and a *strong sense of commitment* to the work (see Figure 4.2).

Nurses also need certain *practical* skills. For example, a hospital nurse might:

- take temperatures, blood pressure and respiration rate;
- give injections;
- administer medicines;
- clean and dress wounds;
- bandage and splint limbs;
- administer blood transfusions and drips;
- do routine tasks such as making beds, ensuring patients are comfortable, or escorting them to other departments (such as X-ray or the operating theatre);

and many, many other jobs.

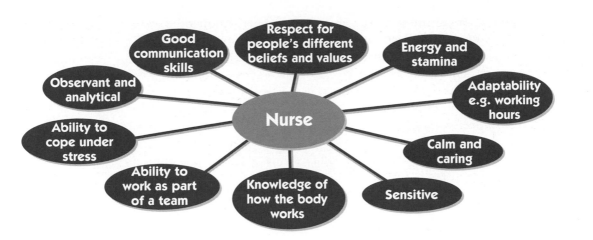

Figure 4.2 *The skills and qualities required of a nurse*

Case study

Serge is a fully qualified nurse on a busy medical ward at his local teaching hospital. When he arrives at work he meets with the other nurses to discuss the care given to the patients during the night. He is part of the Blue Team and has responsibility for a certain number of patients. This morning he will be caring for six patients but will have a care assistant to help him.

First, he gives tablets, which have been prescribed by the doctor, to each patient, and makes sure that each of them has had breakfast. His first priority is to care for Mr Desai, who has a chest infection and needs particular care with his breathing.

After he is satisfied that Mr Desai is comfortable and has easy access to his oxygen mask, if he needs it, he checks the drip on Mr Smith. Mr Smith has had diarrhoea and vomiting for three days and needs extra fluids regularly.

As Mr Smith is quite weak, Serge decides to give him a bed bath with the help of the care assistant.

▶ 1 What information will have been discussed at the meeting with other nurses when Serge first arrives at work?

2 What practical skills will Serge have to use in caring for Mr Desai?

3 Why does Serge decide to have a care assistant with him when he bed baths Mr Smith?

4 What personal qualities will Serge need in being part of Blue Team?

▶ 1 What does the term 'teaching hospital' mean?

2 What are the implications of the hospital being a teaching hospital for (a) Serge and (b) for the patients?

3 What personal skills must Serge have to deal with nursing in a teaching hospital?

Nurses not only have to be fully aware of their patient's medical history, conditions and treatments but also need to plan a programme of care which includes taking account of their emotional and social needs, thereby providing a *holistic* system of care. They often provide both patients and relatives with reassurance and are also health educators, explaining what lifestyle changes are needed to improve health and hopefully prevent further illness. Nurses provide an overall service to their patients that means more to the patients than if they simply performed practical tasks.

Checkpoint

A **holistic** approach means looking at all the different needs a patient may have – for example, their medical condition and treatments, whether there is anyone to look after the patient when they go home from hospital, whether the patient understands what is wrong with them, and understanding the reasons why the patient may be upset.

Nurses also work as part of a team, which includes many other health professionals depending on the area the nurse works in. The team may include other nurses, doctors, social workers, health care assistants, pharmacists and physiotherapists. This is known as a *multidisciplinary team*, which basically means a team that is made up of different health professionals (see Figure 4.3).

In primary care the team is typically made up of a GP, a practice nurse, a practice manager, a health visitor, a district nurse, a health care assistant, a social worker and a community psychiatric nurse, and this is known as the *Primary Health and Social Care Team* (PHSCT).

In hospitals there are lots of different areas a nurse may work in. Some of these are listed below:

- Surgical wards – for patients who are having operations.
- Medical wards – for patients who have such illnesses as diabetes, heart conditions or breathing problems.

- Orthopaedic wards – for patients with bone problems.
- Operating theatres.
- Accident and emergency departments.
- Intensive care units.
- Day case areas.
- Outpatient departments.
- Elderly care areas.
- Children's units.

Doctors

Doctors, like general nurses, all undergo the same initial training before they go on to specialise in different areas of medicine. Part of a doctor's job is to diagnose (find out what is wrong) the illness and treat it appropriately. Sometimes there is nothing wrong and the doctor or nurse will need to reassure the patient this is the case. Doctors need to be able to listen to people's problems, to provide advice and to be able to educate patients about their health.

General practitioners (GPs): The GP or family doctor is probably the doctor we are

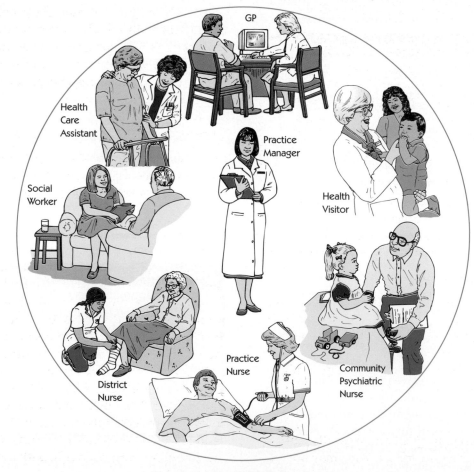

Figure 4.3 A multidisciplinary team

most familiar with as the GP is usually the first doctor we go to see when we are not well. The GP works in local surgeries or health centres and will examine the patient, and may do certain tests to establish what is causing the problem. The GP will then either prescribe suitable treatment or refer the patient to the hospital for further tests, to the hospital consultant when necessary or to other agencies for specialist services.

Consultants: Depending on the patient's needs, the patient may be referred on to one of a number of doctors who specialise in one particular area. These are known as consultants and usually work in the hospital (secondary care). Below are some examples of different types of consultants:

- Paediatrician – specialises in children's diseases.
- Oncologist – cancer specialist.
- Cardiologist – heart specialist.
- Surgeon – performs operations.
- Pathologist – examines blood and tissue specimens and provides a diagnosis.

Activity

Write a list of the skills and qualities needed by a GP *and* by a nurse. Then divide your page in two, putting the heading 'Similarities' at the top of one column and the heading 'Differences' at the top of the other. Put the skills you have identified into the correct column.

1 Do GPs and nurses need similar skills for their work with patients?
2 Do they need similar qualities?

Physiotherapists

A physiotherapist provides exercises and other treatments to improve mobility, to relieve pain and to prevent permanent physical disability as a result of injuries or disease. They can work in a range of different settings in both hospitals and the community.

Dieticians

Dieticians help to prevent and treat diseases caused by poor eating habits. They may advise individual patients on a one-to-one basis or work with groups of patients with the same problem (for example, groups of diabetic patients or heart disease patients who will need similar dietary advice). They work in community settings, in hospitals and sometimes in schools.

Pharmacists

Pharmacists dispense prescribed medicines. They advise doctors and other health professionals on the selection of the safest and most effective drugs. Pharmacists also educate patients on the proper use of both prescription and non-prescription drugs.

Occupational therapists

Occupational therapists help patients with disabilities to develop, recover or maintain the basic skills needed to work or perform the activities of daily life. They treat elderly patients with, perhaps, mobility problems or who may have suffered a stroke. They help patients with severe arthritis or others with physical disabilities or memory problems. They usually specialise in either the physical or mental health care of patients but do occasionally work in both. They work in different settings, such as hospitals, day centres and the community.

Speech and language therapists

Speech and language therapists help people who have speech problems due to hearing loss, brain damage, stroke or other conditions.

Health care assistants

Health care assistants are now increasing in numbers in general practice and their main areas of work are usually to support the practice nurse role. The health care assistant would ideally hold an NVQ (National Vocational Qualification) in care, and tasks would typically include clerical support for the practice nurse, ordering of stock, maintenance of supplies and some computer work e.g. data input and audit information. The health care assistant may also receive training for the taking of blood samples, blood pressure recording, testing of urine samples and checking patients' height and weight.

Check your knowledge

1 What is the difference between direct and indirect care?
2 Name three areas of specialised nursing.
3 What is the difference between a quality and a skill?
4 What is meant by the phrase 'a holistic system of care'?
5 Name three different wards a nurse might work on and explain what each one specialises in.
6 What do the initials PHSCT stand for?
7 List five tasks a doctor might do.
8 What is a consultant?
9 Name three areas in which a consultant might work and say what the specialism is for each.
10 What is a therapist?
11 Name three different types of therapist.
12 What is the name of the qualification you can gain while doing a job – a qualification that is *about* that job?

Direct provision of social care

People who work in social care may be employed by public, private or voluntary organisations. They may undertake residential work, day care work or 'fieldwork'. *Fieldwork* is the term used when a worker operates from a base (usually an office) but goes out to meet people, sometimes in their own homes. As with health care, many other people are employed in jobs that support the direct provision of care (such as clerks and catering staff) but who may not come into direct contact with the clients.

Care assistants

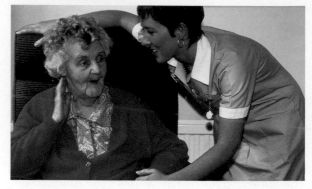

Care assistants often provide social care. Most are employed by local authorities but they are increasingly being employed in the private sector as local authorities move away from the direct provision of services to the purchase of private care services. Care assistants work in a variety of settings, such as residential homes, day centres, day nurseries or in people's own homes. Numerous other people are also employed in jobs that are concerned with people's social welfare (see Figure 4.4).

Care workers assist people who require help with every day tasks, such as getting up, washing, bathing, going to the toilet, dressing, shopping and housework. Sometimes care assistants will help people to learn new skills such as budgeting. They may also help set up activities for their clients that will help them improve or maintain their independence, as well as providing friendly advice and a listening ear. Obviously these tasks vary

Social workers	Care workers	Counsellors	Others
Children and families	Residential care	People with AIDS	Community workers
Older people	Day care	Bereavement	Housing officers
People with disabilities	Home care	Drugs and alcohol	Instructors
People with learning disabilities	People with disabilities	Family work	Liaison officers
People with mental health problems	People with learning disabilities	General counselling	Probation officers
Medical social workers	People with AIDS	Marital problems	Social work assistants
Palliative care social workers	Children and families	Students	Wardens
People with AIDS		Teenagers	

Figure 4.4 A few of the main jobs in social care

according to the individual client: care assistants can work with children and young people, people with physical or learning disabilities and with older people. As care assistants work in a variety of settings their working hours can vary greatly. Some may be required to work shifts, or over weekends and at bank holidays.

Skills and qualities: Care assistants must be able to work with people from all sorts of backgrounds, religions, cultures and of different ages. They will need to be able to work alone and as part of a team. Maturity and common sense are very important. They must also have the right attitude and personality to be able to work with frail people, people with disabilities or people who have difficulty doing everyday tasks. Patience, tolerance and the ability to encourage clients to do for themselves those things they are able to do are very important.

Social workers

The majority of social workers are employed by local authorities although some may be employed by the health services or by voluntary organisations, such as the National Society for the Prevention of Cruelty to Children (NSPCC). The role of the social worker is to help people of all ages who need support with various aspects of their lives. These problems may be connected to low incomes, poor housing, difficulties due to illness, disability, old age or relationships. Social workers often work in teams that specialise in working with particular client groups, such as children and families, older people, people with physical disabilities, people with learning disabilities or people with mental health problems.

When appropriate, social workers meet their clients and families to assess the needs of individuals and families. They then set up and co-ordinate the services required to meet those needs. For example, a young man who has had a road traffic accident that results in him having to use a wheelchair may need someone to help with personal care, household tasks and may need special transport to get about. Sometimes the team includes other professionals such as occupational therapists, home carers and clerks.

Some social workers specialise in areas of work such as fostering or helping people who are drug or alcohol dependent. They often provide ongoing emotional support to the people they work with. Most work a 36-hour week, but they are required to be flexible in their working hours, which can sometimes involve evening and, occasionally, weekend working.

● Snapshot

Anthony is a social worker specialising in the care of older people. His clients are referred by GPs, health visitors, the hospital and sometimes by friends and family of the older person.

Albert has been referred by a hospital to the social services department where Anthony works. Albert was in hospital being treated for an illness caused by drinking too much alcohol (alcohol abuse). Anthony plans to help Albert cut down on his drinking to avoid serious problems in the future. Anthony knows that Albert has not claimed the benefits he is entitled to and has been using his small savings to pay for his drinking instead of paying his bills and buying food. His electricity supply has been cut off. Anthony is dealing with that before Albert goes home.

Anthony knows that Albert has a son and daughter somewhere but does not think they have much contact with their father.

Skills and qualities: Social workers deal with all sorts of people, from different backgrounds, religions, cultures and of different ages. They therefore need to respect individuals' personal beliefs, identities and the choices they make. They also need to be very good communicators, both verbally and in writing. Keeping records and writing reports is an important aspect of the social worker's role. To assess people's needs they must be able to build up a rapport with people, collect and analyse large amounts of complex information, explain the options available to meet people's needs and negotiate with others in order to obtain the services necessary to meet those needs.

There are often conflicting demands made on social workers' time. Therefore they must be able to prioritise the tasks they need to do and to be capable of working under pressure.

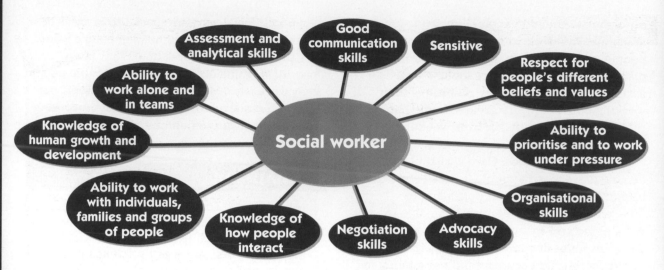

Figure 4.5 The skills and qualities required of a social worker

Much of the work can be emotionally demanding, but they must come to understand their clients' problems without getting involved at a personal level. Social workers must be strong enough to deal with a lack of co-operation from some of their clients while still trying to help them (see Figure 4.5).

Direct provision of early years services

Local authorities, voluntary organisations and private agencies are involved in the provision of day care services and playgroups for children aged 5 years and under, and they may also provide out-of-school 'clubs' for children between the ages of 5 and 8 years. The main jobs in early years services include nursery nurses, childminders, and play and playgroup leaders. They also include 'nannies' and au pairs (who are employed directly by parents, often through agencies) and child care professionals such as educational psychologists.

Other professionals involved in providing appropriate health care services for babies and young children include paediatricians, midwives, health visitors, nurses who specialise in working with ill children, speech therapists, physiotherapists and play therapists.

As in health and social care, there are also many people in jobs that provide support to those giving direct care but who may not come into direct contact with the clients (see Figure 4.6).

Health care	Social care and early years education	Support staff
Midwives	Play leaders	Managers
Health visitors	Play therapists	Administrators
Paediatric nurses	Social workers	Secretaries
Nannies	Nannies	Cooks
Nursery nurses	Nursery nurses/ Nursery teachers	Cleaners
Speech therapists	Au pairs	
Physiotherapists	Psychologists Childminders Specialist teacher assistants	

Figure 4.6 A few of the main jobs in early years services

Nursery nurses

Nursery nurses can work in a variety of settings, such as day nurseries, residential nurseries, school crèches, hospitals or in the child's own home. They may work as part of a team or alone with one or two children or a group of children. They take responsibility for the overall care of the children in their charge.

Nursery nurses can be involved in many care tasks, such as feeding, washing and toileting. They are also responsible for planning activities and play following the guidelines set out in the Early Learning Goals. These provide guidance on what children should be able to do at the ages of 3, 4 and 5 years. From school year 1 onwards the children's learning is planned according to the requirements of the National Curriculum.

Hi, I'm Jodie, and I work at Riverside Playgroup. I qualified last year and this is my first job. I work with children in the 3–4 years group. There are eight at the moment. My title is nursery nurse.

We usually start the day with a song and then I set up activities for them to do. We have a theme each month: it is autumn colours this month (September), so we do lots of work on colour, trees, season changes, and songs and stories with the theme of autumn.

I have one structured activity in the morning, so the children will all be able to take something home. Today it was bubble painting with autumn colours – I had to make sure they 'blew' the paint not drink it up!

I have a sort of checklist to help me make sure we cover a range of activities over a two-week period. It is important to give the children a wide variety of activities. Most of the activities can be included in the Early Learning Goals. We have fun! The children are always curious and are great to be with. I am tired at the end of the day though.

Skills and qualities: These are shown in Figure 4.7.

Activity

What tasks do nursery nurses perform as part of their routine work with children? What tasks do hospital nurses perform as part of their routine work with children? Draw the table below and put the tasks into the correct column.

Similar roles of a nursery nurse and a hospital nurse	Different roles of a nursery nurse and a hospital nurse

Write a job description, a person specification (which states the skills and qualities applicants for the job should have) and an advertisement for a job as a nursery nurse in a private day nursery.

Jobs providing indirect care

To care for their clients effectively, health and social care workers who provide direct care very often need the help of support services. The people who work in these supportive roles may never have any direct contact with patients/clients but, without them, the care

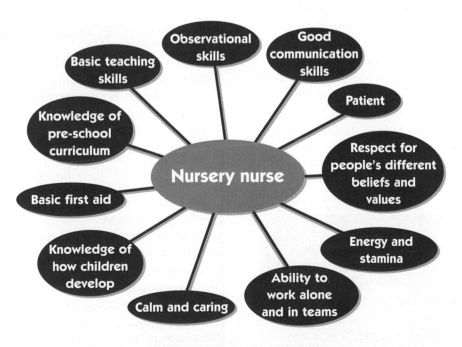

Figure 4.7 The skills and qualities required of a nursery nurse

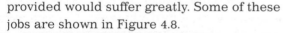

Job	
Ambulance drivers	Managers
Porters	Administrators
Catering assistants	Secretaries
Cooks	Clerks
Domestic staff	Receptionists
Gardeners	Record keepers
Caretakers	ICT officers
Laboratory	Finance officers
technicians	Supplies officers
Radiographers	Personnel officers
Drivers	

Figure 4.8 A few of the jobs indirectly involved in health, social and early years services

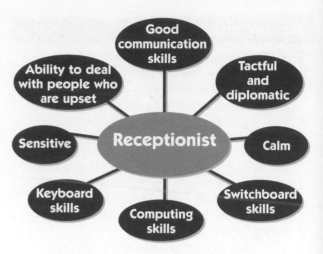

Figure 4.9 The skills and qualities required of a receptionist

provided would suffer greatly. Some of these jobs are shown in Figure 4.8.

Administration staff are required in all the care-providing organisations, whether it be local authority social service departments, GP practices or local hospitals. Services like catering, sterilisation and laundry are essential services for hospitals.

Receptionists

Receptionists are to be found working in many health and social care units and their roles vary according to the setting where they are employed. However, the receptionist's basic tasks remain the same and they usually involve operating the telephone switchboard and greeting people as they arrive at the unit. Sometimes they are also required to do general clerical tasks or to take on administrative or secretarial duties. They must also be able to use a computer for sending out letters, keeping the unit's information up to date and so on.

Skills and qualities: These are shown in Figure 4. 9.

The effect of changes in services and service provision on care workers

As services and service provision change, so do the job roles of care workers and some of the skills needed for those jobs. For example:

- In the past few years, complementary therapies (e.g. aromatherapy, homeopathy and acupuncture) have become more widely accepted. These therapies are often used alongside conventional medicines and treatment. This use of complementary therapies has resulted in a rise in the need for workers to provide these additional services.

Activity

Choose one of the job roles you have just read about in this chapter. Construct your own spider diagram of the skills and qualities needed for that job.

▶ **1** Which skills do you think are most important?

2 Why do you think this?

▶ Contact the care setting where a person with the job you have chosen for the activity above might work. Ask if it is possible to go to interview a person with that job. Ask if you can tape the interview. On the basis of the interview, prepare a short presentation on the skills needed to do that job, including a visual image to illustrate your main points.

Activity

▶ Research what is involved in the complementary therapies mentioned in the paragraph above and how a client would go about accessing these services in your local area. *Hint:* Your local telephone directory might be useful here.

▶ Pick one of these therapies and produce an information sheet on what the benefits of this therapy are, the problems it would help, how much it costs and other useful facts.

- As new technology continues to develop, the equipment used becomes increasingly sophisticated and technical staff are required to operate and maintain these types of equipment.
- Information technology is now being used to record service users' records, which means members of staff must acquire the necessary computing and technical skills.
- Because there are not enough doctors, some nurses are now doing tasks that once only doctors used to do, so they have had to learn the practical skills to carry out such tasks.
- When new illnesses, diseases and viruses appear, care workers have to respond accordingly. They have to learn about them and how to cope with them. With the advent of problems such as the HIV virus and AIDS care, for example, workers have had to adopt universal guidelines for dealing with blood and body fluids.

Interpersonal and communication skills

Interpersonal skills are those skills that enable us to interact with another person – in other words, those skills that allow us to communicate successfully with another person. Good communication skills are vital to care workers because they help them to:

- develop care relationships in which they understand and meet the needs of others (covered in more detail in Chapter 5);
- provide information;
- receive information; and
- report on the work they do with clients.

Activity

With a partner, write down as many different reasons as you can think of why it is absolutely vital that everyone, no matter what his or her situation, needs to be able to find some way of communicating with others. Then write down as many different ways of communicating with others you can think of.

Care workers have to communicate with many different people, as shown in Figure 4.10.

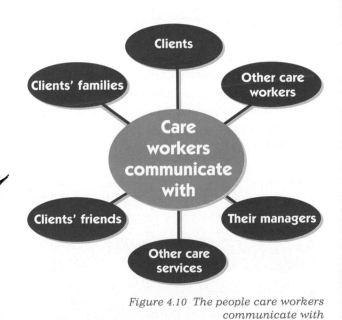

Figure 4.10 The people care workers communicate with

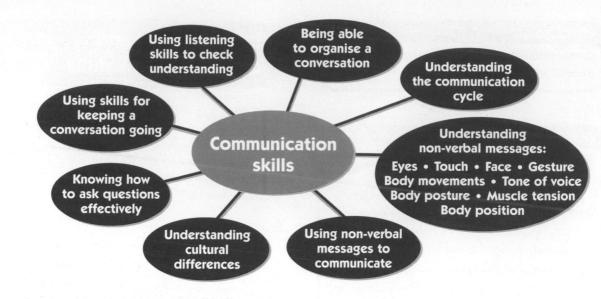

Figure 4.11 The communication skills needed for care work

The diagram shows "Communication skills" at the centre, connected to:
- Using listening skills to check understanding
- Being able to organise a conversation
- Understanding the communication cycle
- Understanding non-verbal messages: Eyes • Touch • Face • Gesture • Body movements • Tone of voice • Body posture • Muscle tension • Body position
- Using skills for keeping a conversation going
- Knowing how to ask questions effectively
- Understanding cultural differences
- Using non-verbal messages to communicate

Effective communication skills

Care workers have to develop a range of communication skills, which include those shown in Figure 4.11. Effective communication skills can help to establish and support positive relationships with colleagues, clients and their families because they enable care workers to:

- understand the needs of others;
- form relationships with clients;
- show respect towards clients and other members of staff; and
- meet the clients' social, emotional and intellectual needs.

Being an effective carer involves learning about the individual people you work with. Learning about other people involves listening to what they have to say and understanding the messages people send with their body language. It is not always easy to get to know people. We need the skills of being able to listen, of being capable of sustaining a conversation and of interpreting other people's body language correctly.

Non-verbal communication

The proper term for body language is 'non-verbal communication'. This refers to the messages we send out without putting them into words. When people are sad they may signal this emotion with eyes that look down or away – there may also be tension in their faces and their mouths may be closed. The shoulder muscles are likely to be relaxed but the person's face and neck may show tension. A happy person will have 'wide eyes' that make contact with you – his or her face will smile (see Figure 4.12).

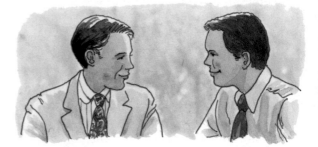

Figure 4.12 We signal our emotions through the expressions on our faces

Most people are able to recognise such emotions but skilled carers must go one stage further and understand the messages they are sending out with their own bodies when working with other people.

Non-verbal messages

Some of the most important body areas that send out messages are shown in Figure 4.13.

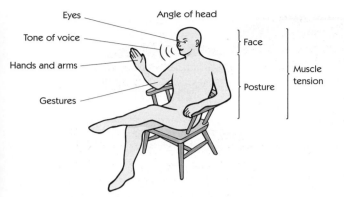

Figure 4.13 Areas of the human body that send out non-verbal messages

The eyes

We can often tell what other people's feelings and thoughts are by looking at their eyes. Our eyes get wider when we are excited, or when we are attracted to or interested in someone else. A fixed stare may send the message that someone is angry. In European culture, to look away is often interpreted as being bored or not interested.

The face

Our faces can send very complex messages and we can read these easily, even in diagrammatic form (see Figure 4.14).

Tone of voice

If we talk in a loud voice with a fixed tone people think we are angry. A calm, slow voice with a varying tone may give out the message that we are being friendly.

Body movement

The way we walk, move our heads, sit, cross our legs and so on sends messages about whether we are tired, happy, bored or sad. When people are excited they might move their arms and hands about more.

Posture

The way we sit or stand can send messages (see Figure 4.15).

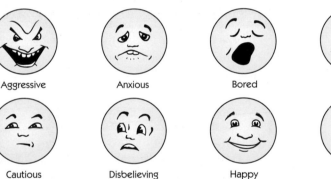

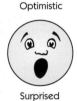

Aggressive	Anxious	Bored
Cautious	Disbelieving	Happy

Joyful	Negative	Optimistic
Relieved	Sad	Surprised

Figure 4.14 Facial expressions that send out messages

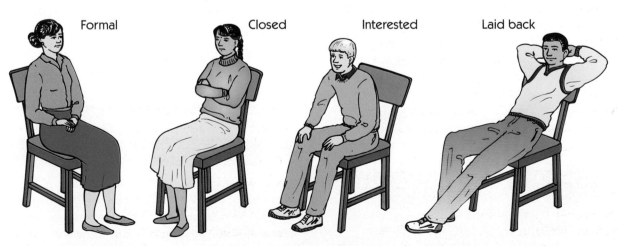

Formal   Closed   Interested   Laid back

Figure 4.15 Our body posture can send out messages

Muscle tension

The tension in our feet, hands and fingers can tell others how relaxed or tense we are. If people are very tense their shoulders might stiffen, their face muscles tighten and they might sit or stand rigidly.

Gestures

Gestures are hand and arm movements that can help us to understand what someone is trying to say. A thumb stuck in the air says everything is fine.

Touch

Touching another person can send messages of care, affection, power over that person or sexual interest. The social setting and other body language usually help people to understand what a particular touch might mean. Carers should not make assumptions about touch: even holding someone's hand might be interpreted as an attempt to dominate them.

Face-to-face positions

Standing or sitting eye to eye with someone might send the message of anger or formality. A slight angle will create a more relaxed and friendly feeling (see Figure 4.16).

Appearance

The way in which people dress also sends messages to others. Different cultures have different ways of dressing that show they belong to that culture. Some groups of people may dress in a certain way to show what kind of music they like. Similarly, people with particular jobs may wear a uniform to make them easily identifiable.

Activity

In small groups, agree on three different messages you want to convey (such as 'I'm not interested in you in anyway') and produce a freeze frame to deliver that message to the rest of the group. Discuss your three messages quietly so that other groups do not know what you are trying to portray before you do your freeze frame. Try to make your messages as interesting and difficult as possible.

If you have access to a digital camera, record each freeze frame to make a display of them.

Checkpoint

A **freeze frame** is a frozen image made by actors to show a real-life situation.

Activity

Try to convey with non-verbal communication a situation between a client and a care worker where a care worker wants the client to do something that will benefit the client, but the client does not want to do it. Do this in a series of freeze frames.

If you have access to a digital camera, record each freeze frame to make a display of them.

Written communication

Care workers also need to be able to communicate with the written word. This could be by *writing* something themselves, such as a letter to refer a client to a different service, a record of a client's condition and treatment or

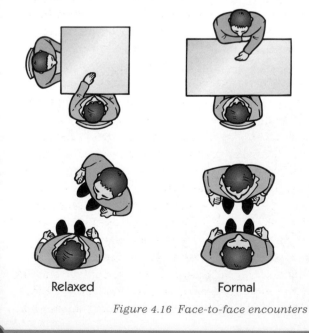

Relaxed   Formal

Figure 4.16 Face-to-face encounters

entitlement to a particular benefit, or filling in a form to help a client receive a particular treatment or benefit. This means they need to be able to use different written forms of presenting information, such as business letters, memos, short reports or application forms. They need to be able to make their meaning clear by structuring the material and by using headings, subheadings and paragraphs, as well as by writing clearly and using a level of language that is appropriate for the person the document is going to. For example, there is little point including lots of complicated, technical words in a letter to a person who has no idea what the terms mean. It is important to use punctuation correctly and to check spellings.

Care workers also need to be able to *read* information provided by other care workers. They need to be able to identify the main points of what they have read and to summarise the information accurately and concisely. They need to be able to find information from a variety of sources, such as letters, textbooks, articles or the Internet. They also need *ICT* (information and communication technology) skills to be able to update client records, to prepare reports and to find out information.

The communication cycle

Communication is not just about giving people information. When we talk we go through a process (or 'cycle') of:

- hearing what the other person says;
- watching the other person's non-verbal messages;
- having emotional feelings;
- beginning to understand the other person; and
- sending a message back to the other person.

Listening skills

Skilled listening involves:

- looking interested and ready to listen;
- hearing what is said;
- remembering what is said; and
- checking understanding.

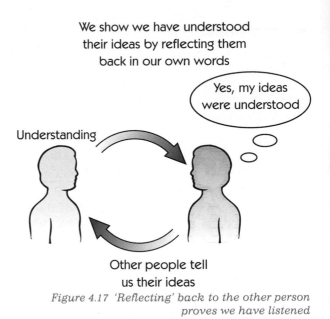

We show we have understood their ideas by reflecting them back in our own words

Yes, my ideas were understood

Understanding

Other people tell us their ideas

Figure 4.17 'Reflecting' back to the other person proves we have listened

Checking our understanding

Checking our understanding involves hearing what the other person says and asking the other person questions. Another way is to put what the person said into our own words and to say this back to him or her to see whether we did understand what he or she said (see Figure 4.17). Good listening is hard work. However, people who are attracted to work in care usually enjoy learning about other people and their lives.

Keeping a conversation going

Once we have started a conversation we must keep it going long enough to meet our purpose and the emotional needs of others. Skills that help us achieve this are taking turns, using non-verbal communication to show interest, the skilful use of questions and using silence at the appropriate moments.

If we are trying to get to know someone, we will probably listen more than we will talk. The person we are talking to will give us clues as to when it is our turn to talk by slowing down the rate at which he or she speaks, changing his or her tone of voice and looking away. He or she might then stop speaking and look directly at us. We will then be ready to ask a question or say something that keeps the conversation going.

Showing interest means giving the other person your full attention, by eye contact, smiling, hand movements and gestures and slight head nods, while talking to signal that we understand.

Asking questions

Some of the questions we ask will not encourage people to talk: these are closed questions because there is only one simple answer. For example, if you ask someone 'How old are you?', the reply you will most likely receive will simply be that person's age and nothing else. Open questions 'open' up the conversation. The person is encouraged to consider his or her reply. For example, 'How do you feel about the food here?' should get the person talking a little more.

Silence

Pauses in a conversation can be embarrassing – it can look as if we are not listening or interested in what is being said. However, sometimes a silent pause can mean 'let's think'. Silent pauses do not always stop the conversation as long as our non-verbal messages demonstrate to other people that we respect them and are interested in them.

The effects of poor communication skills

If care workers do not have or develop good communication skills, the effectiveness of their care work will be reduced and care relationships will be damaged. If a client feels, for example, as though his or her care worker does not listen to her and avoids eye contact, the client will not respond well to suggestions made by that care worker and will not like or respect him or her. This will not help the client to feel good about herself or her situation and so will reduce the client's feelings of well-being.

Differing communication needs of client groups

Babies and children

Babies and children might be apprehensive or worried if they have to go, for example, to see the doctor or the dentist. It is therefore important the care worker talks in a kind, friendly way and is calm and reassuring even

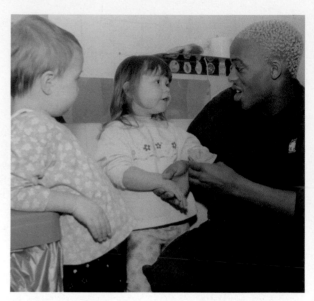

Care workers should try to sit at the same level as children

when something is seriously wrong. Children will feel intimidated by someone talking to them in a formal way and using words they do not understand. The care worker should also sit down at their level rather than towering over them. Sometimes, exaggerating non-verbal communication can be useful when communicating with young children (for example, stretching your arms as far as you can when saying something is really big).

Adolescents

Again, someone talking very formally will more than likely intimidate an adolescent. However, adolescents will expect a care worker to explain things to them clearly yet not in a patronising manner, as though they were not intelligent enough to understand. They will also not like a care worker invading their personal space by getting too close to them unless the care worker explains to them that this is necessary, for example, in order to examine them. It is also easy for a care worker to look disapprovingly at a young person because he or she thinks that young person is dressed in a rather bizarre way. This might make the young person feel the care worker doesn't like him or her. It is important a care worker avoids such non-verbal communication so as not to damage the care relationship.

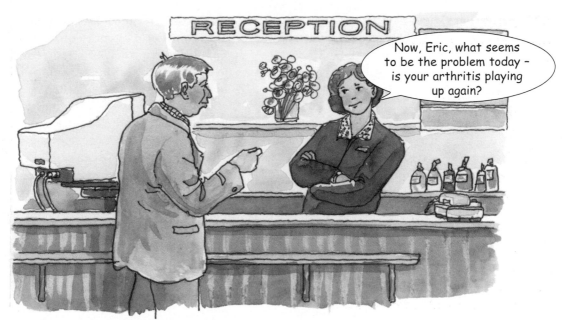

How would you describe the receptionist's manner towards the patient?

Checkpoint

Personal space is the space around a person in which a stranger (someone that person does not know very well) or someone he or she does not like is not welcome. He or she would feel uncomfortable if any such person entered that space. Only those people the person knows well may enter that space.

Older people

Older people might not like to be spoken to in an over-familiar and informal manner. They may prefer not to be called by their first names by a care worker who is much younger than themselves or whom they do not know very well. Also, some people have a tendency to speak loudly and very patronisingly to older people, assuming that, just because they are older and perhaps not as physically active as they were, that they are lacking in intelligence and/or are slow to understand.

Disabled people

People with a visual disability may need to have letters and other written information provided in Braille, so they can read it for themselves, or communicated verbally instead of non-verbally. They might also want to sit close to the care worker so they can touch the care worker's face in order to recognise him or her.

Those with a hearing impairment might want to face the care worker, with the care worker positioned in good lighting so they can see the care worker's face clearly. This will help them to see the care worker's expressions and will also help them to lip-read. It might also be necessary to use pictures or to write messages. Those who can hear with the use of hearing aids or who are just a little hard of hearing will not want to be shouted at as though they are unintelligent. They will want to be spoken to normally or just loud enough in a quiet room. People who can use sign language should have access to a professional translator or interpreter.

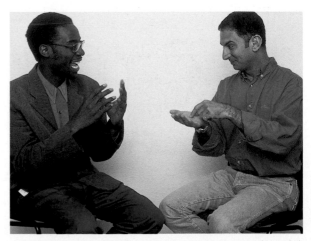

Using sign language to communicate

Care workers should sit down when talking to someone in a wheelchair so that their faces are at the same level, rather than looking down, which can be intimidating or uncomfortable if the person in the wheelchair has to tilt his or her head up all through the conversation. Again, it is important not to talk loudly and slowly or to talk over the person's head to whoever is accompanying the client, as if the person in the wheelchair does not understand just because he or she cannot walk.

Those with learning difficulties may struggle to understand unfamiliar words or ideas. The care worker needs to empathise with the client and try to find a way to explain things simply and clearly, perhaps using diagrams and signs. It is also important to speak calmly and patiently so the client does not get flustered and confused.

Checkpoint

Empathise means trying to imagine being in the other person's place so you can understand more readily how he or she feels.

People who speak a different language and/or are of a different culture

Information in leaflets, reports, letters, application forms, signs and so on need to be provided in a variety of languages so that those who speak a different language can understand the information. It might be necessary to use pictures and signs if an interpreter is not available. For a client to provide information, it might be necessary for an interpreter to be available. It is also important for care workers not to use slang, jargon or dialect when speaking to someone who understands only a little English or who speaks English as a second language. The care worker should try to find a different, simpler way to say things and should speak in short, clear sentences.

It is also necessary for care workers to remember that, in some cultures, it is considered disrespectful to look directly at the person you are talking to. Hence, when clients look down most of the time, this should not be interpreted as meaning they are being dishonest or are feeling sad.

What if it is not possible to communicate with a client?

Sometimes, when people have a very serious learning disability or an illness such as dementia, it is not possible to communicate with them. In such situations care services will often employ an advocate – someone who speaks for someone else. For example, a volunteer might try to get to know someone who has dementia and will try to communicate this client's needs and wants as he or she understands them. Advocates should be independent of the staff team so they can argue the client's rights without being constrained by what the staff think is easiest or cheapest to do.

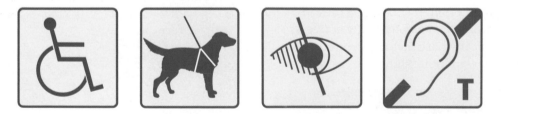

Examples of signs that can be interpreted by people from different cultures

Check your knowledge

1 Health care roles involve working with which people?
2 Social care roles involve working with which people?
3 Who do early years roles involve working with?
4 Give at least five examples of indirect care roles you might find in a hospital.
5 Name three main jobs in early years services.
6 What does a social worker do?
7 Why does a receptionist need to be sensitive?
8 Why does a care worker need good communication skills?
9 State five different ways in which we give out non-verbal messages.
10 What do we mean by the phrase 'the communication cycle'? Why is it called a cycle?
11 What four things does a good listener do that makes him or her a good listener?
12 Why do we say that communication is a two-way process?
13 Name five ways to keep a conversation going.
14 What is meant by a closed question? Give an example (other than the one given in this chapter).
15 What is meant by an open question? Give an example (other than the one given in this chapter).

Practice activity

Copy the table below and put each of the following jobs into the correct column, without looking back in the chapter unless you are really stuck:

- receptionist
- nurse
- ambulance driver
- social worker
- nursery nurse
- physiotherapist
- dermatologist
- health visitor
- midwife
- occupational therapist
- care assistant
- dietician
- dentist
- radiotherapist
- anaesthetist
- secretary
- cleaner
- au pair
- surgeon
- childminder

You may think some of them should go in more than one column and you would be quite right!

Health care	Social care	Early years

Can you sort the above jobs into examples of (a) direct care and (b) indirect care?

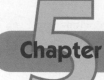

Chapter 5

The value bases of care work

Key issue

What values do care workers promote through their work?

In this chapter you will learn that health and social care services are all aiming to help people develop or maintain their independence. You should understand the balance that services have to achieve between getting involved in people's lives or not, including the risks associated with both action and inaction.

You should understand the values that are an essential feature of all care practice. You will appreciate and understand that care practitioners use guidelines and codes of practice to empower clients by:

- promoting anti-discriminatory practice;
- maintaining confidentiality of information;
- promoting and supporting individuals' rights to dignity, independence, health and safety;
- acknowledging individuals' personal beliefs and identities;
- protecting individuals from abuse;
- promoting effective communication and relationships; and
- promoting individualised care.

You will learn how these values are reflected in the behaviour and attitudes of care workers and how these values are incorporated into the codes of practice of different care professions, and the policies, procedures and contracts of employment of care organisations.

Be prepared

You will need a copy of the charter your local medical centre has produced for an activity at the end of this chapter. You will also need a copy of the booklet *Your Guide to the NHS*, available from doctors' surgeries, walk-in centres, medical centres, hospitals and various other public places.

The aim of health and social care services

All health and social care services aim to help people either to develop or maintain independence. An example of someone needing to develop independence could be a young child who has a bad dose of an illness such as polio, which might leave his legs paralysed. He will be helped to learn to walk, if possible, or to cope with being in a wheelchair so that he can develop as much independence as possible in order not to be dependent on his parents or anyone else, and to lead an independent adult life.

An example of someone needing to maintain her independence is an adult who suddenly has a stroke and is left perhaps with impaired speech or not able to move one side of her body and is afraid to exert herself in case it happens again. This person has to be taught how gradually to build up the amount of exercise she does, not to be afraid to take regular exercise and to change her diet.

Checkpoint

Independence means not having to rely on someone else to do things for you.

The balance between action and inaction

One challenge facing the care services is to achieve the right balance between getting involved in people's lives or not. It might be that if a service does not take a certain action, both individuals and other members of society could be at risk. For example, an elderly woman with a failing memory might be very independent and determined to continue to live in her flat on her own, despite the advice of a care worker that she should be living somewhere where she is supervised. If her carers don't take any action it might be that she puts the chip pan on, forgets about it and sets fire to her flat, putting herself and those who live in flats adjoining hers, as well as the fire personnel who come to tackle the blaze, at risk.

Similarly, if a care worker gets too involved in a person's life he or she can also put people at risk. A care worker who calls round more regularly than is necessary and is seen to be interfering can cause resentment and unnecessary stress to a family. An example of a care worker taking action that could put an individual or group of people at risk would be the case of a social worker who is rather overzealous and who refers a family because he or she has seen a child who has a large bruise near the top of his leg. If the child has had accidents before (as most children do) and has a medical record that shows other examples of bruising, it might be that the child is considered to be at risk and is taken away from the family for a time. The bruises might all have been caused by the child being a bit accident prone, but by the time this is proved the family and the child concerned will have suffered and the health and well-being of all will have been put at risk.

The care value base

All care work is about improving the client's quality of life by meeting people's intellectual, emotional and social needs, as well as their physical needs. One way of doing this is for care practitioners to *empower* their clients.

Checkpoint

Empower means giving someone the ability to do something for him or herself.

Care practitioners empower clients by promoting certain values, which are important to both the care practitioner and the client. These values form the basis for a set of principles that help care workers to give the kind of care each individual client requires. These principles form the basis for all care work and are sometimes referred to as the care value base. This base describes the kind of attitude towards care you would appreciate if you were being cared for as a patient or client. The guidelines care practitioners follow in order to ensure that clients know what quality of care to expect are based on this set of principles. The form these guidelines take will be discussed later in this chapter.

Checkpoint

A **value** is a belief about what is important in life, is something you hold dear and what you believe is morally right. A value does not usually change and is important to both individuals and society. Your attitudes may often change but your values are more deeply held, more permanent and affect your actual behaviour. Society is based on a set of shared values. This is a shared agreement about values that makes it possible for us to live a well ordered and predictable social life, without people (usually) breaking the unspoken rules of how to behave towards each other. One example of a value is the sanctity of life – that is, that someone's life is sacred and should not be taken. Another value is the belief that everyone should be treated fairly.

A **principle** is a basic guide to follow in life as to the right way to behave – your own personal code of conduct. This is based on values. For example, you should try to treat everyone fairly because you believe it is the right thing to do and that it is important to behave that way.

Activity

In a group, list all the values you feel are important in care practice. To do this, imagine you are ill or have a problem and are in need of care. How would you expect to be treated? How do you think your carers would expect you to treat them? Then try to agree on the six most important points on your list. If you have time, present your six most important points attractively on either sugar paper, a flipchart or on a computer. You will be asked to present your points to the rest of the class so you should work out how you are going to share out the work so that you all take part in the presentation.

The values that are an essential feature of all care practice

The care values attempt to define the key principles that should guide how carers behave. These are shown in Figure 5.1.

1 Promoting anti-discriminatory practice

No two people are the same and, because people are different, it can be easy to think that some people are better than others or that some views are right while others are wrong. We must remember that different people see the world in different ways, and that our way of thinking may seem unusual to someone else (see Figure 5.2). This difference between people is called *diversity* and we should value it.

> **Checkpoint**
>
> **Discrimination** means treating people or groups of people differently in comparison to other people or groups of people.

Unfair discrimination is when people or a group of people are treated unfairly or unequally in comparison with other people or groups of people. When people discriminate unfairly against someone else we say they are prejudiced against that person.

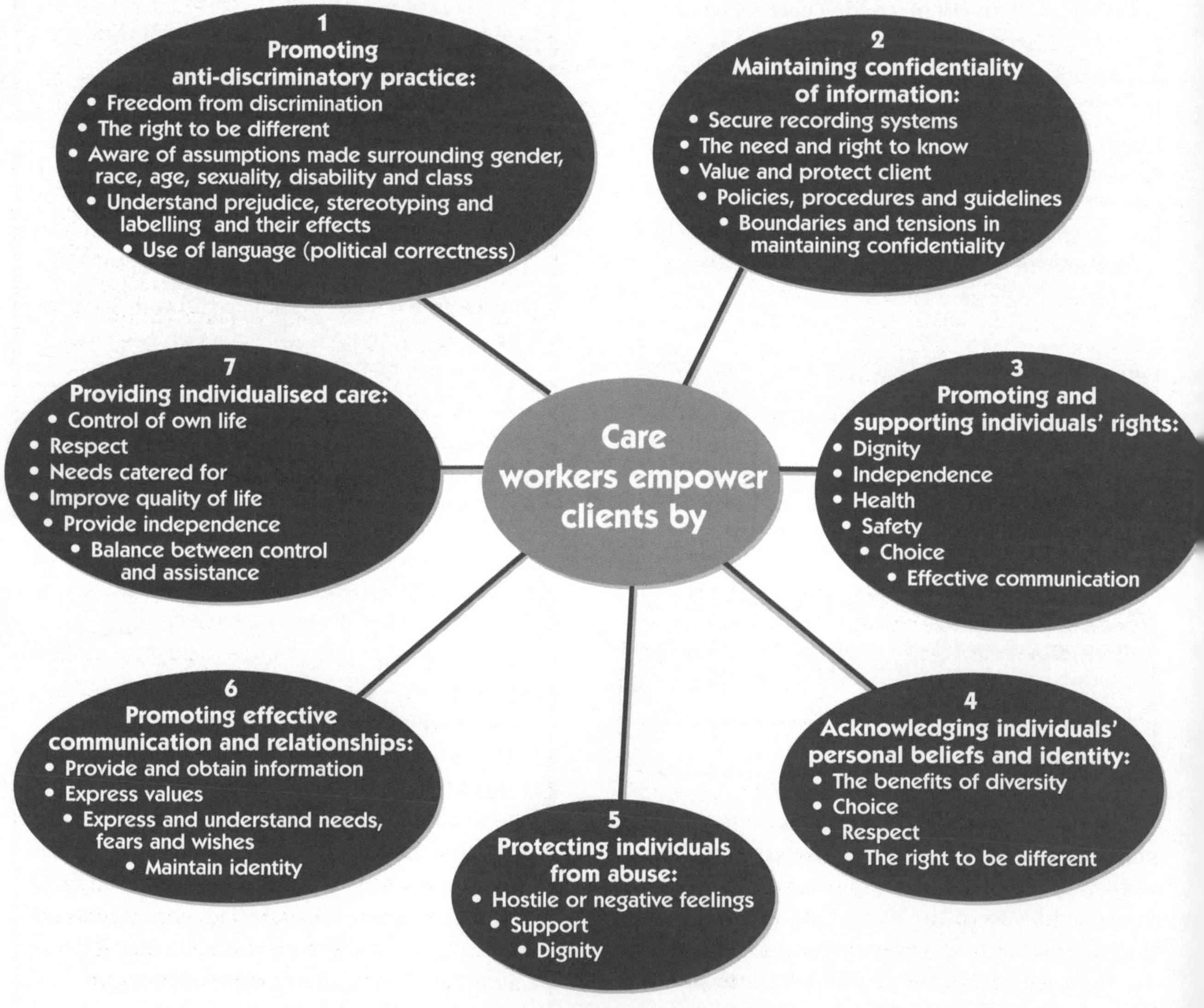

Care workers empower clients by

1 Promoting anti-discriminatory practice:
- Freedom from discrimination
- The right to be different
- Aware of assumptions made surrounding gender, race, age, sexuality, disability and class
- Understand prejudice, stereotyping and labelling and their effects
- Use of language (political correctness)

2 Maintaining confidentiality of information:
- Secure recording systems
- The need and right to know
- Value and protect client
- Policies, procedures and guidelines
- Boundaries and tensions in maintaining confidentiality

3 Promoting and supporting individuals' rights:
- Dignity
- Independence
- Health
- Safety
- Choice
- Effective communication

4 Acknowledging individuals' personal beliefs and identity:
- The benefits of diversity
- Choice
- Respect
- The right to be different

5 Protecting individuals from abuse:
- Hostile or negative feelings
- Support
- Dignity

6 Promoting effective communication and relationships:
- Provide and obtain information
- Express values
- Express and understand needs, fears and wishes
- Maintain identity

7 Providing individualised care:
- Control of own life
- Respect
- Needs catered for
- Improve quality of life
- Provide independence
- Balance between control and assistance

Figure 5.1 Care values are an essential feature of all care practice

Difference	Possible discrimination
Age	People may think of others as being children, teenagers, young adults, middle aged or old. Hence discrimination can creep into our thinking if we see some age groups as being 'the best' or if we make assumptions about the abilities of different age groups
Gender	In the past, men often had more rights than women and were seen as more important. Assumptions about gender still create discrimination problems
Race	People may understand themselves as being black or white, as European, African or Asian. People also have specific national identities, such as Polish, Nigerian, English or Welsh. Assumptions about racial or national characteristics lead to discrimination
Class	People differ in their upbringing, the kind of work they do and the money they earn. People also differ in the lifestyles they lead and the views and values that go with levels of income and spending habits. Discrimination against others can be based on their class or lifestyle
Religion	People grow up in different religious traditions. For some people, spiritual beliefs are at the centre of their understanding of life. For others, religion influences the cultural traditions they celebrate – for example, many Europeans celebrate Christmas even though they might not see themselves as practising Christians. Discrimination can take place when people assume that their customs or beliefs should apply to everyone else
Sexual orientation	Many people consider their sexual orientation as very important to understanding who they are. Gay and lesbian relationships are often discriminated against. Heterosexual people sometimes judge other relationships as 'wrong' or abnormal
Ability	People may make assumptions about what is 'normal'. Hence people with physical disabilities or learning disabilities may be labelled as 'not normal' or others may have stereotypical views about what they are capable of doing
Health	People who develop illnesses or mental health problems may feel they are valued less by others; they may feel discriminated against
Relationships	People choose many different lifestyles and have different emotional commitments, such as marriage, having children, living in a large family, living a single lifestyle but having sexual partners or being single and not being sexually active. People live in different family and friendship groups. Discrimination can happen when people think that one lifestyle is 'right' or best
Presentation and dress	People express their individuality, lifestyle and social role through their clothes, hairstyles, make-up and jewellery. While it may be important to conform to dress codes at work, it is also important not to make stereotypical judgements about people because of the way they dress

Figure 5.2 The dangers of discrimination

Checkpoint

Prejudice means a bias or preconceived opinion against a person or a group of people.

If someone is rude, hostile or offensive to someone because that person is different, this is known as *direct discrimination*. For example, some football fans chant at certain football players when they run out on to the pitch because of the colour of their skin. This discrimination is heard by all and easy to prove.

Indirect discrimination is harder to prove because it is usually shown in people's attitudes to one another – for example, by not respecting someone's opinions in the workplace or by the careless use of language and tone of voice when referring to a certain person or group of people. When some people speak to someone who is hard of hearing or elderly, they often speak in a patronising way because they assume being deaf or elderly means being intellectually less capable, instead of realising that these people simply have a hearing disability or are of a particular age.

Positive discrimination is when a decision is made to pick someone for something *because* that person belongs to a certain group of people. For example, when advertising auditions for a particular show,

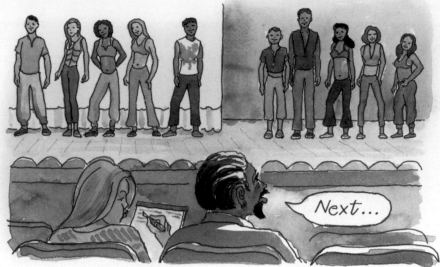

An example of positive discrimination

the casting director might ask for dancers to be of a certain minimum height or of a certain ethnic origin.

Activity

Take a few minutes to write down whether you would rather be male or female and why. Be prepared to put your point of view forward in a class discussion.

Care workers have to adopt an anti-discriminatory approach in their work. This means recognising and responding to the individual needs of clients rather than treating everyone the same. Care workers need to be aware of:

- the assumptions that are made about others;
- the different forms of prejudices people have;
- the different forms of discrimination that occur;
- the ethnic and social backgrounds of their clients; and
- the correct use of language so as not to cause offence.

Checkpoint

The correct use of language, or **political correctness**, means not using words to identify people in an offensive way.

Care workers also need to encourage an anti-discriminatory attitude in those they come into contact with. This might mean challenging the attitudes of some clients.

There is much legislation concerning equal opportunities and anyone feeling he or she has been discriminated against can take his or her case to the Equal Opportunities Commission.

Checkpoint

Equal opportunity means everyone has the same chance to obtain or achieve something as everyone else, for example a job.

The effects of discrimination

Discrimination in all forms has permanent and extremely damaging effects (see Figure 5.3).

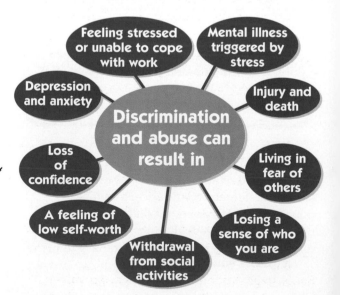

Figure 5.3 The effects of discrimination and abuse

2 Maintaining confidentiality of information

Keeping information confidential is very important in care work, and confidentiality is an important right of all clients (see Figure 5.4). It is important for the following reasons:

- **Trust:** If you know your carer will not pass on things you have said you will be more likely to tell your care worker what you really think and feel.

- **Self-esteem:** If your carer keeps things confidential this shows the care worker respects and values you and that he or she believes that what you have to say matters. Your self-esteem will therefore be higher than if your private details had been shared with others.

- **Safety:** You may have to leave your home empty at times and if your carer tells someone else this, he or she may be tempted to break in or pass the information on to someone else who may break in. Care workers must therefore keep personal details confidential to protect their clients' property and personal safety.

- **Professionalism:** A professional service that claims to maintain confidentiality must be seen to keep private information confidential. Maintaining confidentiality is part of a care worker's professional code of conduct.

- **Legality:** There are legal requirements to maintain the confidentiality of personal records.

- **Discrimination:** Confidential information passed on to the wrong people might result in the client being discriminated against or put in danger. If care workers were to pass on information to friends, neighbours or other members of the public, clients may feel they have lost control of their lives. For example, someone with mental health problems that are kept totally under control by medication might become the subject of gossip and even seen as a threat to neighbours, resulting in resentment and possible abuse of the client.

Sometimes, when serious risks are involved, it is important to tell a manager about a client's

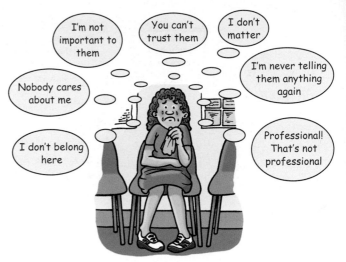

Figure 5.4 The confidentiality of the things clients tell you is of vital importance

personal details This is known as 'keeping confidentiality within boundaries'. For example, if clients:

- are at risk of danger to their physical or mental health in that they might harm themselves in some way;
- pose a risk to the safety of others, including care workers; or
- have broken, or are going to break, the law

it is necessary to breach confidentiality.

Therefore care workers should not promise that they will keep all conversations confidential but should tell clients that there will be times when it might be necessary to share information with colleagues and other authorities in the situations mentioned above.

Checkpoint

Confidential means information that has been passed on as a secret. It has only been entrusted to the person(s) it has been communicated to.

A **code of conduct** is a set of guidelines or rules a person has to follow or stick to.

3 Promoting and supporting individuals' rights

People have the right to their own beliefs and lifestyles, but no one has the right to damage the quality of other people's lives. This means

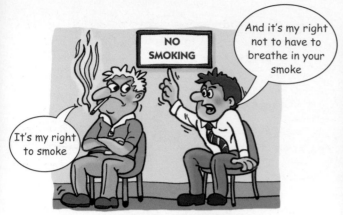

Figure 5.5 *We all have rights but we also have responsibilities to others*

Rights	Responsibilities
Not to be discriminated against	Not to discriminate against others
To have control and independence in their own lives	To help others to be independent and not to try to control other people
To make choices and take some risks	Not to interfere with others or put others at risk
To maintain their own beliefs and lifestyles	To respect the different beliefs and lifestyles of others
To be valued and respected	To value and respect others
A safe environment	To keep things safe for others
Confidentiality in personal matters	To respect confidentiality for others

Figure 5.6 *The rights and responsibilities of people receiving care*

that rights often come with responsibilities towards other people.

The easiest way to understand this is to think about the issue of smoking. Adults have a right to choose to smoke even though smoking usually damages health and often shortens a person's life. Smokers have a responsibility to make sure their smoke is not breathed in by other people (see Figure 5.5).

Government legislation, codes of practice, employers' policies and national training standards outline the rights clients have when they are receiving health and social care services (see Figure 5.6). These rights include the following:

- Freedom from discrimination (see above).
- A right to independence – although we all think of ourselves as independent there are times in our lives when we need another person's help. In care settings we can increase clients' independence by giving them control and choice over certain aspects of their care, and so increasing their self-esteem.
- The right to be respected and to retain one's dignity – clients must be treated with respect. When helping clients eat, wash, dress or use the toilet it is vital we allow them to retain their sense of self-worth and dignity.
- Health, safety and security – all clients have the right to feel safe and secure when they are receiving care. When working in care it must be part of our daily routine to assess the safety of all situations.
- Confidentiality (see above).

Activity

A care home manager was concerned that it was taking too long for his clients to be woken up, dressed and washed and given breakfast. Many of the clients had mobility problems so needed to use a commode (portable toilet) in their own bedroom. The manager decided the solution was to give the clients their breakfast on trays while they were sitting on their commodes.

▶ 1 How would you feel if you were one of these clients?
2 Which of the rights clients have when they are receiving health and social care are (a) being met (if any) and (b) not being met?
3 What are the hygiene issues here?

▶ 1 Imagine you are a relative of one of the clients and the client tells you about what is happening. In a small group, discuss all the issues involved. Then role play the scene when you go to see the manager about the situation. Try to be assertive rather than rude.
2 Imagine you are a care worker in this care home. You are reluctant to upset the manager as you need to keep your job, but feel strongly that this is an unacceptable practice. Write down exactly what you could say to him that is tactful but makes the point without sounding threatening.

4 Acknowledging individuals' personal beliefs and identity

In order to learn about other people's cultures and beliefs, we must take great care to listen to and observe what other people say and do. We may feel our own culture and beliefs are being challenged when we realise there are so many different lifestyles. Such feelings may block our ability to learn about others.

Skilled carers must get to know the people they work with so that they will not make false assumptions about them. Individuals may belong to the same ethnic group but they might have different religions, so it is impossible for us to know all the differences that might exist among individual clients.

If you are open to other people's life experience and differences, and value diversity, it will enrich your life. Employers are also likely to want to employ people who value diversity for the following reasons:

- Effective non-discriminatory care depends on all staff valuing diversity.

- People who value diversity will form good relationships with their colleagues and with the clients.
- People who value diversity are likely to be flexible and creative.
- Diverse teams often work together more effectively. If people have different interests and skills it is more likely the team will do all the work required and the people in the team will enjoy working together.

> **Checkpoint**
>
> To value diversity means to respect and value the cultures and beliefs of other people.

In care settings, everyone should receive a service of equal quality that meets his or her own personal needs. That is not, however, the same as everyone receiving the same service. Treating people as individuals, taking into account their different beliefs, abilities, likes and dislikes, is at the heart of caring for others (see Figure 5.7).

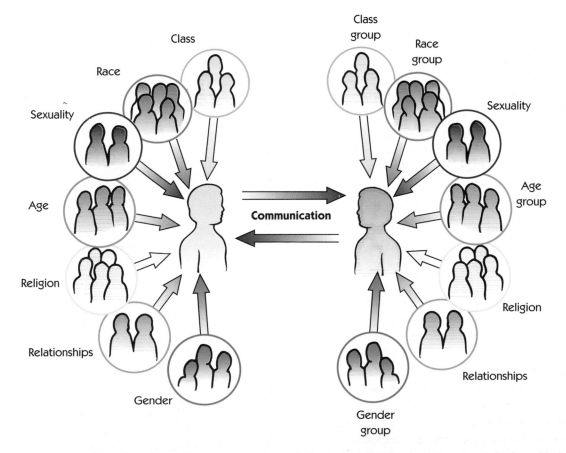

Figure 5.7 *The groups a person belongs to will influence his or her beliefs and behaviour*

A care practitioner needs to acknowledge an individual's personal beliefs and identity by accepting the person as he or she is, even if the practitioner does not share those beliefs. For example, if a patient needs to pray at a certain time of day the practitioner should allow the patient to do so, even if the practitioner would rather get on with a treatment or consultation at that time. If a hospital patient is Jewish and only eats kosher food at home, it is only right that the hospital should obtain kosher food for him to eat while he is in hospital. This will make him feel that his identity has been acknowledged rather than being ignored, improving his sense of well-being and, hopefully, aiding his recovery.

5 Protecting individuals from abuse

Abuse can take several forms:

- **Physical abuse:** Hitting, pushing, kicking or otherwise physically assaulting a person.
- **Sexual abuse:** Interfering with a person's body in a sexual way.
- **Verbal abuse:** Insults, put-downs, name-calling or otherwise assaulting a person verbally.
- **Neglect:** Ignoring a person or not giving him or her the help he or she needs and that others receive.
- **Exclusion:** Stopping a person getting the help or the job he or she needs.
- **Avoidance:** Deliberately avoiding contact with a person.
- **Devaluing:** Letting a person see that he or she is thought of as less valuable than others by denying him or her care that others receive, or ignoring that person's ideas and opinions.

Abuse might happen because of frustration with the person, because of a loss of temper, a desire to exert power over someone else, discrimination or prejudice due to certain groups or individuals being different from the person who is being abusive, or because of many other reasons.

It is very important that care practitioners are vigilant and look out for signs of abuse in their clients. Physical abuse is easier to spot because of the risk of bruises or other unexplained injuries, but other forms of abuse are less easy to notice or prove. A person who is being abused might have mood swings or become withdrawn and quiet, and care workers are always on the lookout for such signs (look back at Figure 5.3).

Case study

Cecil

One family support worker had a nickname – he was known as 'Cecil', short for Cecil B. de Mille, the film director. Cecil was known for regularly phoning the schools, social workers and GP surgeries of the families he visited every time there was any event, incident or change with the families he visited. Cecil always started his conversation with 'I'm just keeping you in the picture' – hence the nickname!

However, with the G family, it was thanks to being 'kept in the picture' by Cecil that the social worker was made aware of the mother's new boyfriend. When his details were checked out, it was discovered that he had lived with another family where the children were on the Child Protection Register. When this information was put together with the teacher noticing that one of the children had become much quieter recently, alarm bells began to ring and the children were carefully monitored, both at home and at school.

1. What was Cecil doing that was important?
2. What might have happened if the information had not been passed on?
3. Why was Cecil in a good position to keep everyone informed?

There are many support organisations to offer advice and to help protect against different forms of abuse. Childline, for example, is a national charity, as is the National Society for the Prevention of Cruelty to Children (NSPCC), and both have a 24-hour telephone helpline for children who are in trouble or danger. The NSPCC aims to prevent child abuse and neglect in all forms. The Samaritans are another organisation that has a 24-hour telephone helpline that provides emotional support for people of all ages in times of crisis. Organisations such as Survivors UK offer counselling for men who have been sexually abused, and Action Against Abuse of Women and Girls aims to support groups that help females who have been subjected to sexual abuse, domestic violence, forced prostitution and other forms of abuse.

Anyone who has been abused or suspects someone else is being abused can contact his or her local police station who have specially trained Child Protection Team Officers. Child Protection Teams work with social workers from the relevant social services departments and/or representatives from other care agencies. All police officers and social workers employed on child protection matters have to receive joint training in what is very complicated and sensitive work.

6 Promoting effective communication and relationships

The need for care practitioners to promote effective communication was covered in Chapter 4, and now is a good time to turn back to the end of that chapter to read the sections on communication again. It is important that care practitioners communicate effectively with their clients so that relationships can be formed that empower the clients to feel that their opinions about their care are valued, that they are respected and that they can take part in the decision-making about their own care (see Figure 5.8). It is through relationships that we express who we are, how we are feeling, what we think, our opinions and our needs.

Case study

Caroline

Caroline has always worked very hard at school and is about to take her GCSEs. Her parents are both very successful in their own careers and have little time to spend with her, except to push her to do as well as they have. She is lonely at home, being an only child, and has been encouraged to take school friends home.

She revised thoroughly for her mock exams and was delighted when she got 98 per cent in one of her exams, thinking that at last her parents would praise her. When she proudly told her father he looked disappointed and demanded that she try harder in the real exam, saying she was careless to drop any marks. She was very upset and rang a telephone helpline as she felt she couldn't take any more pressure.

Caroline was worried she shouldn't be using the helpline when other people had what sounded like much worse problems, such as being physically abused or not knowing when they were going to eat again.

However, the counsellor on the line was very supportive and assured her that everyone's problems are listened to and taken seriously.

▶ 1 Explain why Caroline was right to use the helpline.
2 What effect are Caroline's parents having on the way she sees herself?
3 What will happen to Caroline if she doesn't get help soon?
4 What advice do you think the counsellor would give her?

▷ 1 With a partner, role play the conversation between Caroline and the counsellor. If you are the counsellor, try to use the communication skills covered in Chapter 4.
2 Helpline counsellors do not know where the caller is calling from or the full name of the caller. What could the counsellor do if Caroline threatened to kill herself to find out where she is and so get help to her?

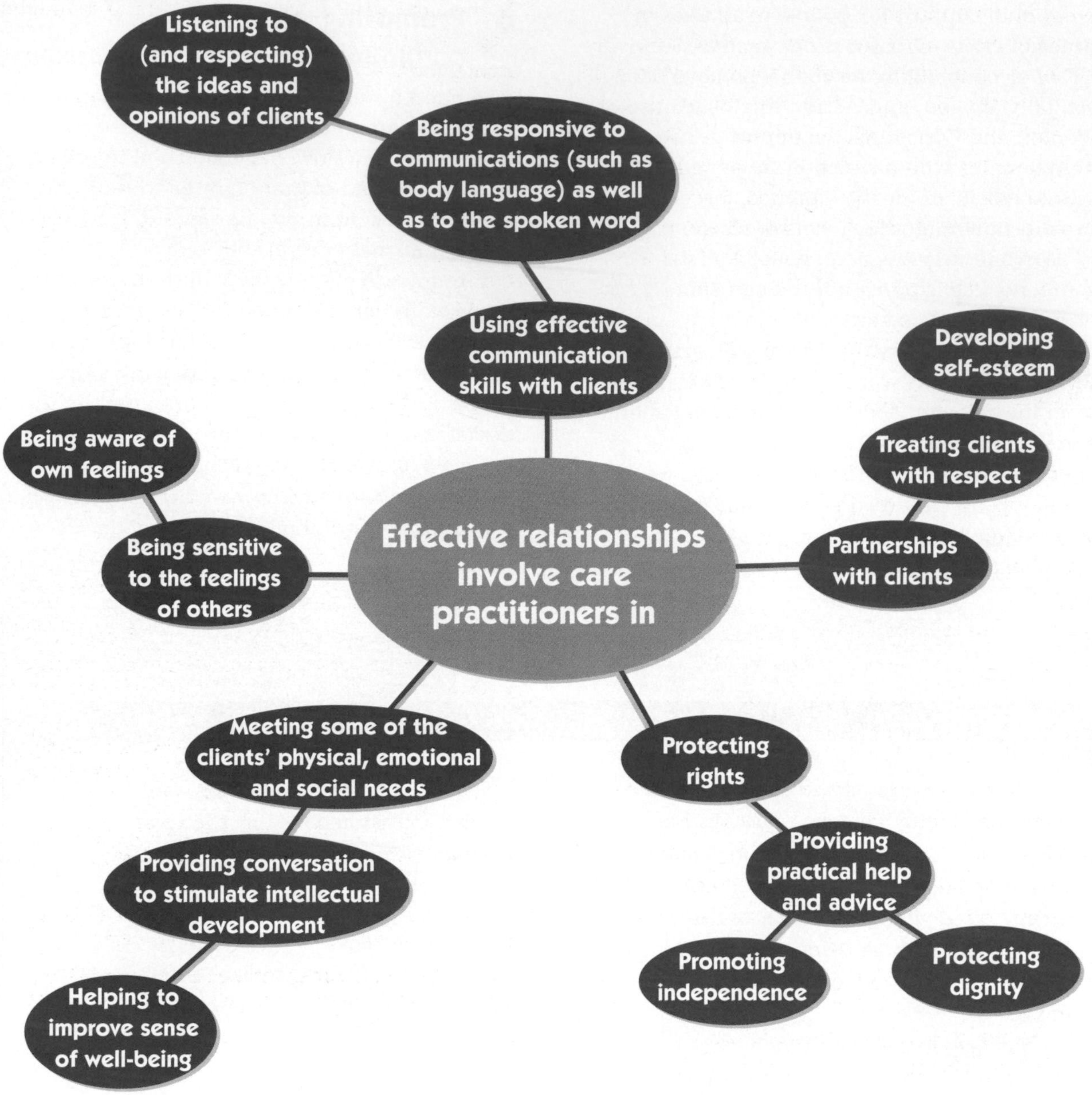

Figure 5.8 *Effective relationships enable care practitioners to meet many needs*

7 Providing individualised care

It is important that clients have control of their own lives. A client needs help from care practitioners but it is important that the practitioner strives to achieve the correct balance. Clients need to express their own opinions and make informed choices so that they feel in control of their own care. All clients have their own set of needs and the good care practitioner makes sure as many of these needs are met as possible, and that clients feel they have the attention they need. If clients feel they are receiving individualised care, they will feel valued. This will improve their sense of well-being, and enhance the chances of the client responding well to the care.

For example, an elderly person may wish to live in his own home for as long as he can. A social worker will make an assessment of what support will be needed or wanted by visiting and talking to the person concerned about the different types of care available. The social worker will help the person make a decision and arrange for the services to be provided so he can stay at home until this is no longer possible.

Another example of the importance of providing individualised care is that of providing food in hospitals. If everyone was made to eat exactly the same because it is easier for the kitchen staff, many patients would become steadily more ill. Some patients might be on a very low-calorie diet to lose weight before a particular operation; another might be on a wheat-free diet because she is allergic to wheat; another might have Muslim beliefs and so does not eat pork; and so on. It is vital that the needs of each individual are catered for.

Guidelines in care settings

All care settings have guidelines which tell both care practitioners and their clients about the quality of care that is expected and how it will be provided. You need to understand the difference between the different sorts of guidelines – namely, codes of practice, policies, procedures, charters and contracts of employment.

Codes of practice

Codes of practice help to define the quality of care clients can expect if they receive care services and they can be used as a basis for measuring the quality of care provided. All care professions have codes of practice (see Figure 5.9).

For example, *Home Life: A Code of Practice for Residential Care*, first published in 1984, has a checklist of 218 recommendations for monitoring the quality of social care. Many of these have now been built into regulations which inspectors check before a residential

home can be registered, or for a home to remain registered. The first ten recommendations (which concern staff qualities) are shown in Figure 5.10. Another code of professional

STAFF

148 Staff qualities should include responsiveness to and respect for the needs of the individuals.

149 Staff skills should match the residents' needs as identified in the objectives of the home.

150 Staff should have the ability to give competent and tactful care, whilst enabling residents to retain dignity and self-determination.

151 In the selection of staff at least two references should be taken up, where possible from previous employers.

152 Applicants' curriculum vitae should be checked and for this purpose employers should give warning that convictions otherwise spent should be disclosed.

153 Proprietors should consider residents' needs in relation to all categories of staff when drawing up staffing proposals.

154 Job descriptions will be required for all posts and staff should be provided with relevant job descriptions on appointment.

155 In small homes where staff carry a range of responsibilities, these must be clearly understood by staff.

156 Any change of role or duty should be made clear to the member of staff in writing.

157 Minimum staff cover should be designed to cope with residents' anticipated problems at any time.

Figure 5.10 Home Life: A Code of Practice for Residential Care (reproduced with permission from the Centre for Policy on Ageing)

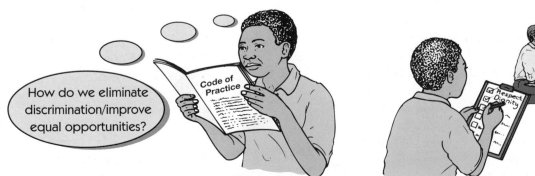

Figure 5.9 Some codes of practice mainly give advice and guidance; others can be used to measure the quality of care

conduct (for nurses, midwives and health visitors) is shown in Figure 5.11.

Codes of practice often advise workers on how to behave. For example, the Equal Opportunities Commission has published a code to help eliminate sexual discrimination, and the Commission for Racial Equality has issued a code that gives guidance on the elimination of racial discrimination. Similarly, the Department of Health has published a

Code of professional conduct

As a registered nurse, midwife or health visitor, you are personally accountable for your practice. In caring for patients and clients, you must:

▶ respect the patient or client as an individual

▶ obtain consent before you give any treatment or care

▶ protect confidential information

▶ co-operate with others in the team

▶ maintain your professional knowledge and competence

▶ be trustworthy

▶ act to identify and minimise risk to patients and clients.

These are the shared values of all the United Kingdom health care regulatory bodies.

4 As a registered nurse, midwife or health visitor, you must co-operate with others in the team

4.1 The team includes the patient or client, the patient's or client's family, informal carers and health and social care professionals in the National Health Service, independent and voluntary sectors.

4.2 You are expected to work co-operatively within teams and to respect the skills, expertise and contributions of your colleagues. You must treat them fairly and without discrimination.

4.3 You must communicate effectively and share your knowledge, skill and expertise with other members of the team as required for the benefit of patients and clients.

4.4 Health care records are a tool of communication within the team. You must ensure that the health care record for the patient or client is an accurate account of treatment, care planning and delivery. It should be consecutive, written with the involvement of the patient or client wherever practicable and completed as soon as possible after an event has occurred. It should provide clear evidence of the care planned, the decisions made, the care delivered and the information shared.

4.5 When working as a member of a team, you remain accountable for your professional conduct, any care you provide and any omission on your part.

4.6 You may be expected to delegate care delivery to others who are not registered nurses or midwives. Such delegation must not compromise existing care but must be directed to meeting the needs and serving the interests of patients and clients. You remain accountable for the appropriateness of the delegation, for ensuring that the person who does the work is able to do it and that adequate supervision or support is provided.

4.7 You have a duty to co-operate with internal and external investigations.

Figure 5.11 Extract from the Nursing & Midwifery Council's Code of Practice (reproduced with permission)

guide to the professional behaviour expected of social workers, doctors and the police when working with people who are mentally ill. These codes do not provide checklists to help in the assessment of qualities. Rather, they provide guidelines for service managers when they are devising policies and procedures staff must follow.

Codes of practice also provide practical guidance to protect workers and employers in particular circumstances, for example, workers infected and affected by HIV/AIDS. The International Labour Organisation (ILO) has produced a code of practice, adopted by the ILO Governing Body in June 2001, which gives principles for policy development (as well as practical guidelines) in the key areas of:

- HIV/AIDS prevention;
- the management of the impact of HIV/AIDS on the world of work;
- the care and support of workers infected and affected by HIV/AIDS; and
- the elimination of stigma and discrimination on the basis of HIV status.

The code was produced because the majority of those infected by HIV are workers in the productive prime of their lives. This means that HIV/AIDS affects the cost of labour and can affect the income of many workers. Labour costs are rising because of increased absenteeism, and illness can result in workers leaving their jobs so that valuable skills and experience are lost. In some countries this is a real threat to social and economic progress. The code therefore establishes principles that include no termination of employment because of HIV status and the need for prevention programmes, as well as care and support to protect workers with or without HIV/AIDS and their employers.

Most professional bodies therefore have a code of conduct or code of practice that explains the values that guide people who work in that profession.

Policies

A policy is different from a code of practice in that it is set in a particular care setting in a particular place. A code of practice for nursery

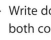

Activity

Compare the Home Life (Figure 5.10) and the NMC (Figure 5.11) codes. There are similarities among them but there are also differences because social workers have slightly different responsibilities from nurses.

▶ Write down three points that are similar in both codes of practice. Why do you think they are there?

▶ Pick out the lines in each code of practice that support each of the following values:

1 Promoting anti-discriminatory practice.
2 Maintaining confidentiality of information.
3 Promoting and supporting individuals' rights.
4 Acknowledging individuals' personal beliefs and identity.
5 Protecting individuals from abuse.
6 Promoting effective communication and relationships.
7 Promoting individualised care.

How will these protect vulnerable people?

nurses will apply to all nursery nurses working in any care setting. If the nursery nurse works in a hospital, however, the policy that tells her how to deal with a particular situation in that particular hospital might be different from that followed by a nursery nurse in another hospital elsewhere in the country. Each care setting has its own policies, depending on its specific needs and situation.

Procedures

A procedure is a list of steps to follow in order to complete a particular task in an acceptable way. Procedures are written so that they incorporate the care values that form the care value base. One example of the many procedures that nurses follow is how to give the patient a bed bath. This will be written so that, when followed correctly, the patient is cleansed with as little embarrassment as possible.

Charters

Recent governments have produced a series of charters that outline the standards people can expect from a wide range of services. These charters are like codes of practice but the government designs them. The Citizen's Charter, in particular, sets out the quality we can expect from public services. The charter contains information about the services and gives advice about how we can seek redress (chase up our rights) if a service does not fulfil all the stipulated standards. An important section of the Citizen's Charter was the Patient's Charter but this has now been superseded (replaced) by *Your Guide to the NHS*, published in 2001 (see Figure 5.12).

Many GPs are now producing practice charters that give information about the standards of service provided by their particular health centres. These cover such information as opening times, test results collection, how to get a repeat prescription, facilities for people with disabilities and out-of-hours treatment.

The Department of Health requires all local authority social services departments to publish community care charters. These explain what users and carers can expect from the community care services provided in that area and they also set out their services' commitments and standards.

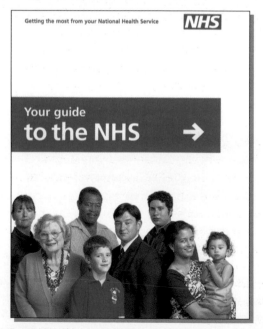

Figure 5.12 Your Guide to the NHS

Contracts of employment

Contracts of employment set out the details of the terms and conditions of employment (see Figure 5.13). Incorporated within them will be the values covered earlier in the chapter as these apply to someone who is employed in a care sector. For example, Figure 5.14 shows an extract from a specimen 'Practice nurse contract,' which sets out to protect the individual's right to health and safety.

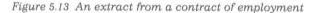

Figure 5.13 An extract from a contract of employment

Checkpoint

- A **code of practice** contains advice and guidelines on the delivery of quality care. They apply to all workers in a certain professions, wherever they are based.
- A **charter** is like a code of practice but these are produced by the government. Charters set out the rights to a quality of service people might expect.
- A **policy** is a code of practice adapted for a specific care setting in a particular place.
- A **contract of employment** is a document that sets out the terms and conditions of employment. A contract of employment is legally binding for both the employee and employer.

1.13 It is the practice's policy to provide a safe and healthy workplace, and to enlist the support of all employees towards achieving this end. It is recognised that overall responsibility for health and safety rests with the employer. However, employees should be fully aware of the potential health and safety hazards in the practice environment. The main hazards that staff should be aware of are:

a safe working environment: for example, trailing leads or exposure to chemicals such as glutaraldehyde; high workloads; poor communication; long hours; fire precautions; heating; lighting; ventilation; and regulations for workstations, screens and keyboards

safe equipment: slides, autoclaves, and electrical equipment must be adequate for the job and properly maintained

safe systems of work: procedures for the safe disposal of clinical waste, and for spillages of substances such as mercury or body fluids. In dispensing practices, dispensers must be trained in health and safety aspects of formulation and special handling precautions

free use of personal protective equipment: for example, powder free latex gloves with a protein level lower than 50ug/g

information: written employer's safety policy where there are more than five employees

immediate first aid: arrangements must be in place for first aid in the event of an accident, and a trained staff first aider, and a first aid box

welfare: exposure to passive smoking, access to immunisation such as hepatitis B, and access to occupational health advice

consultation: nurses are entitled to be consulted about anything in the practice that has an impact on health and safety

accidents: if an accident occurs a record must be made in an accident book. Certain categories of accident must be reported to the Health and Safety Executive and these are defined in the Reporting of injuries and dangerous occurrences regulations (1995) (4).

Figure 5.14 Extract from 'Guidance on Employing Nurses in General Practice' (2002), reproduced with permission from the Royal College of Nursing.

Check your knowledge

1 What is the aim of all health and social care services?

2 Give an example of the dangers of a care service not taking action in a particular situation. Try not to use the ones given in this chapter.

3 Why is it unwise for a care worker to get too involved in a client's life?

4 What is meant by the term 'the care value base'?

5 What does the word 'empowering' mean?

6 What is the difference between a value and a principle?

7 Why is it important to have the set of key values that all care workers try to base their work on?

8 Give the name of a kind of discrimination and give an example to show what it means.

9 Give three reasons why it is important to maintain confidentiality if you are a care worker.

10 How might acknowledging the personal beliefs and identity of an individual affect the work of a hospital nurse when he or she has to look after someone who is Muslim?

11 If a school bully calls his victim names, what kind of abuse is this?

12 What is a policy?

13 Why is it important that care practitioners communicate effectively with their clients?

14 Why do the care services try to provide individualised care?

15 What is the difference between a charter and a code of practice?

Practice activity

You are on a placement in a residential nursing home and have noticed that one of the care assistants is 'less than polite' to one of the residents, who speaks hesitantly because of a stammer. The care assistant interrupts the client and often makes choices for the client 'because we haven't got all day'. How would you handle the situation?

1   At coffee time, argue with the assistant about the rights and wrongs of the assistant's behaviour.

2   Talk with the client about how the client would like the situation to be handled, offering your support if wanted.

3   Go straight to the manager and tell him or her about the incident.

▶ Discuss the pros and cons of each of these three approaches. Which is the best course of action? Is there a better way to deal with the situation?.

▶ Look at the core principles in *Your Guide to the NHS* or in Figure 3.7 in Chapter 3. Which principle(s) are they failing to meet in this care establishment?

Assessment

Your syllabus states that you need to produce a report of your investigation into one local provider of health, social care or early years services. Your report must show:

(a) who provides the services, how they are organised and paid for and where they are located
(b) how the services meet the different needs of the people who use them
(c) your understanding of the skills and values required for care or early years work and the jobs which workers do
(d) how people access the services they need and the things which may prevent them from obtaining services.

You need to go and visit your chosen service provider, for example, a local nursery and a residential home. If you can spend time there helping on some form of work placement, it will help you to collect the information you need for this assignment. It is a good idea to complete a work placement diary so that you record the information in note form while it is still fresh in your mind.

Assessment task

1. Choose two clients who have different needs, for example, people of different ages or abilities or an able-bodied person and a disabled person.
2. Choose two workers who have obviously different roles.
3. Present your work logically and in clearly identifiable sections, such as:

    - Introduction (background)
    - Methodology (how you collected your information)
    - Information gathered (the main body of work)
    - Summary (conclusion, what you have found out)
    - Recommendations (suggestions for realistic and justified changes to improve the services provided)
    - Source details (where you got your information, bibliography of books used)

Total marks possible	Mark Band 1 To achieve grade FF, you need to:	Mark Band 2 To achieve grade CC, you need to:	Mark Band 3 To achieve grade AA, you need to:
(a) 14 marks available	1 – 6 marks Give a basic description, using limited sources such as books and leaflets, of the local provider of health, social care or early years services you have chosen. Include where it is, the times it is available, whether it is private, public, voluntary or not-for-profit, and where it gets its money. Show that you understand the difference between statutory services and other services.	7 – 10 marks Give a clear description, using both first hand information and sources such as books and leaflets, of the type of care the local provider of health, social care or early years services you have chosen delivers and how it fits into the national framework. Give examples of the client group and say where the organisation is and whether it operates in the private, public, voluntary or not-for-profit sector. Make clear where the funding for the services comes from and show how the funding is linked to those targets. Make sure you clearly label any diagrams used, using a key when appropriate.	11 – 14 marks Use at least three sources to describe in detail the type of service provision, location of services and the sector (public, private, voluntary or not-for-profit) in which the organisation operates. Explain the relevant sources of funding, comparing it with those for other sectors. Explain how local and national provision can vary, giving reasons for this. Present your evidence in a variety of ways. Show how the local provision, national framework, government health targets, population profile and funding of the services are linked.
(b) 10 marks available	1 – 4 marks With guidance from a teacher identify the main needs (at least their physical needs) of two different people who use the services you have picked. State how the service is organised and delivered so that the two people actually get the services and how their care needs are met. The two people can be either actual people with their names changed or fictional.	5 – 7 marks Identify and fully explain the needs of two different people who use the services you have picked. As well as physical needs show that you understand the emotional or psychological effects of illness and disability by describing them clearly. Explain how the services are organised and delivered in order to meet these needs. Show that more than one service may be needed to meet all the needs of your chosen two clients and that these may be provided by different organisations or sectors.	8 – 10 marks Identify and clearly explain the physical, psychological, emotional and social needs of two different people who use the services. Say how their needs may vary over time and predict any of their likely future needs. Explain how the provision is organised and delivered in order to meet their needs. Identify any gaps and make suggestions for improvement. Show clearly that you understand that it is necessary for services to work together to fully meet the needs of your two chosen clients.

Total marks possible	Mark Band 1 To achieve grade FF, you need to:	Mark Band 2 To achieve grade CC, you need to:	Mark Band 3 To achieve grade AA, you need to:
(c) 13 marks available	**1 – 5 marks** Using mainly books and leaflets give a basic description of two main job roles within the chosen organisation. The workers must have different roles. Describe how the basic skills and the qualities required for those roles are gained by describing the route to such a career, including the opportunities for training and gaining qualifications. Also show how the values necessary for care work are incorporated into the work of the two workers described, giving an example.	**6 – 9 marks** Use both primary and secondary sources of information to accurately describe two main job roles within the organisation you have chosen. Show that you understand the skills and qualities needed. Describe the activities your two workers carry out with individuals, how these activities help to meet the client needs and how this links with the level of responsibility which the roles require, such as giving medication. Show that you understand the routes to training and qualifications for the roles you have chosen and show the similarities and differences within and between the roles. Show using examples how the appropriate values are applied and contribute to individual care and what is likely to happen to clients if a worker fails to do this. Show the links between values and the independence and empowerment of clients.	**10 – 13 marks** Use a wide range of information sources to give a full and accurate description of two job roles within your chosen organisation. Explain how the full range of activities and skills carried out by the chosen workers enable client needs to be met, including non-physical needs, using several examples. Show how skills and knowledge are acquired during training and through qualifications. Provide a detailed description of how all the values necessary for care work are implemented by workers in the organisation. Show you understand how important these are and give relevant examples. Identify and give examples of the potential conflicts encountered by your two workers when promoting values such as the rights of individuals.
(d) 13 marks available	**1 – 5 marks** Explain the different ways in which people can access the services they need, giving examples of each method of referral. Describe the main things that may stop them from obtaining services, such as physical or geographical barriers. Say how easy or difficult the various referral processes are and say why you think this.	**6 – 9 marks** Use a variety of information sources, including those who actually use the service, to clearly explain the different ways in which people can access the services they need, and include more than one service provider. Describe the range of things which may stop them obtaining services, including those such as embarrassment or fear, and suggest ways to overcome these barriers. Say how efficient or otherwise the different referral procedures are and say why you think this.	**10 – 13 marks** Use a wide range of information sources to explain the different ways in which people can access the services they need. Describe in detail the range of things which may stop them from obtaining services and give at least two clear examples to illustrate your points regarding access to local services experienced by individual people. Make an accurate and thorough evaluation of the effectiveness of relevant procedures, suggesting realistic and justified ways of improving access to local services. Show that you recognise the multi-agency nature of the responsibilities relating to access and the implications of widening access to services as linked to local and national provision.

Unit 2

Promoting health and well-being

Introduction to Unit 2

In this unit you will learn about:

- definitions of health and well-being;
- common factors that affect health and well-being and the different effects they can have on individuals and groups across the lifespan;
- methods used to measure an individual's physical health; and
- ways of promoting and supporting the health improvement of an individual or small group of people.

The knowledge you gain from this unit will help you to look after your health and well-being and understand ways of promoting health and well-being for others.

What you will learn

If you choose to pursue a career in health and social care, you need to be able to identify lifestyle practices that put a person's health at risk, and how you can help that person get the information he or she needs to change his or her lifestyle. It is also important you consider the various aspects of your own health now so that you can prevent problems developing either now or later on in your life.

Assessment

This unit is assessed through portfolio work. Your overall result for this unit will be a grade from G to A*.

Chapter 6 Understanding health and well-being

Key issue

What are health and well-being?

By the end of this chapter you will have learnt that there are several different ways of thinking about *health* and *well-being*. You will find out about the following:

- Health and well-being can be described as the absence of physical illness, disease and mental distress. This is a **negative** definition of health and well-being.
- Health and well-being can be described as the achievement and maintenance of physical fitness and mental stability. This is a **positive** definition of health and well-being.
- Health and well-being are the result of a combination of physical, social, intellectual and emotional factors. This is a **holistic** definition of health and well-being.

You should also be aware that ideas about health and well-being change over time and vary between different cultures.

How can we define health and well-being?

Health can be described in negative and positive ways. The word 'health' means different things to different people. The word health comes from the old English word *helthe*, meaning 'the state of being hale, sound, or whole, in body, mind, or soul.'

Negative definition

You might think health means not having any illnesses, injuries or diseases. However, this is a negative view of health because it is based on *not* having anything wrong with you.

Checkpoint

A **negative** definition of health and well-being is the absence of physical illness, disease and mental distress.

Positive definition

The World Health Organisation takes a more positive view when it describes health as 'a state of complete physical, mental and social well-being and not merely the absence of disease or infirmity' (WHO, 1946). This is a very general definition because a person's health can change from day to day. It also includes mental and social well-being, which many people would not think to include if they were asked to write down what is meant by the word 'health'.

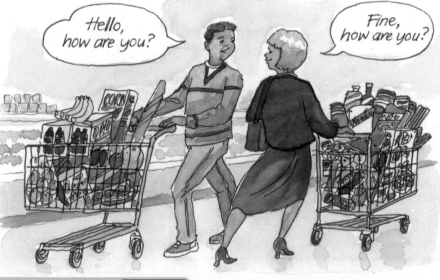

Hello, how are you?

Fine, how are you?

What, then, is meant by well-being? It is the way people feel about themselves. If you feel good about yourself and have good relationships with others, you are more likely to have a high level of well-being. You are the person who can best judge your own sense of well-being.

Holistic definition

A holistic approach means looking at all parts of something. For example, if you look at every aspect of a person's health and well-being you are taking an holistic approach. Our health is affected by everything and everyone around us, and it changes all the time. Our basic health needs do not change as we pass through the various life stages, but different people do need different kinds of support, depending on their particular situation or life stage. Figure 6.1 shows a hierarchy of needs, designed by the psychologist Abraham Maslow in the 1930s.

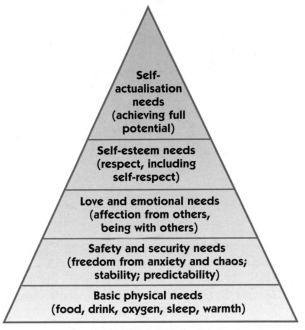

Figure 6.1 *Maslow's hierarchy of needs*

In this case, the most basic needs we all have to survive are positioned at the bottom of the pyramid to show they are the most important and are supporting the other health needs. The most complicated needs are at the top. Since Maslow suggested this hierarchy of needs, health and well-being professionals have decided there are four main basic health needs all human beings have. They are physical, intellectual, emotional and social needs.

well as possible. They include mental
stimulation, education and employment. If we
do not have enough to keep our minds active
we become bored, (sometimes boring!) and fed-
up (see Figure 6.4).

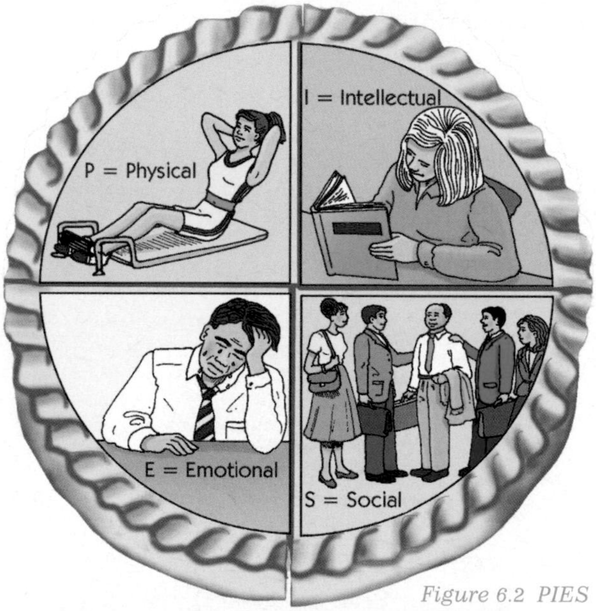

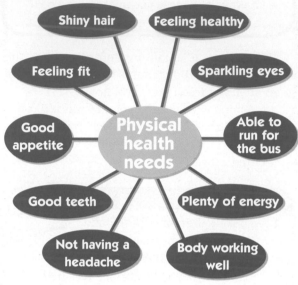

Figure 6.3 Physical health needs

P = Physical
I = Intellectual
E = Emotional
S = Social

Figure 6.2 PIES

Physical aspects of health and well-being

Physical needs are all the needs we have to
keep our bodies working as well as they can.
Even though everyone's body is unique there are
certain physical needs we all have. They include
food, water, shelter, warmth, clothing, rest,
exercise and personal hygiene (see Figure 6.3).

Intellectual aspects of health and well-being

Intellectual needs are all the needs we have
which develop and keep our brains working as

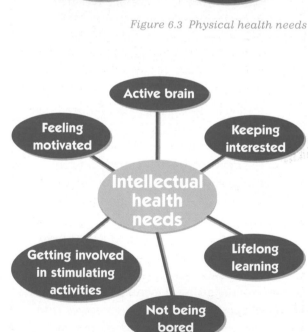

Figure 6.4 Intellectual health needs

▶ Write a list of all the things you could do to stimulate your brain (e.g. reading, watching television). Compare your list with those of the rest of your group and add any you didn't think of to your list. Which of these could you find time to do?

▷ One way of improving intellectual health is to read. In a group, find out who reads books regularly and who doesn't. Discuss why you think it is that some people only read when they are made to and others get a lot of pleasure out of reading. Decide what and who influences them.

Then repeat the exercise but discuss going to the theatre instead of reading.

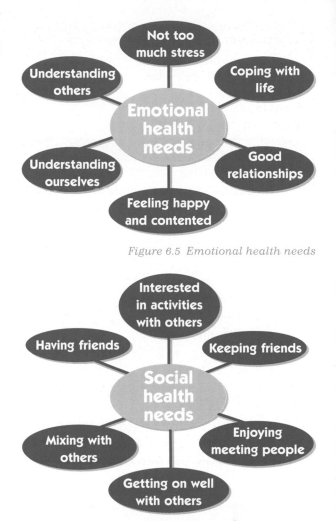

Figure 6.5 Emotional health needs

Figure 6.6 Social health needs

One way to keep mentally healthy as we grow older is to keep doing and learning a variety of things. Medical research has shown that people who use their brains regularly are more likely to keep 'their wits about them' for longer, as well as live longer and have more fulfilling lives. It is important for carers to recognise the importance of intellectual health and to help clients to keep interested in their world.

Emotional aspects of health and well-being

Emotional needs are those that make us feel happy and relaxed, such as being loved, respected and secure. We need to be able to feel, express and recognise different emotions in order to cope with different situations that arise in life (see Figure 6.5).

Social aspects of health and well-being

Social needs are those that enable us to build and enjoy good relationships and friendships. These include opportunities to mix with others and an appropriate environment (see Figure 6.6).

▶ We need certain social skills in order to develop good relationships with others. Write down as many as you can think of (e.g. listening skills). Compare your list with a partner's to see if you have forgotten any.

▷ Think of someone whom you think has very few social skills. Do not tell anyone else who you are writing about – this could cause offence, which is not a good social skill! Write a list of ways in which that person behaves that make you think that. Then write a list of ways in which that person could learn social skills.

What is there about his or her lifestyle that makes that person the way he or she is?

For us to be accepted in society is important for our social health. We need to recognise the rules of our society so that we can be a part of it. This means behaving and responding to others in a way that is acceptable to them.

Check your knowledge

1 What is the difference between the terms 'health' and 'well-being'?
2 What are the three ways of defining health and well-being?
3 How does the World Health Organisation define health?
4 What item of food helps us remember what the four basic health needs of people are? How does it do this?
5 Name five things all people need, whatever their age, for their physical health needs.
6 Give an example of what is meant by an 'intellectual need'.
7 What are the three social health needs people of any age have?

What are the health needs of different groups of people?

Although there are certain needs all client groups have, other needs vary. You need to know what the needs of each group are. The different groups of people you need to know about are described in Chapter 1. To recap:

- Babies and children aged 0–11 years.
- Adolescents aged 11–18 years.
- Adults aged 19–65 years.
- Older people aged 65+ years.
- Disabled people – people who are not ill but who have special needs because of a physical or mental disability.

Babies and children

Figures 6.7 and 6.8 show the PIES for babies and children separately. As you can see, there is no difference in physical needs, not much difference in intellectual and social needs but the most difference in emotional needs as people develop from babies into children.

Physical needs	Intellectual needs	Emotional needs	Social needs
Warmth	Play	Bonding with carer	Develop routines
Shelter	Stimulation	Love	Meet people
Balanced diet	Toys	Encouragement	Play with others
Protection	Experiences	Laughter	Explore their
Good hygiene	Picture books	Value	environment
Sleep	Television		
Exercise	Role modelling		

Figure 6.7 PIES for babies

Physical needs	Intellectual needs	Emotional needs	Social needs
Warmth	Play	Respect	Develop routines
Shelter	Role modelling	Love	Meet many people
Balanced diet	Stimulation	Encouragement	Play and learn
Protection	Advanced toys	Laughter	with others
Good hygiene	New experiences	Value	Explore their
Sleep	Books	Dignity	own environment
Exercise	Television	Learning independence	Use social facilities
	Education	Self-esteem	

Figure 6.8 PIES for children

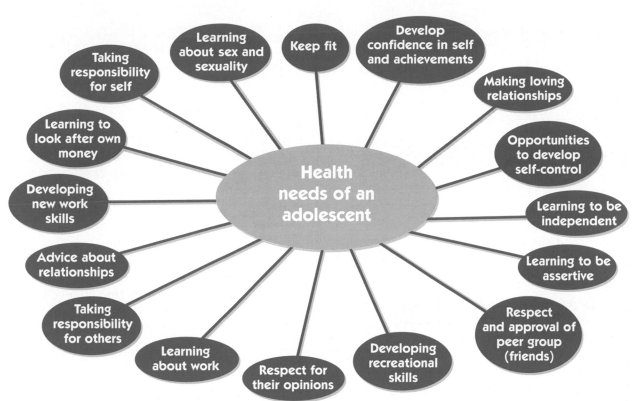

Figure 6.9 Health needs of an adolescent

Adolescents

Adolescence is one of the most difficult periods of life. It is when you usually go through puberty and start to change into an adult. Your reproductive organs start to function and changes in hormone level mean that emotions become confused and you may feel under a lot of stress. The health needs of an adolescent are shown in Figure 6.9.

Activity

Draw a table like the one shown below. Write down your own PIES in each column.

Physical needs	Intellectual needs	Emotional needs	Social needs

Now write down who provides each of these for you.

Adults

The health needs of adults are as varied as they are for younger people. In any age group

the importance of different health needs changes with time. Health care workers need to be in tune with their clients' health needs at any time so they can help to meet the changes as they arise (see Figure 6.10).

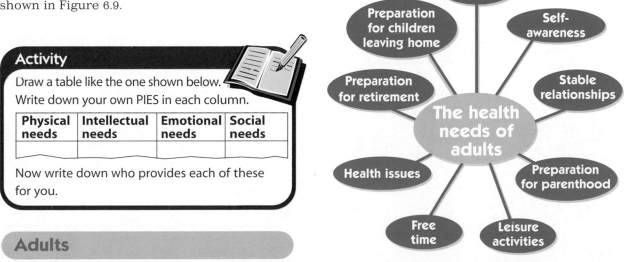

Figure 6.10 The health needs of adults

Older people (65+ years)

The changes that occur for many older adults as they retire are life changing. However, for many it is an experience to look forward to, with time to travel or do the other things they have not had time to do while at work. Sadly, some older adults are not able to be as active in their retirement as others because they are not as healthy as they used to be. They may also lose a partner and friends through old age. Figure 6.11 shows some of the PIES for older people, and Figure 6.12 shows some of the milestones in the journey through an adult's life.

Activity

Learning from others

Try to talk to an older person (not one of your teachers – they're not old enough yet, whatever you think!) about his or her life and how it has changed from when he or she was a child. Tell the person you are doing a course that will help you become a health and social care worker. Make notes of what he or she tells you and prepare a brief talk about that person for the rest of your group. Do not repeat anything this person tells you in confidence. Be very polite and do not push him or her into talking about something he or she does not want to talk about.

Disabled people

Disabled people have special needs that are usually either inherited and present from birth or acquired as a result of an accident or illness. These conditions affect their health and well-being. Disabled people have to adapt their lifestyles to cope with everyday situations (for example, picking something up or going to the toilet). When a person becomes disabled through illness or an accident, it will alter the person's personal relationships and friends; family and work colleagues will all need to adjust to take account of the person's disability. Whatever the condition, the disabled person's basic health needs are those that able-bodied people have, within whichever age group they fall. They are, however, likely to have needs that become especially important to them, as shown in Figure 6.13.

Learning difficulties

Some people have learning difficulties, which means the learning and development of intellectual needs are slowed down. This could be due to:

- being born with some disability or being injured by the process of being born;
- a loss of sight, hearing or speech;
- an accident which affects the brain;
- a disease such as Alzheimer's, which affects memory and gets gradually worse;

(continued on page 96)

Physical needs	Intellectual needs	Emotional needs	Social needs
Warmth	Books	Respect	Leisure facilities
Shelter	Television	Love	Opportunities to mix
Balanced diet	Newspapers	Encouragement	with others
Safe surroundings	Conversation	Feel valued	Information about
Good hygiene	Education	Dignity	leisure activities
Sleep		Independence	Access to facilities
Exercise		Self-esteem	and activities
Convenient health		Supportive relationships	
facilities		Support in times	
Comfort		of distress	
Practical help		Financial security	

Figure 6.11 Some PIES for older people

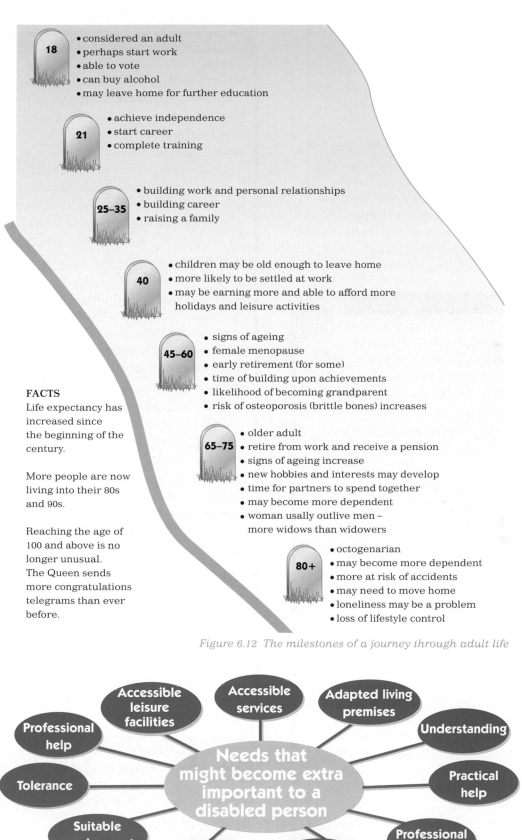

18
- considered an adult
- perhaps start work
- able to vote
- can buy alcohol
- may leave home for further education

21
- achieve independence
- start career
- complete training

25–35
- building work and personal relationships
- building career
- raising a family

40
- children may be old enough to leave home
- more likely to be settled at work
- may be earning more and able to afford more holidays and leisure activities

45–60
- signs of ageing
- female menopause
- early retirement (for some)
- time of building upon achievements
- likelihood of becoming grandparent
- risk of osteoporosis (brittle bones) increases

65–75
- older adult
- retire from work and receive a pension
- signs of ageing increase
- new hobbies and interests may develop
- time for partners to spend together
- may become more dependent
- woman usually outlive men – more widows than widowers

80+
- octogenarian
- may become more dependent
- more at risk of accidents
- may need to move home
- loneliness may be a problem
- loss of lifestyle control

FACTS

Life expectancy has increased since the beginning of the century.

More people are now living into their 80s and 90s.

Reaching the age of 100 and above is no longer unusual. The Queen sends more congratulations telegrams than ever before.

Figure 6.12 The milestones of a journey through adult life

- Accessible leisure facilities
- Accessible services
- Adapted living premises
- Professional help
- Understanding
- Tolerance
- Practical help
- Suitable employment
- **Needs that might become extra important to a disabled person**
- Professional support
- Appropriate facilities
- Access to education and training

Figure 6.13 The needs that might become extra important to a disabled person

- a disorder in the brain, such as a brain tumour;
- the side-effects of drugs being given to help some physical problem; or
- substance abuse, such as taking drugs or sniffing glue.

Carers working with clients with learning difficulties have to encourage and teach their clients, and have to be sensitive to the fact that, for people who have lost some of their skills through having, for example, a stroke which affects their speech and mobility, the world will be confusing and distressing. It is also distressing for their family and friends.

Case study

Doris

Doris is in the early stages of Alzheimer's disease and is very forgetful, but she has good days when she remembers almost everything and is articulate and friendly. She is 85 and rather infirm. She lives in a residential home, which she finds very boring. She gets upset when one of her carers talks to her very slowly and loudly and doesn't bother listening to what she says in reply any way.

▶ 1 Why is the carer's behaviour towards Doris inappropriate?

2 How should he modify his behaviour?

3 What activities could the residential home organise that would keep Doris stimulated?

▶ 1 What do you think Doris can do about this situation? Give reasons for your answers.

Check your knowledge

1 What health needs are changed if a person has an accident and can no longer move around without a wheelchair?

2 How do the health needs of a child differ from those of an older person who has retired from work?

3 Name five health needs of an adolescent.

4 Why are the health and well-being needs of homeless people difficult to provide?

5 Why is job security important for the health and well-being of an adult?

Case study

Gareth

Gareth is 39 years old. He is very bright and has a job that involves flying all over Europe, sometimes to two or three countries a week, to solve problems with computers being used, for example, to run stock exchanges. It is a challenging but enjoyable job. He spends a lot of evenings in hotels during the week and often orders from room service because he does not want to sit in the hotel dining room on his own. He returns to his apartment in a very popular and picturesque European city at the weekends and works in the office nearby when he is not having to visit other countries. He has a good social life with people he has met at work.

Gareth's family only see him when he comes back to England at Christmas unless they fly out to see him. They worry about the fact that he has not met anyone to marry and settle down with yet. They think he has a glamorous life but very often the only parts of the countries he sees when he flies round Europe are the airport, the building containing the computer system he has gone to sort out and the view from his hotel window at night. In his summer holiday he flies to the South of France to lie on a beach in the sun or to Paris or America to stay with friends.

1 Write down Gareth's physical, intellectual, emotional and social needs.

2 Which of the needs you have identified are being met?

3 How are they being met?

4 Which of Gareth's needs are not being met?

5 Make some suggestions as to how these needs can be met, taking into account his busy lifestyle.

How have ideas about health and well-being changed over time?

Ideas about health have changed in two main ways: firstly, the accessibility of services and their funding; and, secondly, the methods of providing health care.

Accessibility and funding

National health care

A Labour government (between 1945 and 1951) established an extensive health and welfare system. They passed the National Health Service Act 1946 which resulted in the health care system that went into effect in 1948. The Act said that citizens had the right to free health care regardless of income.

Before this many people had not been able to afford health care. However, the new system proved to be too expensive for the government so some charges were brought in for items such as prescriptions, dentures and glasses.

Tax revenue pays for most of the system's cost and the rest comes from national insurance, paid by employers and employees. Fees for items such as prescriptions and glasses have continued to rise, although certain groups of people (including children, pregnant women, the unemployed, those over 60 and those disabled in the armed forces) do not have to pay fees. Even though hospital care is free to all, some choose to pay for private health care in return for faster treatment and more comfortable conditions.

Another Act, the NHS and Community Care Act 1990, tried to make health care more efficient and less expensive by encouraging competition. It did this by allowing hospitals and other health care establishments to become trusts and control the money they receive from the government themselves, instead of the local health authorities controlling their funds for them. The idea was that local health authorities, who are responsible for providing health care for the public using government money, would then 'buy' health care for their patients from these trusts. Doctors who were not based in hospitals were also encouraged to manage NHS funds themselves.

The government is striving to make health care more accessible and free to all by 2004.

Activity

In small groups, discuss why giving establishments and practices their own funds to manage health care services encourages competition.

Welfare

Welfare is another word for well-being. It means being in a satisfactory state of health and having enough money to live on. Welfare services in Britain are meant to meet the needs of those in difficulty from birth to death. Local authorities use funds provided by the government from taxpayers to meet these needs. People such as the disabled and the unemployed receive weekly cash benefits.

The National Insurance Act 1946 built on and expanded earlier welfare legislation and increased benefits for a number of services, such as unemployment insurance, pensions, maternity and widows' benefits, sickness insurance and death grants. Today there are also allowances for families with children until they are 16 (or 18 if still in full-time education).

The government has also helped people with housing. Early in the twentieth century it started to build public housing for those who could not afford to buy their own houses, which are now known as council houses. Those who did not have enough money to pay the full rent were helped out with benefits. In the 1980s, the Conservative government allowed tenants to buy their council houses if they wished and private landlords to own public housing developments.

There have been many other policies, legislation and procedures put in place over the years to help the health and well-being of people. There are too many to mention here but they include areas such as equal opportunities, the sick and disabled, race relations, health and safety, education, carers and services and many more. Details of charters and codes of practice can be found in Chapter 5.

How have methods changed?

There are many ways in which the methods of providing health care have changed. One example is in the use of antibiotics. Penicillin was the first antibiotic to be discovered and many others quickly evolved. They were seen as a cure-all and were given out very readily by doctors even for colds, which are caused by a virus and do not respond to antibiotics. However, because of this, bacteria have adapted and found ways to survive the effects of an antibiotic and have become *antibiotic resistant*.

This has serious consequences because it means that antibiotics are becoming less effective at fighting infections. Although there are other antibiotics being developed, they may not be as effective, may have more side-effects and eventually fewer antibiotics might be discovered. Some bacteria are resistant to several antibiotics already.

The government is now so concerned about this it has launched a national public education campaign on antibiotic resistance. The aim of the campaign is to raise public awareness of the problem and what people can do to help contain it. The four areas they are concentrating on are as follows:

1 Stopping the prescription of antibiotics for simple colds and coughs.
2 Stopping the prescription of antibiotics for viral sore throats.
3 Limiting the prescription of antibiotics for conditions such as uncomplicated cystitis in fit women.
4 Limiting the prescription of antibiotics over the telephone.

Leaflets and posters are being used to promote the idea that by only using antibiotics when they are really needed (for example, for a kidney infection, pneumonia or meningitis), they are more likely to work. They are also delivering the message that antibiotics don't actually work on viruses such as the common cold.

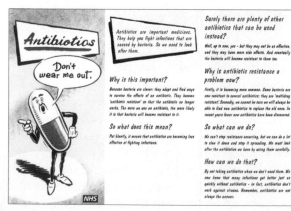

Another example of how methods have changed is in baby care. Mothers used to be told to lie their babies on their stomachs to sleep after they had been fed so that, if they were sick, they would not choke. However, research has shown that 60% more babies who were put on their stomachs died from sudden infant death syndrome (SIDS), or cot death, than those who were put on their backs, probably because of the heat produced from having the baby's face down to the mattress. Mothers are now told to lie their babies on their backs.

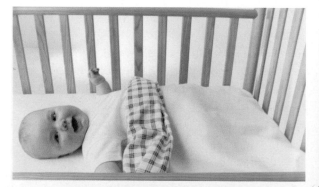

How do ideas about health and well-being vary between different cultures?

Great Britain is a multicultural society. This means the people who live here are from many different nationalities and backgrounds, which have varying religious and cultural beliefs and traditions. It is important that the different needs of different groups of people are respected and known, even if not agreed with. This is important not only in everyday life but also in situations where people are being cared for in hospitals and other care establishments.

What do we mean by 'culture'?

Before you can learn how ideas about health and well-being vary between different cultures, you need to understand what we mean by the word 'culture'. Culture is the pattern of behaviour and thinking people living in a group learn, create and share. Such a group of people live and think in similar ways. A people's culture includes their beliefs, language, style of dress, their food and how they cook it, religion and the rules they live by.

A culture is:

- **founded on the ability to communicate using language**, for example babies are born with an 'inbuilt' basic structure of language with which they learn the language spoken by the people around them;
- **shared**, for example almost all the people living in a particular country celebrate many of the same holidays and wear similar clothes; and
- **learned**, for example people have to learn to abide by the rules of a society. People inherit many physical features and have certain behavioural instincts, but culture is learned from other members of a group.

The way in which a person develops is therefore influenced by the values, traditions, way of life and beliefs of the particular society or group into which the person is born and brought up. Because most cultures do not exist in isolation, they tend to interact with people of different cultures (for example, many people around the world use the same technology, such as telephones and cars). The ability to exchange ideas and resources is usually of benefit to those concerned, but the basic way of life of each culture is usually adhered to by members of that culture.

It is important that, in any health and social care setting, opportunities are provided to allow people of different cultures and religious beliefs to maintain them, as shown in Figure 6.14.

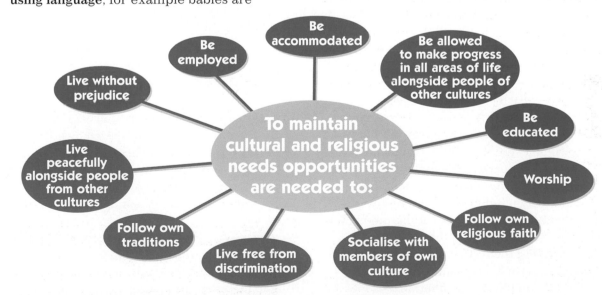

Figure 6.14 The maintenance of cultural and religious needs

Some examples of ways in which ideas about health and well-being vary between cultures are given in the following section. They cover just some of the factors that affect health and well-being.

Medical practices

There are some sorts of medical care that are believed in by some cultures but not by others. One example is that of Jehovah's Witnesses, who believe the Bible is the word of God and that the Bible says that blood is special. Although they value life highly and seek good medical care, including medicines, they will not violate what they believe the Bible is telling them. They do not, therefore, have or allow blood transfusions, believing that to take in blood is as unethical as cannibalism.

In many African societies girls are circumcised as they enter adolescence. This involves removing part or all of the external parts of the reproductive organs. It is a painful practice and can be harmful to the women but, in these societies, the practice is important because it is deeply rooted in their culture. Muslim baby boys are circumcised when they are only about two days old and many Jewish boys are circumcised when they are still babies.

Food production

The way in which a particular culture produces its food is one way in which their health can be affected. For example, the Hanunoo of the Philippines cut down a patch of forest, burn the plant material to release nutrients into the soil and plant gardens to grow food in. After about three years they move to another patch of forest and allow their old gardens to return to forest. This gives a healthy environment in which to live as no pollution has been produced.

Food production in large developed societies such as the USA depends on expensive machinery, automated systems, chemicals for fertilisers and pest control, and large amounts of fuel. This costs more, produces a more polluted, less healthy atmosphere in which to live but gives people the chance to work in areas that are not related to producing food.

Diet

Diet affects the health and well-being of people and varies considerably from culture to culture. This has to be considered when a person is admitted to hospital or any other care establishment. For example, Muslims have clear dietary restrictions laid down in the Holy Quran and these restrictions are considered to be the direct command of God. They may not eat pork or any pork products such as sausages, eggs fried in bacon fat, jellies, etc. Adult Muslims also fast during the month of Ramadan.

Other meat and meat products can be eaten as long as the animals concerned are killed according to Islamic law: it is then said to be 'halal', which means allowed. Such an animal must have its throat cut so it bleeds to death and the name Allah must be said over the animal. Many Muslims therefore stick to a vegetarian diet when they are away from home, as home is one of the few places where they can be sure they are eating halal meat or foods that contain no ingredients that come from pork, as mentioned in Chapter 3. They also wear jewellery that has religious and cultural meaning and cover their heads when praying; strict Muslims cover their heads at all times.

Jewish people also consider pork or shellfish to be unclean and do not eat them. Food that is acceptable in their diet is called 'kosher', and strict Jews have separate areas of the kitchen to prepare meat and milk dishes, as well as separate crockery to eat them from. Meat and milk are not served in the same meal. Kosher foods include barnyard fowl, the meat and milk of cattle, sheep and goats, and fish that have fins and scales.

Dress

Muslim men and women, who adhere to tradition, are expected to show modesty about their bodies, as are Hindus and Sikhs. Muslim women traditionally wear a long loose tunic (*kameez*), very full trousers (*shalwar*) and a long scarf (*chuni*), or a saree. They are worn both during the day and at night. Muslim girls and women who wear western dress usually wear trousers or long skirts to keep their legs covered. They wear gold wedding bangles when they get married (although some now wear a wedding ring), and they may also wear jewellery that has religious or cultural meaning, but none of this should be removed unless absolutely necessary.

Muslim men either wear traditional dress of *kameez* and loose trousers (*pajama*) or western dress. They do not wear gold. They cover their heads with either a cloth cap when praying and at ceremonies such as marriages or funerals, and strict Muslims tend to cover their heads all the time. Most Muslim women do not undress fully unless they are alone, and nudity amongst men can cause offence.

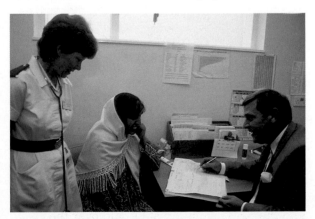
Doctors need to be aware of patients' religious and cultural beliefs

Activity

When a person is admitted to hospital for an operation, he or she is usually provided with a backless hospital gown which leaves the back bare or has a low neckline. Patients also have to remove all jewellery. Write down what problems this will cause a Muslim woman. Write down what you think a hospital can do to ease these problems.

Think about your school uniform, if you have one, including the PE uniform. Write down any possible problems the wearing of such a uniform may cause to a Muslim girl.

Physical contact and cleanliness

Strict Muslims forbid physical contact of any kind between people of the opposite sex unless they are man and wife. This means that being examined by a male doctor or nurse (or being touched by a male ambulance driver) can be very traumatic. It also means that, whenever possible, a Muslim man should be seen by male doctors and Muslim women by female doctors. If it is impossible for a Muslim woman to see a female doctor, it is less shameful to see a non-Asian male doctor than an Asian male doctor. Because it is tradition to use the left hand to wash the genital area, the right hand is used for everything else. Most Muslims find the idea of sitting in their own bath water offensive and either shower or stand in the bath and pour water over themselves with a bowl.

These beliefs apply to Hindu and Sikh people as well. However, Hindu religious practice also involves the removal of any physical pollution, such as urine, faeces, semen, mucus and menstrual blood. Most Hindus take a shower first thing in the morning before they pray and will not eat until they have prayed. People who are bedridden may need help with this.

It is important that carers are aware of the practices of different cultures so they can help to meet their clients' needs and build up a trusting relationship with their clients.

Think about it

Why is it important to hand a Muslim, Hindu or Sikh something with the right hand?

Activity

There are many more examples of ways in which a person's culture affects his or her health and well-being that either your teacher or members of your group may know about.

▶ 1   With a partner, think of how your culture affects your health and well-being.

2   Think about parts of the world where people are fighting against each other because they are of a different culture. How is their health and well-being affected by their culture?

▶ 1   What potential difficulties might arise for a health or social care worker who has to treat someone who has beliefs the worker totally disagrees with?

Check your knowledge

1   What is meant by 'antibiotic resistance'?

2   Why is there a government campaign to increase public awareness of antibiotic resistance?

3   Why is it now considered bad practice to lie a baby on its stomach?

4   Give an example of a culture.

5   What is a culture founded on?

6   Give an example of how a young Muslim child might be affected when he or she starts a new school and stays for school dinners.

7   What is the dilemma facing a doctor who has to treat a child who is a Jehovah's Witness when the child has had an accident and has lost a lot of blood?

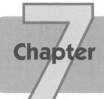

Chapter 7

Factors positively influencing health and well-being

Key issue

What factors contribute positively to health and well-being throughout the lifespan?

In this chapter you will learn that a person's health and well-being is affected by a number of different factors. You will learn about factors that contribute positively to health and well-being, such as:

- a balanced diet;
- regular exercise;
- supportive relationships;
- adequate financial resources;
- stimulating work, education and leisure activities;
- the use of health monitoring and illness prevention services (such as screening and vaccination);
- the use of risk management techniques to protect individuals and to promote personal safety.

You will also learn about the importance of these factors to individuals throughout their lives.

A balanced diet

The word 'diet' refers to our pattern of eating; in other words, the kind and amount of food and drink we eat and drink. Sometimes a person's diet may not be good enough to keep that person's body in a healthy condition. Malnutrition may be caused by not having enough food, eating the wrong types of food, eating too many reformed foods (those that have been processed to remove texture and taste, such as white bread) and eating too much food. The risks associated with a poor diet are covered in more detail in Chapter 8. In this chapter, we will be looking at how to eat a balanced diet and how we need various amounts and types of food at different times in our lives. The food we eat affects the way we feel and look and so is very important to our health and well-being.

Checkpoint

A **balanced diet** is one that contains the correct nutrients in the right proportions to keep your body healthy. **Nutrients** are naturally occurring chemicals found in different foods. Each has a certain part to play in helping our bodies to work properly and a balance of them all is needed to keep us healthy.

Activity

Keep a diary of everything you eat and drink for the next five days. You will need this information to decide whether you are following a healthy diet when you have finished learning about the different requirements for a balanced diet.

The five main groups of nutrients are:

1. proteins
2. carbohydrates
3. fats
4. minerals
5. vitamins.

We also need to eat fibre. This is not recognised as a nutrient as it is not absorbed into our bodies but it is necessary for our digestive systems to work properly. The other very important part of a healthy diet is water (see Figure 7.1).

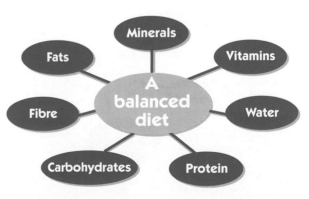

Figure 7.1 *The essential parts of a healthy diet*

Proteins

Protein is needed for the growth and repair of all the cells in the body. In childhood, proteins build the brain, muscles, skin, blood and other tissues. Even when we become adults we still need protein to repair and replace cells that have worn out. Some of the essential chemicals in our bodies are also proteins, such as enzymes, some hormones, haemoglobin and blood-clotting substances. Our diet should contain about 20% protein.

Activity

Look up the definition of the following words in a dictionary or biology book:

- enzymes
- hormones
- haemoglobin
- blood-clotting.

Find out why each is important for our bodies.

Proteins are made up of amino acids. As an adult we need 21 different amino acids but the body can only make 12. We get the other nine from the food we eat.

Most food contains some protein (except for refined sugar, processed fat and alcoholic drinks), and this food contributes to the total protein we eat each day. However, good sources of protein are meat, eggs, milk, fish and cheese. These are all animal proteins, which contain all nine of the amino acids we require from our food. Protein is also found in plant foods such as bread, flour, beans, peas and rice. These do not contain all nine of the needed amino acids but eaten in combinations (such as beans on toast) can provide as much protein as a piece of steak.

Vegetarians get much of their protein from soya products, nuts, cereals and lentils, as well as those plant foods already mentioned. It is much cheaper to eat plant proteins, rather than animal proteins, because it is possible to feed a lot more people from an acre of land used to grow a plant crop than to use that acre of land to fatten up a number of animals for meat.

Our bodies use protein to supply energy if we have not eaten enough carbohydrates. This is not a good thing because it takes away our source of nutrients for growth and repair, and proteins cannot be stored by the body. It is therefore important to eat proteins with carbohydrates (see Figure 7.2).

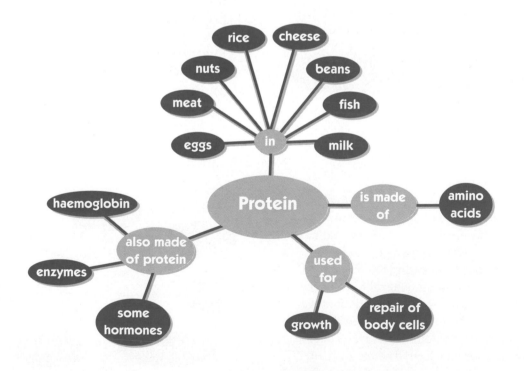

Figure 7.2 Our diet should contain about 20% protein

Check your knowledge

1 Why do we need protein in our diet?
2 Meat contains protein. Why is it not necessary to eat meat every day to get the protein we need?
3 List three animal foods and three plant foods that are rich in protein.
4 Why are foods containing animal protein more expensive than foods containing plant protein?
5 Which foods and drinks contain no protein?
6 What percentage of our diet should be protein?

Carbohydrates

Carbohydrates provide the energy we need to keep us fit and active. Carbohydrate foods can be divided into two main types.

Sugars

These are found in sweets, soft drinks or sugar-containing foods (such as jam, honey, treacle and cakes). These provide the body with a quick boost of energy but are not useful nutrients so are the least useful carbohydrate.

They also cause tooth decay and can make us overweight, as well as possibly playing a part in causing diabetes.

Starches

The starches that are found in bread, potatoes, pasta and rice, for example, are complex (i.e. complicated) and have to be broken down by enzymes in the digestive system. Because of this they provide our bodies with a slow build-up of energy that lasts over a longer period than that supplied by sugars, so they are better for our health. We can eat quite a lot of starchy food without becoming overweight. They are also useful because they:

- contain a variety of other useful nutrients;
- contain fibre (see the section on fibre);
- are relatively cheap to buy and to produce; and
- fill us up so we do not feel as hungry and are so less likely to overeat.

Our diet should contain about 60% carbohydrates, mainly of the starchy food type. From every gram of carbohydrate our bodies absorb we get 17 kJ (kilojoules) of energy (see Figure 7.3).

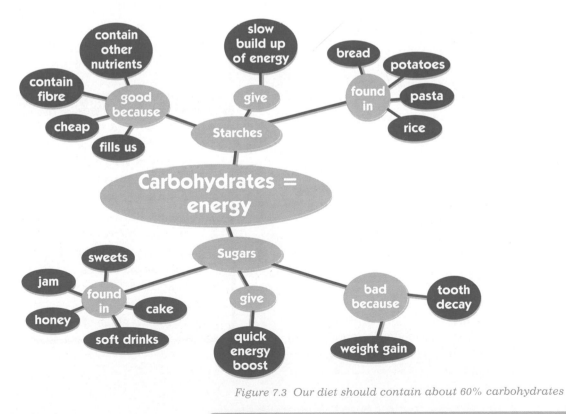

Figure 7.3 Our diet should contain about 60% carbohydrates

Check your knowledge

1   Why do we need to eat carbohydrates?
2   Children often develop a sweet tooth. How could a parent stop this happening?
3   Why are starchy foods better for us than sugars?
4   What percentage of our diet should be carbohydrates?
5   Name three foods made with sugars.
6   Name three foods that contain starches.
7   What protein breaks down the starches in our bodies? (Hint: you may have to read the section on proteins again to answer this.)
8   How many grams of carbohydrate must we absorb into our bodies to get 51 kJ of energy?
9   State three other ways in which carbohydrates are good for you, other than for providing energy.

Fats

Fats are another source of energy for all our activities, such as breathing, walking and talking. Fats may come from animal or plant foods. Those from animal foods are usually hard, such as lard, butter or suet. Those from plants tend to be soft and reach us in the form of oils, although some oils may be hardened to make margarine.

Although every gram of fat we absorb gives us 35 kJ of energy, which is twice that provided by one gram of carbohydrate, it is more dangerous for us, contributing to heart attacks, strokes, and muscle and joint disorders through us carrying too much weight. If we eat too many fats they are stored as fat. Obesity and heart disease are much less common in less developed countries because their people eat less fat in their diets.

There are two main types of fats: saturated and unsaturated (see Figure 7.4).

Saturated fats

Saturated fats are found in such foods as:
- red meats (e.g. beef, lamb and pork);
- products such as dripping, suet and lard;
- dairy products such as milk, butter and cheese; and
- chocolate.

They contain a high level of cholesterol and should only be eaten in small amounts.

Unsaturated fats

Unsaturated fats are found in such foods as:

- oils, such as vegetable, sunflower and soya;
- oily fish such as mackerel;
- nuts; and
- soft margarine.

These fats do not raise cholesterol in our bodies so are better for us, in small amounts.

Fat in small quantities is needed to help our bodies to work properly. Fat is a good food because it:

- is a concentrated form of energy;
- can contain vitamins A, D, E and K;
- provides us with a layer of fat under the skin which insulates us from too much heat or cold;
- provides a layer of fat around some of our organs (such as the kidneys) to protect them from damage;
- helps us feel full for longer because it stays in the stomach for quite a long time;
- provides us with the raw materials to make new cell membranes and certain hormones; and
- adds flavour to our meals.

Fat should form 20% of our diet at the very most.

Check your knowledge

1   Why should we not eat a lot of fat?
2   Give three reasons why fat in reasonable quantities is a good food.
3   Name three fats that come from animals.
4   Name three fats that come from plants.
5   Look up the meaning of the word 'membrane' and explain why fat in small quantities is important for the cells that make up our bodies.
6   What is the difference between saturated and unsaturated fats?
7   What percentage of our diet should be fat?

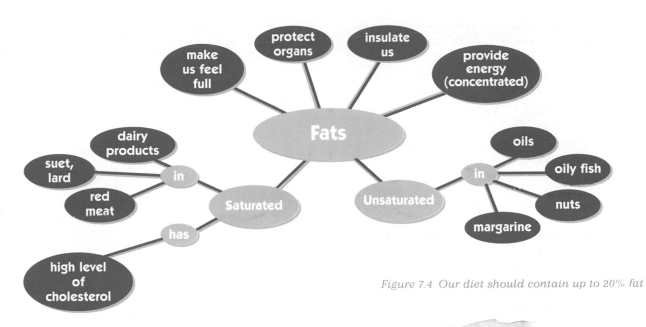

Figure 7.4 *Our diet should contain up to 20% fat*

Minerals

Minerals are chemical elements (such as fluorine and calcium) which are needed by our bodies in small amounts to perform various tasks (see Figure 7.5). There are many of them and some of the main ones are listed in Figure 7.6.

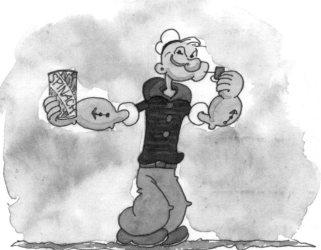

Mineral	Function	Source
Iron	Prevents anaemia – iron forms the red blood cells that carry oxygen around the body; lack of it leads to feeling tired, depressed and an inability to concentrate	Liver, kidney, spinach, eggs, black pudding, dried fruits
Fluorine	Helps prevent tooth decay	Tea, seafood, some tap water
Calcium	Gives strong bones and teeth	Cheese, milk, eggs
Phosphorus	Gives strong bones and teeth	Cheese, milk, most proteins
Iodine	Helps the thyroid gland to function properly	Fish, water, milk
Sodium	Helps muscles to work properly (found in all body fluids)	Salt, cheese, bacon, kippers
Zinc	Helps wounds to heal	Meat, dairy products
Potassium	Found in body fluids	Milk, cheese, eggs, cereal

Figure 7.5 *The tasks minerals perform in our bodies*

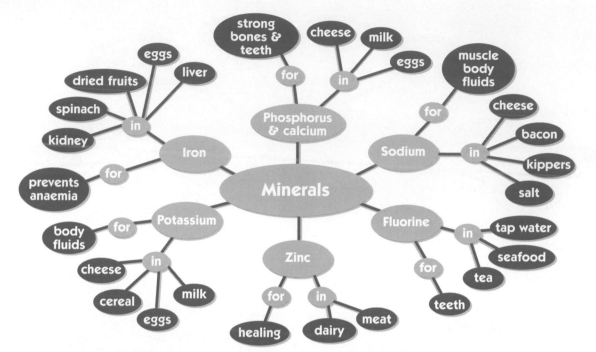

Figure 7.6 Our diet should contain minerals in small amounts

Check your knowledge

1 Minerals occur naturally in the air and soil. Name three ways in which they get into our food.
2 Why is fluorine put in drinking water in some areas of the country?
3 What foods should you eat to make sure your skin heals well?
4 Why do we need to eat foods with iron in them?
5 Why do we need to eat foods with calcium in them?
6 Do you think young women or young men are more likely to suffer from anaemia? Why do you think this is?

Vitamins

Vitamins are essential for a balanced diet but are only needed in very small amounts (see Figure 7.9). There are four main vitamins, which are divided into two groups (see Figures 7.7 and 7.8).

Vitamin	Function	Source
A	Helps children grow, helps eyes to see in dim light, keeps lining of throat, lungs and stomach moist, protects our skin	Dairy products, oily fish, carrots, green cabbage
D	Helps form strong bones and teeth, promotes growth	Fish, margarine, cheese, butter, eggs

Figure 7.7 Vitamins that dissolve in fat and that are found in fatty foods

Vitamin	Function	Source
B	Release of energy from foods, helps nervous system, helps children grow, keeps mouth and tongue infection free, prevents digestive disorders	Brown flour, potatoes, vegetables, meat, eggs, cheese, milk, liver, yeast, bread, cereals
C	Helps body resist infection, keeps gums healthy, helps wounds and fractures to heal, helps give a healthy skin	Citrus fruits, (e.g. lemons, oranges), red currants, green vegetables, tomatoes

Figure 7.8 Vitamins that dissolve in water and that cannot be stored in the body

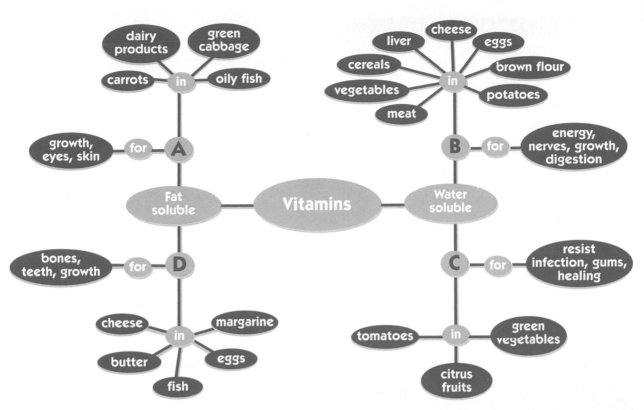

Figure 7.9 *Our diet should contain vitamins in very small amounts*

Check your knowledge

1 Why do you think vitamins that are water-soluble cannot be stored in the body?

2 Given that vitamins B and C cannot be stored in the body, what do we need to do each day to make sure we get all the vitamins we need?

3 Vitamin C is easily lost from food during storage and cooking. How can you make sure this loss is as small as possible when preparing food?

4 Which vitamin do you need to:
- See well?
- Have a healthy skin?
- Grow well?
- Keep your lungs moist?
- Keep your gums healthy?
- Have strong bones and teeth?

5 Rickets is a disease caused by a shortage of vitamin D and calcium. Why do you think some families are at risk of developing rickets?

Fibre

Fibre is not counted as a nutrient because it does not give us either energy or the materials needed to build and repair our bodies. It is made up of the cell walls of the food we eat. It is very important, however, because it:

- adds bulk to our food, so making us feel less hungry and less tempted to over eat;

- helps the movement of food through our digestive systems by a process called *peristalsis*, so aiding digestion of our food;
- helps prevent diseases of the bowel, such as cancer, by soaking up poisonous substances that might be harmful if left in the bowel; and
- helps the bowel muscles to work more easily by absorbing a lot of water so that the contents of the bowel can be easily passed out of the body because they are soft. This stops constipation.

Fibre is found in foods such as vegetables, wholemeal bread, cereals (such as rice), pasta, beans and fruit. It is sometimes referred to as roughage as it simply passes through the body and is passed out as waste. It is also known as cellulose or bran. For a healthy diet we should aim to eat more foods that are unrefined (i.e. they have not been processed to remove outer skins). For example, when wheat grains are milled to make white flour, all the outer layer of bran is thrown away, leaving flour that is smooth and white. Wholemeal flour includes most of the bran, so it contains a lot of fibre (see Figure 7.10).

Water

Water is also very important in our diet. About three quarters of the body is made up of water. Water:

- transports materials around the body;
- removes waste substances in urine;
- keeps our body cells and joints moist;
- helps control our body temperature; and
- makes up the main part of our blood and body cells.

We take in a lot of water through our drinks – even milk is mainly water. Most food also contains water and some items, such as lettuce, are nearly all water. We should drink about 2 litres of water a day to stay healthy. We can survive for longer without food rather than without water, but a lack of water leads to dehydration and a strong feeling of thirst (see Figure 7.11).

Healthy eating

Once we know which foods provide each of the essential nutrients we can plan a healthy diet. In 1983 the National Advisory Committee for Nutrition Education (NACNE) produced five dietary goals to follow when planning meals. Figure 7.12 shows these goals, the possible health risks if we do not pursue these goals and how these risks can be reduced.

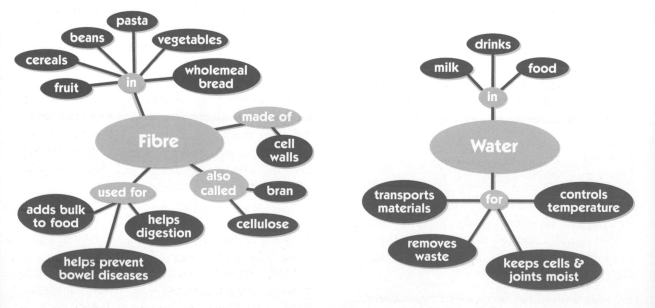

Figure 7.10 Our diets should contain fibre   Figure 7.11 We should drink about 2 litres of water a day

Goal	Health risk	Change from	To
Eat less fat	High cholesterol Heart disease Obesity	Animal fats (e.g. lard)	Vegetable oil (e.g. corn)
Eat less sugar	Tooth decay Obesity	Sweet puddings	Fresh fruit
Eat less salt	High blood pressure	Seasoning with salt	Using herbs or spices
Eat more fibre	Constipation Bowel cancer	White bread	Wholegrain bread
Drink less alcohol	Liver damage Stomach disorders	Alcoholic drinks	Low-alcohol drinks

Figure 7.12 Dietary goals and health risks

Activity

Look at the diary you have made of everything you have eaten and drunk over the last five days. Do you think your diet is balanced? If your school has any computer software that analyses diets, use it to look at your own diet. In what ways could you improve it to make it more balanced?

Plan a day's menu for yourself, making sure each meal is balanced and nutritious. Write down each meal, including drinks and snacks, and explain what each sort of food or drink you have chosen contributes to a balanced diet (for example, cereal for carbohydrates and fibre, with milk for calcium).

How do the nutritional needs of people change throughout life?

Everyone needs a balanced diet but the amount of nutrients a person needs varies from person to person according to his or her:

- age;
- height;
- weight;
- state of the body (e.g. pregnancy);
- gender;
- geographical location (i.e. is it a hot or cold climate?); and
- lifestyle (i.e. is the person very active or fairly inactive?).

However, in general, people do have different dietary needs at different stages of their lives.

Energy needs

The amount of energy needed by individuals is linked to their levels of activity. Although each of us requires a different amount, there are general recommendations for each age group. It is important to balance our food intake to match our energy needs. Otherwise:

- too much exercise + too little food = weight loss;
- too little exercise + too much food = weight gain.

Which foods provide energy?

Most foods are a combination of nutrients and, as can be seen from Figure 7.13, a person's choice of foods can affect whether he or she achieves the right balance. Excess calories taken into the body are stored as fat under the skin, which can lead to obesity.

Babies

Babies need enough nutrients to allow them to grow and develop normally. They are unable to eat solid foods when they are newborn so it is important that, once they stop being breast fed, they get a balance of nutrients in formula milk and, later, in the baby foods they eat.

Children

This is a time of rapid growth so children need plenty of protein, vitamin D and calcium to develop strong bones. They also need fluoride to ensure strong enamel on their teeth to protect them from decay, and iron for red blood cells.

Adolescents

Adolescents need sufficient nutrients to continue to grow and to support their physical activities, such as sports. Their bodies are continuing to change, particularly during puberty, and females will lose, for example, iron during menstruation (their periods). Eating a balanced diet can become harder in adolescence for reasons such as the demands of their busy social life, not liking the food their parents want them to eat, demands on their time due to school and exam pressures, anxiety about relationships and a concern about not becoming overweight.

Food	kJ per 100 g
Whole milk	274
White bread	1,068
Butter	3,006
Sugar	1,680
Roast beef	950
Cod (steamed)	321
Apples	197
Cabbage	66
Crisps	2,222
Chips	1,028
Boiled potatoes	339
Sweet biscuits	1,819

Figure 7.13 Some common foods and their energy values

Adults

The nutritional needs of adults depend on various factors in a person's life. The first is the person's *basal metabolic rate*. This is the amount of energy required for your body to function when lying down, still and warm. This is lower for women than men because women tend to have smaller body masses. Any movement increases the number of kilojoules needed.

The second factor is the person's *occupation*. Different jobs require different levels of energy output and therefore different amounts of kilojoules are needed to sustain the people who do these jobs. Occupations are classified into the following groups:

- **Sedentary:** office workers, teachers, pilots, shop workers.
- **Moderately active:** postmen and women, nursery assistants, care assistants, hospital porters.
- **Very active:** miners, farm labourers, builders.

The third factor is the amount of *activity* a person undertakes outside work – the amount of exercise you take can affect your energy needs. The next factor is the *state of your body* – certain conditions such as pregnancy and breast feeding require an increase in energy intake to cope with the extra demands placed on the body.

The final factor is *age* – young children require more energy for their body size than adults as they are growing rapidly and tend to be more active all the time. Ageing people require less energy as activity levels often slow down along with body processes.

Older people

As activity slows the amount of calories eaten should be reduced to prevent obesity. The digestive system also slows so food needs to be easily digestible, such as fish. Poor teeth may cause problems with eating so food needs to be softer and well cooked. Diet should be high in calcium and vitamin D to help prevent decalcification (removal of calcium) of the bones and teeth. Protein is important to maintain and renew cells, fibre levels need to increase to prevent constipation caused by the slowing of the digestive system and reduced mobility, and iron is needed to prevent anaemia.

Disabled people

Whilst the nutritional needs of people with a disability might be no different from other groups of people of the same age, those who have reduced mobility might find weight gain a problem, just as able-bodied people with a sedentary lifestyle might do.

The nutrient triangle

A quick way to check that a meal is balanced is to look at the nutrient triangle shown in Figure 7.14, which divides the main nutrients into three groups.

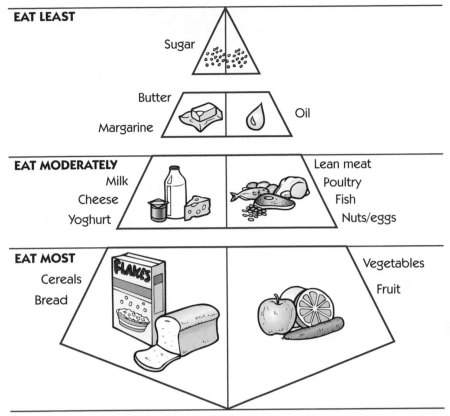

Figure 7.14 The nutrient triangle

EAT LEAST
Sugar

Butter
Margarine
Oil

EAT MODERATELY
Milk
Cheese
Yoghurt

Lean meat
Poultry
Fish
Nuts/eggs

EAT MOST
Cereals
Bread
FLAKES

Vegetables
Fruit

A healthy lifestyle

A healthy lifestyle is one that is balanced – not only in terms of diet but also as regards getting the right balance of activity and rest. Each person is different and we all live on differing amounts of activity and rest. Activity includes work and recreation (both of which we will look at later in this chapter), as well as exercise.

Regular exercise

Figure 7.15 shows how you feel after exercise. Taking exercise is an important part of keeping healthy, and there are many different ways to do so (see Figure 7.16). A person can become fit by exercising about three times a week for 20 minutes. Current medical experts tell us that if we do something energetic every day for a total of at least 30 minutes we can improve our health and well-being.

If you only exercise occasionally and try to exercise too hard, you shock your body and can easily damage your muscles. You should exercise gently at first and build up gradually to harder and longer activity. This way your limbs, heart and lungs get used to the extra pressure on them.

Most exercise is a combination of two types:

1 **Aerobic**, which exercises the heart and lungs, such as walking, running and swimming.
2 **Anaerobic**, which stretches muscles, such as yoga.

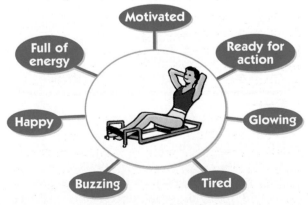

Motivated
Full of energy
Ready for action
Happy
Glowing
Buzzing
Tired

Figure 7.15 Your feelings after exercise

Exercise	Strength	Stamina	Suppleness	Kcal/min
Badminton	**	**	***	5–7
Cycling (hard)	***	****	**	7–10
Golf	*	*	**	2–5
Dancing (disco)	*	***	****	5–7
Ballroom dancing	*	*	***	2–5
Swimming (hard)	****	****	****	7–10
Walking briskly	*	**	*	5–7
Climbing stairs	**	***	*	7–10

*Fair **Good ***Very good ****Excellent

Figure 7.16 The effectiveness of different forms of exercise

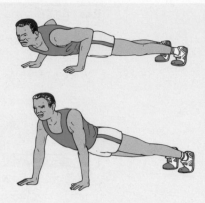

Strength – the ability to exert force for pushing, pulling and lifting. Strong muscles protect against strains and sprains

Benefits of regular exercise

The benefits of each form of exercise are often rated according to how much the exercise improves strength, stamina and suppleness, along with many other factors (see Figures 7.17 and 7.18).

The importance of regular exercise throughout life

It is important that exercise plans are designed to suit a person's lifestyle and personal circumstances, such as age, general agility and income. We will look at this in more detail in the next chapter. However, there are many forms of exercise that generally healthy members of each client group either automatically do or can attempt. For example, babies gain in strength as they try to move their bodies from one place to another by pressing down on their hands to lift their heads up, then rolling over, then crawling and, eventually, pulling themselves to a standing position ready for learning to walk.

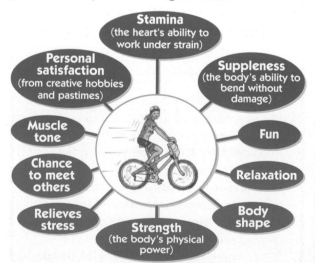

Figure 7.18 The many benefits of exercise

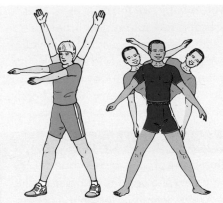

Suppleness – the ability to bend more freely, to stretch and turn through a full range of movement

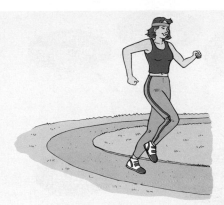

Stamina – the ability to keep going – walking, swimming, running and so on – and to acquire the reserves to make sure everyday tasks are well within the individual's ability

Figure 7.17 How exercise can improve our bodies

Activity

▶ Copy out and complete the following table using the examples given in Figure 7.16. You might find you use the same form of exercise for different age groups.

Client group	Exercise for stamina	Exercise for strength	Exercise for suppleness
Babies			
Children			
Adolescents			
Adults			
Older people			
Disabled people			

▶ Think about as many different types of athletes as you can (e.g. high-jumpers, weight-lifters and gymnasts). Draw a table that shows:

- whether they need mainly stamina, suppleness or strength, or a combination of these; and
- suggested exercises for each athlete.

Check your knowledge

1 Name three activities that are examples of mainly aerobic exercise.

2 Your heart is an example of a muscle. Read the definitions of stamina, suppleness and strength and decide which of the exercises shown in Figure 7.16 is the best type of exercise for your heart.

3 Look at this figure again. Which is the best exercise to do to improve stamina, suppleness and strength, all at the same time?

4 Why is it important for older people to keep up their strength?

5 Give an example of three different types of activity an older person would have difficulty with if he or she did not do exercise that kept him or her supple.

6 Why is it important for an older person to have stamina?

7 Many activities combine aerobic and anaerobic exercise but not many are only anaerobic. Why is this?

Sleep and rest

Sleep and rest are both very important to health and well-being. The human body is like a rechargeable battery. It cannot keep going without recharging itself. It does this through sleep and rest (see Figure 7.19).

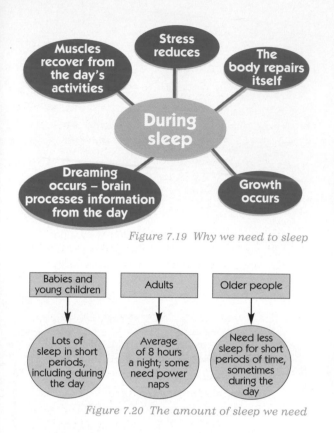

Figure 7.19 *Why we need to sleep*

Babies and young children	Adults	Older people
↓	↓	↓
Lots of sleep in short periods, including during the day	Average of 8 hours a night; some need power naps	Need less sleep for short periods of time, sometimes during the day

Figure 7.20 *The amount of sleep we need*

The importance of sleep

Figure 7.20 shows the amount of sleep we need. There are two different types of sleep.

Non-rapid eye movement sleep

This is when you first fall asleep and lasts for about two hours. Your whole body is quite relaxed, your heart beats more slowly, your breathing slows down and your eyes stay still. The body shuts down to vital functions only.

Rapid eye movement sleep

This is deep sleep during which your eyes make rapid movements and your brain is very active. Your heart and breathing are faster and your muscles are completely relaxed. You dream during this type of sleep.

Supportive relationships

Childhood

Relationships have an important influence on health and well-being. Relationships start to form as soon as a baby is born. The distance from the mother's breast to her face is just the distance at which a newborn baby can focus its eyes, so it begins to recognise its mother as it breast or bottle feeds and a relationship starts to develop. In the first two years of life a child's personality starts to develop, as does its ability to form relationships. A child has to learn how to behave in order to be accepted by others in society.

Checkpoint

Socialisation is the process by which social rules become part of a person's own personality. The rules are no longer imposed on the person but form a self-imposed basis for the normal way of life. The person has learned to conform to the rules of society, so gaining acceptance and respect from others.

Adolescence

When you become an adolescent you become less reliant on your family, become more independent and spend a lot of time with your peers (i.e. others of your own age). There is pressure to behave as members of your peer group and you tend to develop friendships with others who behave and act in the way you do. You and your friends support each other and, if you have strong friendships, your well-being is improved as you gain confidence and feel comfortable with others. This is a time when children often disagree with their parents as they develop their own views but usually still agree on the important issues in life.

Adult

As an adult your relationships change. You might become an employee, someone else's life partner and maybe a parent. You probably won't live with your parents any more, although you still visit them regularly. You might live in a new part of the country because that is where you have found the job you want. If you have learned to build good loving relationships during childhood, new relationships will form more easily.

You will be learning a lot more about relationships in Unit 3. For now it is important to realise that supportive relationships contribute positively to health and well-being.

Case study

Lynette

Lynette was the middle of three children. Her parents were both professional people and were very busy. Her father used to read her stories at night but, because her parents both had work to do at night, she spent a lot of time reading, watching TV or doing homework. She did not receive a lot of affection from her parents although they were proud of her achievements at school and she grew up wanting for nothing as her parents were relatively well off. She was very close to her two sisters and had three close friends at school.

She is now married to Peter, who has recently been made redundant. As Lynette has just returned to work after time off to have children and has a good job, Peter now stays at home and looks after their two children, Mark aged 1 and Susie aged 4. Her parents and sisters all live close by.

1 What physical, intellectual, emotional and social needs did Lynette's parents provide for her?
2 What more could her parents have done to make sure she developed loving and secure relationships as she got older?
3 How do you think her two sisters affected her ability to make good relationships with others?
4 How has her upbringing helped her in her relationship with Peter?
5 How do you think she coped when Peter was made redundant?
6 How do you think she is likely to bring up her own children?

When you have written down your opinions discuss them with a partner to see if you have had similar ideas.

Prepare two role-plays to show what your group thinks could have happened when Peter told Lynette he had been made redundant, one in which she reacted very supportively and one in which she is very negative about the situation. Which do you think was more likely to happen, considering Lynette's upbringing?

Adequate financial resources

Income is the amount of money that goes into a household. This may be from the money earned by people working in that household and/or from other sources such as welfare benefits, investments, pensions, etc.

In 1998 the National Minimum Wage Act made it statutory that all workers in the UK who are not of compulsory school age be paid at least the national minimum wage. This is £3.60 per hour at the time of writing and can be increased from time to time by the Secretary of State. Because of the minimum wage and welfare benefits, most households have at least enough money for basic food, clothing and housing.

Income has a major effect on our health and well-being. People who can afford to buy a variety of healthy foods can choose to eat a healthy diet and so are likely to be more physically healthy and less likely to be ill. Someone who can afford to go to places like the cinema is less likely to be bored and more likely to have opportunities to socialise with friends, and so have some of his or her social and intellectual needs met. When a family has adequate financial resources, there is likely to be less stress because they are not worrying about money. Family members will be less irritable and emotional needs are more likely to be met (see Figure 7.21).

Checkpoint

Statutory means required by law. Welfare benefits are provided by the state to help to improve the standard of living of people who are in some sort of need.

Activity

Look at Figure 7.21. Write down each of the factors shown and describe how they each help our physical, intellectual, emotional and social needs. Are there any other factors you can think of? If so, add them to your list.

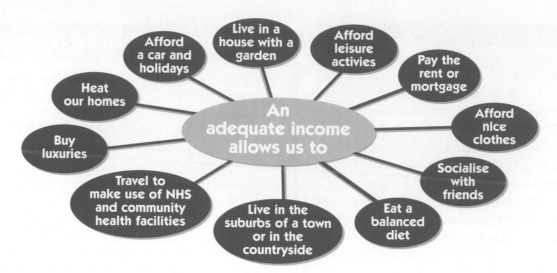

Figure 7.21 The importance of an adequate income

Stimulating work, education and leisure activity

Work

Health and well-being can be seriously affected by work. Work allows a person to use expertise he or she already has and to develop new skills and knowledge, which can be stimulating. Work provides our income and so gives us financial security and a better standard of living. It also gives us an opportunity to socialise and gives our days a routine, so giving us confidence and self-esteem.

The type of work we do also affects our health and well-being. A person in a high-powered job will usually receive a salary that reflects the pressure he or she is under. However, such a person may find that, although he or she can afford a magnificent house, he or she never has time to be there and the pressure he or she is under may similarly threaten the person's health and mental state. People in very low-paid jobs are under pressure for different reasons. Trying to make ends meet is extremely stressful when someone is on a limited income.

It can be argued that the more satisfaction a job gives someone, the less stress he or she will be under. On the other hand, work itself is not without its problems (see Figure 7.22).

There are, however, risks associated with work, such as employment-related accidents, repetitive strain injury and stress in such occupations as teaching, the emergency services and nursing (see Figure 7.23). There are also problems that arise from, for example, racial, sexual, cultural and age discrimination.

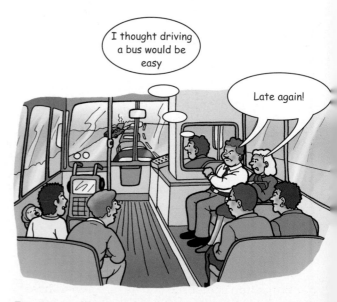

Figure 7.22 All types of work can put people under stress

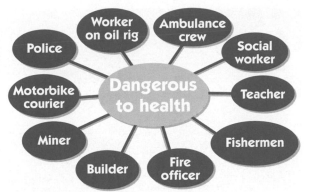

Figure 7.23 Some of the jobs that can be dangerous to health

Education

Learning is something we do from birth. A young child starts to learn how to socialise with its family and the process continues at nursery or playschool and school. The intellectual needs of a child are also partly met at school by the intellectual stimulation provided and, by law, a child is entitled to formal education between the ages of 5 and 16 years. The opportunities for education are not the same for everyone and some children start school before the age of 5 and leave before the age of 16 for a variety of reasons. Likewise, the education a young person receives varies depending on a number of factors, as shown in Figure 7.24.

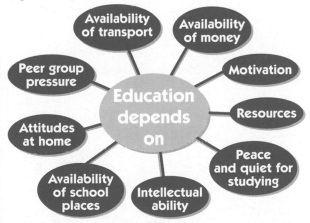

Figure 7.24 Factors that affect our education

Your educational achievements will affect your health and well-being in a number of ways. It will affect your outlook on life. For example, our education sometimes turns us against those things our upbringing told us were right and proper, be it our political views, our taste in music or simply those things that constitute a good square meal. Education will also determine what further education you might choose and the job you will be able to choose, and that job in turn will affect your income and your standard of living. A good education can help you to make sound life choices and so will affect your health and well-being.

Leisure activity

Leisure or recreational activities include physical activities (such as sport) and less physical activities (such as watching television, reading or meeting friends). Different people like to relax in different ways, depending on their situation (for example, having a disability or being elderly) and interests. Relaxation is a time to do something different and is very important to our health and well-being as it gives us a break from work, can provide intellectual stimulation, makes us feel good, keeps us interested in life, gives us a chance to socialise with others and helps us cope with stress.

People with disabilities

A disability can be anything from being visually impaired to having limited movement due to a medical condition (such as multiple sclerosis), an accident or simply being obese.

One thing many people with a disability have in common is their treatment as a result of the attitude of others towards their disability. For example, able-bodied people often talk over disabled people rather than addressing them directly.

Whilst some people with disabilities may be unable to take part in certain activities, they still have the same needs for recreation as anyone else. Sometimes people will be less embarrassed if they take part in activities with people with similar disabilities, but this can lead to a loss of certain opportunities to socialise. Special arrangements have to be made in certain circumstances for a person's disability; for example, able-bodied people running a marathon alongside people in wheelchairs would be dangerous and would not be fair competitively. It is therefore important that facilities and time are allocated for people with disabilities.

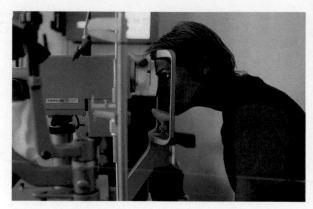

Health monitoring involves regular check-ups

Use of health monitoring and illness prevention services (such as screening and vaccination)

Health monitoring

To monitor someone's health is to make regular checks to see if he or she is remaining healthy. Monitoring is also used to check the progress of someone who is already ill or is in poor health. For example, a doctor can monitor a client's high blood pressure by getting him or her to visit the surgery for a blood test every week for a period of time. The doctor can then take action if the client's condition gets worse.

Health screening

Health screening is a way of checking to make sure certain parts of our bodies are working well. For example, a check-up at the dentist is called oral (mouth) health screening. Other examples of health screening include coronary heart screening to let a client know if he or she needs to change his or her lifestyle to prevent

the client developing heart disease, and screening for breast, cervix and testicular cancers.

Vaccination

Another form of prevention is vaccination. Vaccination works by a weakened form of a disease being injected into the body. This causes the body to produce antibodies, which then protect against the disease if the body comes into contact with it again.

Babies are vaccinated against a range of diseases, such as mumps, measles and rubella (German measles) (see Figure 7.25).

Age	Disease
8, 12 and 16 weeks	Diptheria, whooping cough and tetanus – a combined injection often called the 'triple vaccine' Polio – taken by mouth Hib – injected
12–15 months	Measles, mumps and rubella – a combined injection known as the MMR
3–5 years	Diptheria and tetanus – a combined injection Polio – taken by mouth MMR

Figure 7.25 Vaccinations for infants

Vaccinations are also used to protect travellers to certain countries from diseases such as yellow fever. Another vaccination we often hear about is the flu vaccine.

All these screening and preventative services are free of charge or inexpensive.

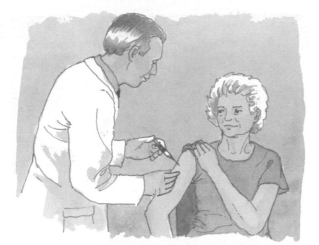

- are diabetic;
- have a respiratory disease such as asthma;
- live in a nursing or retirement home; and
- are taking certain medicines such as steroids or anti-cancer drugs.

Flu can be a serious illness, killing between 3,000 and 4,000 people every winter in the UK. Vaccination can not only prevent this but can also protect people against the unpleasant symptoms of flu.

Use of risk management techniques to protect individuals and promote personal safety

Risk management techniques are used in all areas of work. In the area we are interested in, it is to do with reducing the chance of clients of the care services being harmed and providing a safe working environment for the care workers.

Checkpoint

A **hazard** is anything that has the potential to harm someone in some way. A **risk** is a chance or possibility of danger, loss, injury or some other bad consequence. Hence a risk is a measure of how likely a hazard is to cause harm.

Risk management

Risk management involves several processes.

Identifying a risk

Identifying a risk might include, for example, spotting the chance of someone tripping over wires from a machine to the electricity supply.

Assessment of the risk

This means estimating the extent of the risk (often on a 1–5 scale) and the likelihood of it happening. In the example of the risk of tripping over wires, it might be a risk of 3 that someone might trip up and of 3 that it will happen again. This might be a moderate risk.

Activity

▶ Carry out some research on the topic of strokes by looking in books and leaflets or on the Internet. Design a leaflet containing information on:

- what a stroke is;
- who is most at risk of having a stroke; and
- the monitoring and screening services available to help prevent someone having a stroke.

Your leaflet should be written in simple language so that everyone can understand it and be colourful with plenty of illustrations to encourage people to read it.

▶ Find out about vaccinations given to people travelling abroad. You need to present the information about the diseases each one provides protection against and how it works in a form that makes the information easily understood by those who are not doing this extension activity.

Part of your role as a health and care worker is to encourage clients to make use of the screening and monitoring services available to help maintain their health and well-being.

Vaccination is recommended for anyone who has difficulty fighting infection, such as those people who:

- are aged 65 and over;
- have heart disease;
- have kidney trouble;

Controlling the risk

This means deciding what can be done to reduce the risk. In the example of the wires, taping them down to the floor or re-routing them might reduce both the risk and the likelihood of an accident happening again to 1. This then becomes a low risk, which is considered more acceptable than a moderate risk.

Monitoring how effectively the risk is being controlled

This means making sure the precautions taken to reduce the risk remain in place.

Reassessing the risk

This means looking at the risk again to see if it can be reduced still further. In the example of the wires, it might be that if a room is rearranged, the machine concerned could be positioned against a wall right in front of an electrical supply so the wires are behind the machine and the risk of tripping over them is reduced to 0.

This process is cyclical (goes round in a circle) and continuous.

Unsafe practices in the workplace

Workplaces are subject to various inspection systems and must comply with a wide range of legislation. This includes the Health and Safety at Work Act 1974 (HASAW), the key features of which are shown in Figure 7.26. What HASAW basically means is that both the employer and the employee share responsibilities for health and safety and that any organisation employing more than five people must have a written policy statement on health and safety (see Figure 7.27).

There has also been more recent legislation: a general framework for workplace health and safety in the European Community in the form of a series of directives on health and safety matters, adopted by the European Council of Ministers in 1989. The one that affects care settings is called the Workplace Regulations, which applied from 1996 and says that employers have to make workplaces suitable for the individuals who work in them. They must pay particular attention to the needs of disabled people, pregnant workers and other vulnerable groups.

- **Employers must make all reasonable efforts to ensure the health, safety and welfare of all their employees by informing you:**
  - how to carry out your job safely without risk to yourself and others
  - of risks identified with the job that may affect you
  - what measures have been taken to protect you from the identified risks
  - how to use these measures
  - how to get first aid treatment
  - what to do in an emergency
  - by leaflet or poster about the Health and Safety at Work Act and the local Health and Safety Executive's address

- **Employers must provide free of charge:**
  - adequate safety training
  - clothing or equipment required to protect you while at work

- **As an employee, your responsibilities are:**
  - to take reasonable care of yourself and others (including the general public) who may be affected by your work
  - use any equipment provided for you for its intended purpose and in a proper manner
  - not to carry out tasks that you do not know how to do safely
  - let your manager know if you witness anything that is not safe and could place yourself or others at risk
  - to co-operate with employers on health and safety matters
  - inform the appropriate person in the organisation if you have an accident or witness a near miss

Figure 7.26 The key features of the Health and Safety at Work Act 1974

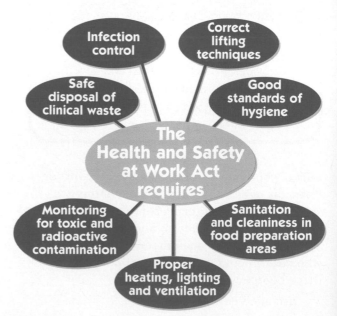

Figure 7.27 How the Health and Safety at Work Act affects care settings

Practice activity

Consider the examples below and decide what the risk is, on a scale of 1–5. Use 5 for the worst likelihood of that risk occurring. Decide what could be done to reduce the risk.

1   The possibility of a door handle dropping off so that no one can get in or out.
2   Someone collapsing in a day care centre for older people and no one knowing what to do.
3   Someone getting the wrong medicine at the pharmacist.
4   The possibility of someone slipping on a wet floor in a busy Citizens Advice Bureau when it has just been mopped.
5   A child tripping up in a playground where there is an uneven gutter around the edge of it.
6   Someone on crutches falling on steep hospital steps.

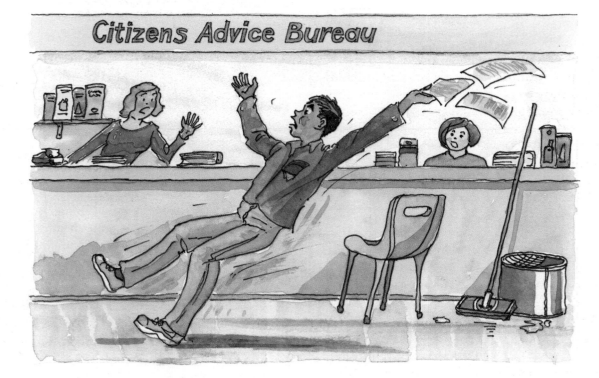

Risks to health and well-being

In Chapter 7 we looked at the factors that contribute positively to health and well-being. Some of those same factors can also damage health and well-being if not balanced or adequate, as can the intake of various substances, unprotected sex, our environment and other aspects of our lifestyle and behaviour. We are now going to look at those factors that put health and well-being at risk.

By the end of this chapter you will have learnt about factors that put an individual's health and well-being at risk. You will be able to identify the lifestyle factors over which people have control and also the genetic, social and economic factors which people may not be able to control. You will learn that health and well-being can be affected by:

- genetically inherited diseases and conditions;
- substance misuse (including misuse of legal and illegal drugs, solvents, tobacco smoking and excessive alcohol intake);
- an unbalanced, poor-quality or inadequate diet;
- too much stress;
- a lack of personal hygiene;
- a lack of regular physical exercise;
- unprotected sex;
- social isolation;
- poverty;
- inadequate housing;
- unemployment; and
- environmental pollution.

You will find out how these factors can affect a person's health and well-being.

Genetically inherited diseases and conditions

In Chapter 6 you learnt that you can have a *disease* such as cancer (with your body changing in some way) but not be aware of it in the early stages, although some form of screening would enable a doctor to see it. Some diseases are *inherited* (i.e. passed on from one generation to another), and the inheritance of characteristics is called *heredity*. The study of how heredity works is called *genetics*.

All human body cells contain thread-like structures called chromosomes. These carry genes that carry coded information to control and develop your body. Each chromosome carries a large number of genes and children have similar characteristics to their parents because of the genes that are passed on to them, as shown in Figure 8.1.

Did you know?

Chromosomes carry the chemical DNA (deoxyribonucleic acid). Each **gene** is a section of DNA which instructs the cell how to make a particular protein. **Proteins** are very important to the functioning and structure of our cells. The position of each gene along the length of a chromosome gives the code that produces the information provided by that chromosome. Changes in a DNA molecule in a cell are called **mutations**. Mutations are more often harmful than good and result in changed characteristics.

When humans reproduce, genes are passed to the next generation so that each generation looks similar to the previous generation. Very rarely a sudden change happens in genes and the offspring are born with something different about them. This change is called a *mutation*. Occasionally a mutation is inherited that is

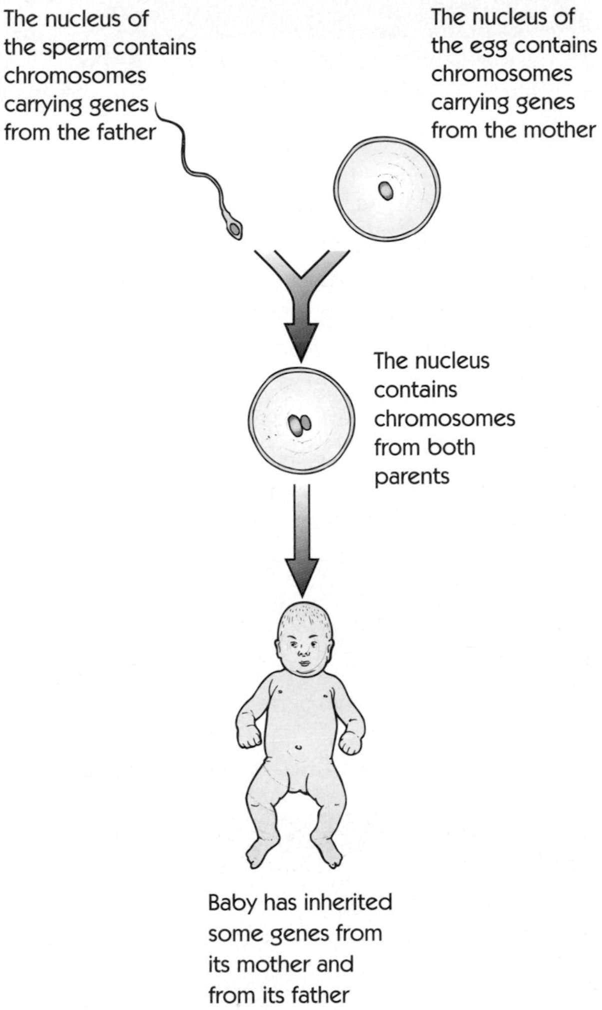
The nucleus of the sperm contains chromosomes carrying genes from the father
The nucleus of the egg contains chromosomes carrying genes from the mother
The nucleus contains chromosomes from both parents
Baby has inherited some genes from its mother and from its father

Figure 8.1 Inherited information

harmful to the individual. For example, when a gene is inherited that results in body cells having an extra chromosome, that child will have Down's syndrome. Some mutations are not necessarily inherited. Some chemicals, such as those in cigarette smoke, and other factors (such as radiation), can increase the chance of a mutation happening. If a mutation occurs in body cells, the cells may start to multiply in an uncontrolled way and so invade other parts of the body. This is how cancer occurs. However, there are over 3,500 diseases that are known to be produced by a defect in a single gene and these are genetically inherited.

In some of these conditions the defective gene is **dominant**, which means that only one parent has to have the gene to pass the disease on to his or her children. One example is myotonic dystrophy, a type of muscular dystrophy that leads to muscle wasting and loss of muscle tone. Another example of a disease that is inherited from just one parent having the gene is Huntington's chorea.

Activity

Huntington's chorea is also known as Huntington's disease and causes jerky and contorted movements of the limbs. There is medication available that is only partially successful at reducing these movements.

▶
1. Which needs of a 35-year-old woman with Huntington's chorea will be met by her continuing to work in an office after she is diagnosed with the disease?
2. What difficulties will she face that will affect her health and well-being, other than the disease itself?
3. How can her working conditions (e.g. the layout of her office) be adapted so that she can keep working as long as possible?

▶
1. Discuss in a small group whether you would want to go on working in this situation and why.
2. There is a 50% chance that someone with the condition will transmit it to an offspring. Genetic counselling is advised if there is a family history of the disorder. Find out what is meant by genetic counselling and discuss whether you would want to take this advice if you were in this position as an adult, bearing in mind that people with the disease most usually develop it between the ages of 35 and 50 years.

In other cases the gene is **recessive**, meaning that both parents have to have the gene before the disease is passed on to their children. The parents may not have the disease but carry the gene. One example of such a disease is cystic fibrosis. This is a common disease and one child in every 2,000 born in the UK has it. It is a disease of the exocrine glands of the lungs, skin and pancreas. Children who have cystic fibrosis produce very thick sticky mucus which can cause blockages in the air passages in their lungs. A child with this disease gets many chest infections and each one leads to more damage to the lungs so that the child becomes even more ill. The infections cannot be prevented but can be treated with strong antibiotics. Children with cystic fibrosis also have to have regular massage to clear their lungs. An uncleared build-up of mucus would mean the child would die. Another example of a disease that is recessive is sickle cell anaemia.

Other defective genes are linked to a particular sex. For example, only males can develop haemophilia, although women can pass it on. Haemophilia is a disease where the blood cannot clot, so if a cut is left untreated the person will bleed to death.

Adults with a genetic disorder in the family may decide not to have any children so that they do not pass the disease on. Such people can have genetic counselling so they can discuss the risks and possible options. For some inherited disorders such as Down's syndrome, screening during pregnancy can reveal the condition in the unborn baby and allow the parents to think about terminating the pregnancy.

There are also techniques now that can change genes and so change characteristics. These techniques are called *genetic engineering*. This can be of great benefit to humans. For example, diabetes is a disease caused because the body cannot make a hormone called insulin. This hormone is very important because it controls the amount of glucose in our blood. People who have diabetes need to be injected with insulin and, because it is a common disease, a large amount of insulin is needed. Some people use insulin obtained from sheep and pigs but others react badly to animal insulin. Genetic engineering means that scientists can now produce human insulin from bacteria, thereby overcoming the problem. It is important, however, for anything produced by genetic engineering to be carefully monitored and not to be released into the natural environment.

Activity

In a group, discuss the answers to the following two questions:

▶ 1   What are the benefits of genetic engineering?
    2   What are the dangers of genetic engineering?

Decide as a group whether you feel the benefits outweigh the dangers or not. You have to decide one way or the other. Appoint a spokesperson to report your group's decision and reasons for that decision to the rest of the class.

▶   An article appears in a newspaper saying that a couple have been given the go-ahead to have a baby specifically for the purpose of trying to get a perfect match for a bone marrow transplant for their son who will die from a genetically inherited disease without such a match being found. Write a letter to the newspaper giving your opinion on this. Try to base any opinions on facts.

Check your knowledge

1   What is the study of heredity called?
2   What do chromosomes do?
3   What causes Down's syndrome?
4   Name two factors that can increase the chance of a mutation happening.
5   Name two diseases inherited from just one parent having a defective gene.
6   What does 'recessive' mean?
7   What are the symptoms of cystic fibrosis?
8   Give an example of a medical benefit of genetic engineering.
9   Insulin, used to treat diabetes, is a protein. Think back to what you learned about proteins in Chapter 7 and try to explain why insulin cannot be taken in tablet form.
10   Why do diabetics have to be careful when they exercise?

Substance misuse

People may use drugs or other substances in a way that feels pleasurable but that may be harmful to their health. Many substances can be misused and these range from, for example, too much coffee causing nervous tension, to an individual who is addicted to crack cocaine (see Figure 8.2). The word 'drug' also covers nicotine and alcohol, both of which are legal in the UK. Choosing to use any drug has an effect on our bodily functions.

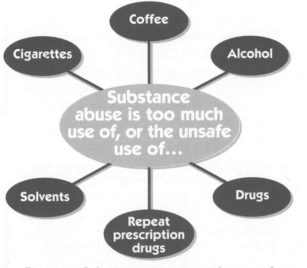

Figure 8.2 *Substance misuse can take many forms*

Drug abuse

Drugs may be obtained in three main ways:

1   From a doctor, via a prescription made up by the chemist. These are known as **prescribed drugs** and are part of a treatment given to combat illness.
2   From chemists or supermarkets, for money. These are known as **over-the-counter drugs**.
3   Illegally. These are **controlled drugs** and are often the type that can lead to addiction or that have dangerous side-effects if misused. Some of these are shown in Figure 8.4 on page 128. Some of these, such as cocaine, are referred to as recreational drugs because they are taken by some people at parties for fun, despite the risks.

Solvent abuse

Solvents are substances used in the manufacture of glue, lighter fuel, petrol, paint, paint thinners and aerosols. People sniff or inhale them to get 'high' on the solvents they contain. Some of the effects are shown in Figure 8.3. It is against the law in the UK for children under the age of 18 to buy certain substances that may be misused.

Developing a tolerance to any drug can mean that more is needed each time to get the same effect. This means increased costs and increased risks. Also, most drugs that are misused are not made under safe laboratory conditions. Some drugs are contaminated with other dangerous substances, and so the effects are unpredictable. Some drugs may be deliberately mixed with other substances and some could be far weaker or stronger than those previously experienced.

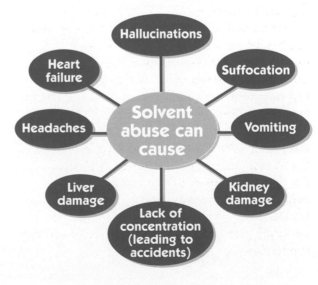

Figure 8.3 *The effects of solvent abuse*

Misused drug	Appearance and use	Effects of use	Possible risks
Cannabis or hash, grass, marijuana, Black Leb, rocky, weed	Like dried herbs, a dark brown block or sticky and treacle-like Usually smoked but sometimes eaten	Feeling of sickness, hunger or worry More alert and talkative Imagines things (hallucinations)	Bronchitis and damage to lungs Raised pulse rate and blood pressure Inactivity and loss of memory Mental illness
LSD or acid, trips, tabs	Blotters and micro-dots that are swallowed	Greater self-awareness Disorientated in time and place Altered hearing, panic Depression and feeling that everyone and everything is against them (paranoia)	Never quite returning to previous normal state and needing more and more to achieve the same effects (tolerance) Flashbacks Anxiety Disorientation and depression
Heroin or H, Henry, smack	White or brown powder that is injected, sniffed up the nose or smoked	Feeling sleepy and coddled	HIV/AIDS and hepatitis B when it is injected Thrombosis of veins or abscess at the injection sites Blood infection (septicaemia) Heart and lung disorders Can be fatal if impure
Ecstasy or E, xtc, M25s, lovedoves, Adam	Flat, round tablets that are swallowed	Confidence, calmness and alertness Thirst, anxiety Symptoms of heat stroke Sexual feelings	Nausea, headache and giddiness Raised body temperature with no sweating Muscular cramps Collapse Mental illness including paranoia
Cocaine, coke, snow or Charlie	White powder that is injected or sniffed	Anxiety, thirst and heat stroke symptoms	HIV/AIDS and hepatitis B when it is injected Thrombosis of veins or abscess at the injection sites
Crack	Crystals that are smoked	Feel on top of the world, could do anything Panic, worry or hostility	Blood infection (septicaemia) Heart and lung disorders Addictive Raised body temperature with no sweating, muscular cramps Lack of appetite (anorexia)
Amphetamines or speed, sulph, whizz	White powder in tablets or screws of paper that are swallowed, sniffed or injected	Palpitations (increased force and rate of heart beat), weakness, hunger Lots of energy and confidence Depression and worry	HIV/AIDS and hepatitis B when it is injected Raised blood pressure and risk of stroke Mental illness Tolerance develops
Solvents or glue, Evo, aerosols, petrol, lighter fluid	Various fluids or sprays that are sniffed	Heightened imagination, depression, happiness or sadness, hostility Fatigue, confusion Liver and kidney damage	Liver and kidney damage Increased risk of accidents during the abuse Heart failure, suffocation, vomiting/choking, death

Figure 8.4 The effects and risks of some commonly misused drugs

Activity

There is a small shop near to a high school that lots of students sneak out to at lunchtimes to buy crisps and sandwiches. Some of them regularly go to stand behind it to smoke. One Year 10 student asks the shopkeeper to sell him six cans of deodorant. The shopkeeper is suspicious about this, because the Intoxicating Substances Act 1985 states that supplying substances the supplier knows can be used to achieve intoxication to someone under the age of 18 years is an offence. He asks the student why a 15-year-old lad would want to buy six cans of deodorant in a light hearted way because he doesn't want to upset the students and lose their custom. The student says that they've got PE that afternoon and he and his mates have all forgotten their deodorant and the teachers will go mad if they don't have any.

▷ 1 What do you think the shopkeeper should do?

2 What do you think should be the punishment for shopkeepers or anyone else who chooses to supply such products in these quantities to young people?

3 Produce a poster showing the products this applies to that shopkeepers could display in their shops. It should also explain the dangers of such substances to young people who might not understand why the shopkeeper shouldn't sell them to them.

▷ 1 Do you think it is a good or bad idea to display lists of these products and the effects they can have? Give reasons for your answers.

Tobacco smoking

Tobacco smoking is the drawing into the mouth, and inhalation of, the smoke from burning tobacco, a plant material. Sounds silly, doesn't it! However, the smoking of tobacco, usually as cigarettes, is legal and more socially acceptable than other drugs, despite there being an increasing opposition to smoking in public places. A large number of environments, both social and work, are now either non-smoking areas or only allow smoking in a certain designated place. This is because smoking is a major cause of ill health, preventable disease and death. All smoking material packaging and adverts now carry a government health warning. Health and life insurance premiums are generally lower for non-smokers. However, many people still do smoke, showing how difficult it is to overcome nicotine addiction and how successful cigarette companies are with their advertising strategies. The hazards of smoking are shown in Figure 8.5.

Checkpoint

Bronchitis is a chest infection and can be caused by cigarette smoke damaging the airways of the lungs so that the tubes become blocked by mucus and easily infected by bacteria.

Emphysema is a condition caused when cigarette smoke destroys the delicate structure of the air sacs in the lungs, preventing the efficient exchange of oxygen and carbon dioxide. It leads to severe shortage of breath and eventually a dependence on oxygen supplies. Smoking causes nine out of ten cases of emphysema.

A **stroke** is the term used when part of the body is disabled, either as a result of a clot in a blood vessel preventing blood getting to part of the brain or by a blood vessel bursting and bleeding into the brain.

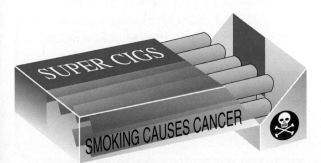

SUPER CIGS

SMOKING CAUSES CANCER

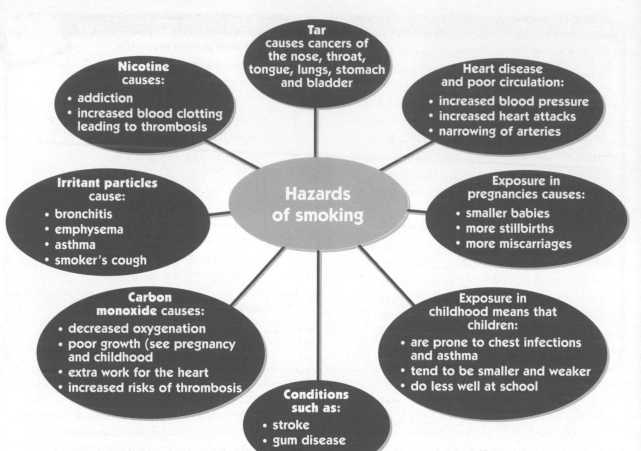

Figure 8.5 The hazards of smoking

Checkpoint

Nicotine is a very powerful, fast-acting and addictive drug. When smoke is inhaled, nicotine is absorbed into a smoker's bloodstream and the effects are felt on his or her brain within seven or eight seconds. Nicotine causes:

- increased heart rate;
- increased blood pressure;
- increased hormone production;
- constriction of small blood vessels under the skin;
- changes in blood composition; and
- changes in metabolism so, hence, a change in appetite.

Carbon monoxide is a poisonous gas which is highly concentrated in cigarette smoke. It combines more easily with **haemoglobin** (the substance that carries oxygen in the blood) than oxygen does, so up to 15% of a smoker's blood may be carrying carbon monoxide round the body instead of oxygen. Because of this reduction in oxygen flow, problems can be caused with:

- the growth of tissues;
- the repair of tissues; and
- the absorption of essential nutrients.

Carbon monoxide can also affect the electrical activity of the heart and can lead to blocked arteries causing heart disease and other circulation problems. About 70% of the **tar** contained in cigarette smoke is deposited in the lungs. Many substances in tar are known to cause cancer. Irritants in tar also cause problems by damaging the cilia (small hairs that line the lungs and help protect them against dirt and infection), producing an increase in mucus and coughing and so a greater tendency to throat and chest infections.

Passive smoking occurs when non-smokers inhale unfiltered smoke from the smokers around them. Such smoke has larger amounts of tar, nicotine and other irritants than those inhaled by the smoker. Some non-smoking, well-known entertainers, such as Roy Castle, have died as a consequence of working for many years in smoky night-clubs and similar places. The foetuses of pregnant women who smoke are also passive smokers.

Half the children in England live in households with at least one smoker and do not have any choice about whether or not they inhale unfiltered smoke, unlike the adult who is smoking. A recent study by the Imperial Cancer Research Fund's health behaviour unit, published in January 2002, shows that passive smoking is far more of a risk in the home than elsewhere. It showed that someone living with a person having 15 cigarettes a day suffered four times more exposure to tobacco smoke than an individual in a smoke-free household. Young people were the most heavily exposed in the home.

In 1964 the first official warning about the health hazards of smoking were given and since then fewer adults have smoked. However, current trends show an increase in women as a proportion of all smokers as more women than men now take up the habit. Smoking among adults has declined steadily but the proportion of young people has remained constant and even gone up over recent years.

Activity

▶ Discuss in your group the reasons why you think young people smoke. Also discuss why you think more women are taking up smoking than men.

▶ Go on the Internet to find out the trend over recent years of the percentage of children in England who regularly smoke. You could try the National Statistics website.

Smoking is very costly in terms of health care and lost working days. There are also massive costs due to homes needing decorating more often, homes setting on fire, litter, smoking breaks at work, etc.

Stopping smoking

It is difficult to stop smoking but when you do the body begins to repair the damage done. When the body is no longer taking in nicotine, tar, carbon dioxide and other poisonous substances generated by smoking, body systems begin to return to normal quite quickly. The benefits of stopping smoking are shown in Figure 8.6.

There are organisations dedicated to helping smokers break the habit, such as QUIT, the Health Education Authority and ASH, to name but a few. They recommend

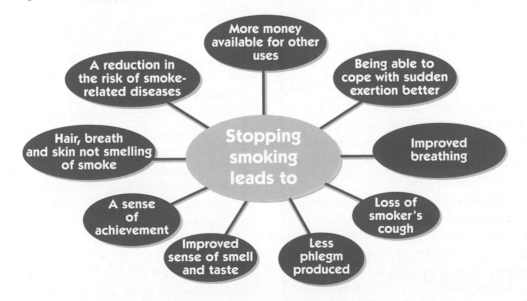

Figure 8.6 The benefits of stopping smoking

nicotine replacement therapy (NRT), such as using nicotine patches, gum, lozenges or a nasal spray – all products that have been scientifically tested. These work by getting nicotine into your system without the tar, carbon dioxide and other poisonous substances in tobacco smoke. Once you can cope without the smoking you can then cut out the NRT.

Did you know?

Ten million people in Britain have stopped smoking and stayed stopped in the last 15 years – that's over 1,000 a day!

Case study

Brenda

Brenda started smoking when she was 18, when a friend offered her a cigarette and she really enjoyed it. She was soon smoking about 25 a day. She tried to give it up many times but found it impossible. Then she had to run to a phone box to get an ambulance for someone who had been knocked down in the street. By the time she had run the short distance there and back she was very out of breath. She was only 24 years old and had always prided herself on being physically fit.

1   What could have been the consequences for the person who had been knocked down if Brenda had had to run any further to get help?

2   How dangerous do you think Brenda's habit is to her health?

3   What facts about smoking do you think will make Brenda realise she needs to give up?

4   What steps would you recommend she takes to try to give up?

5   What timescale would you recommend for each of the steps you have mentioned in question 4?

6   What benefits will Brenda feel if she manages to give up totally?

Drinking alcohol

Unlike smoking, alcohol is a socially acceptable drug. It is addictive and can kill but drinking in small quantities can be both a pleasurable experience and beneficial to health. It has been scientifically proven that a glass of red wine, two or three times a week, can reduce the risk of heart disease.

So what is alcohol? It is a chemical called ethanol that is made when yeast acts on sugar. The yeast uses the sugar to feed on so that it can grow and multiply, and alcohol and carbon dioxide are produced. This process is called fermentation. The alcohol can be further concentrated by boiling the water off to produce spirits.

Why drink alcohol?

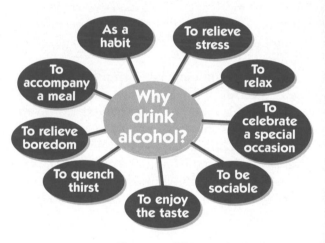

Figure 8.7 Why people drink alcohol

Adults drink alcohol for a number of reasons (see Figure 8.7). Young people are likely to start drinking alcohol because of a number of reasons, such as:

* their friends drink
* to see what drinking is like
* to impress their mates
* they like the taste
* they like the sensation
* boredom
* to overcome shyness.

What happens to the alcohol?

Alcohol passes from the stomach straight into the bloodstream, travelling around the body until it reaches the brain. It affects you very quickly, within a few minutes. As blood passes through the liver, any alcohol in it is gradually broken down by an enzyme so it is the liver that cleans the alcohol out of your body. A little is disposed of either in urine or sweat. The liver gets rid of it at about one unit per hour (for example, half a pint of lager) and, no matter how fast you drink the alcohol or how many cups of coffee you have later, your liver can only work at that speed.

Checkpoint

An **enzyme** is a protein produced by the body to bring about a chemical change.

The effects of alcohol on behaviour

When consumed in large amounts, alcohol can be a major risk to a person's health and well-being. Alcohol is a depressant. It affects the nerves that pass messages round the body by slowing them down, so it can act as a pain killer. The more a person drinks the greater the effect. It also affects the parts of the brain that are responsible for self-control and so can produce the effects shown in Figure 8.8.

Too much alcohol can lead to damaged relationships, unsafe behaviour and accidents. Many fights, domestic violence and injuries

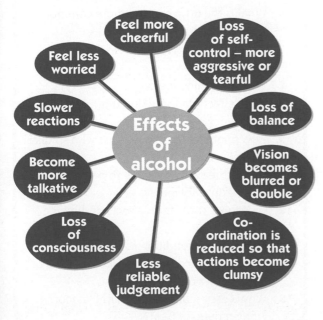

Figure 8.8 The effects of alcohol

result from excessive intake of alcohol. Many people pass out or suffer from memory lapses. This, combined with loss of self-control and judgement, can lead to people doing things they would not normally do, such as having unprotected sex, picking fights, committing criminal offences or doing dangerous things such as drink driving. It can also affect a person's ability to work and to pay bills.

Effects of alcohol on health

Drinking too much alcohol regularly can lead to the following:

- Weight gain and obesity – a pint of beer contains 300 calories, a glass of wine 80.
- Reddened (and eventually permanently mottled) skin.
- Liver damage – light drinking lets the tissue that has been damaged repair itself but heavy drinking kills cells so the liver stops working effectively. This leads to a disease called **cirrhosis**, which can be fatal.
- Stomach problems – gastritis can lead to a lack of vitamins in the body and consequent problems such as malnutrition. For example, a lack of vitamin B in the body can lead to serious mental disturbance.
- Brain damage.
- Heart disease and ultimately heart failure when the heart can no longer pump blood around the body.
- High blood pressure and increased risk of strokes.
- Cancers of the mouth and throat.
- Depression and other emotional problems.
- Bowel and stomach cancer.
- Ulcers.
- Damage to unborn babies.
- Insomnia.
- Reduced sexual function.

Recommended limits

How much you can drink and still stay healthy is measured by the number of units of drink. What a unit is, however, varies according to the kind of alcoholic drink, as shown in Figure 8.9. The limits are:

- not more than 14 units in a week if you are female; or
- not more than 21 units in a week if you are male.

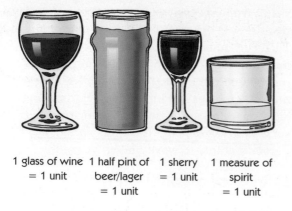

1 glass of wine = 1 unit | 1 half pint of beer/lager = 1 unit | 1 sherry = 1 unit | 1 measure of spirit = 1 unit

Figure 8.9 Recommended limits

If men and women follow this guide there should be no significant risk to their health. However, if the guide is exceeded regularly there is an increased risk to health. Also, the limits can only be used as a rough guide because different brands of the same drink can have very different strengths. One strong pint of beer can contain the same number of units as over two pints of ordinary beer, or just over four whiskies.

To help drinkers judge how strong a drink is, all containers of alcohol show the percentage of alcohol by volume on the label. The higher the percentage the stronger the drink. This percentage is known as the alcohol by volume, or ABV.

You can work out the exact number of units in a drink by multiplying the volume of the drink in millilitres (ml) by the ABV and dividing the result by 1,000.

Worked example

The number of units in a 330 ml bottle of lager at 5% is:

$$\frac{330 \times 5}{1,000} = 1.7 \text{ units}$$

Activity

Work out how many units are contained in the following:

1 A 25 ml pub measure of gin (ABV 37.5%).
2 A 25 ml pub measure of whisky (ABV 40.0%).
3 Half a pint (284 ml) of strong cider (ABV 4.0%).
4 130 ml of low alcohol wine (ABV 0.05%).
5 130 ml of wine (ABV 10%).
6 130 ml of wine (ABV 13%).

Other factors also affect the amount of alcohol in your blood stream, such as the following:

- **Your size:** If you are small you are likely to be more affected by the same amount of alcohol as someone else because you have less blood volume.
- **Your water level:** If you are dehydrated alcohol will affect you more than when your water concentration is normal, so you will be more affected after exercise or in hot weather.
- **Your gender:** Women are usually smaller than men so they have less water and blood in their bodies and so are more easily affected by alcohol. They also have more fat in their bodies and so hold the alcohol for longer because alcohol cannot dissolve in fat.
- **The amount of food in your stomach:** Alcohol reaches your brain more slowly if there is food in your stomach.
- **How often you drink:** Regular drinkers are more used to alcohol and so need to drink more for it to have the same effect.

Check your knowledge

1 What do we mean by 'substance abuse'?
2 Name three different substances that get abused.
3 What are controlled drugs?
4 Write down three effects of solvent abuse.
5 What is the drug cocaine more commonly known as?
6 What are the risks associated with cannabis?
7 What does nicotine cause?
8 What effects can smoking during pregnancy have?
9 How might tar affect someone who smokes?
10 What is passive smoking?
11 Name three aids available to help someone to give up smoking.
12 Give three short-term effects of drinking alcohol.
13 Describe the condition called cirrhosis.
14 What is the recommended limit of units of alcohol for women?
15 Why is the recommended limit less for women than for men?

An unbalanced, poor-quality or inadequate diet

We have already looked at the positive effects of a balanced diet on health and well-being in Chapter 7. However, it is also important to realise the risks of an unbalanced, poor-quality or inadequate diet.

Under-eating

Everyone has different nutritional needs and some people can cope with nutritional shortages better than others. The body is able to adapt to a reduced intake of food but too little food over a long period of time can lead to malnutrition. In extreme cases starvation causes stunting of physical and mental development and wasting of the body. Some diseases can be caused by a shortage of certain nutrients, as shown in Figure 8.10.

Shortage of	Possible effects
Carbohydrate	Protein used for energy so less available for growth and repair
Iron, folic acid or vitamin B12	Anaemia – a decrease in the ability of the body to carry iron around, leading to tiredness, paleness, headaches, pounding of the heart, shortness of breath, pins and needles, giddiness
Calcium or vitamin D	Stunted bone growth and rickets (bones develop badly and legs are bowed). Osteoporosis (a bone-weakening disorder) in women in later life
Sodium	Muscle cramps
Potassium	Heart failure
Iodine	Goitre (swelling of the thyroid gland)
Vitamin A	Poor vision and blindness
Vitamin B1	Depression, tiredness and diseases of the nervous system
Vitamin B2	Sores in the mouth
Vitamin C	Bleeding from small blood vessels and gums, wounds heal more slowly, scurvy
Fibre	Bowel cancer

Figure 8.10 The effects caused by a shortage of certain nutrients

Checkpoint

Malnutrition means the condition caused by not eating the correct balance of nutrients.

Overeating

Excessive amounts of food can also cause malnutrition. If you eat too much from time to time it is unlikely to do you any harm other than to make you feel bloated. If you continually overeat, however, your body will start to store fat under the skin in a thick layer. More importantly, it will store the excess fat on your organs and inside your arteries. Both these are dangerous to our health and could lead to obesity, heart disease or high blood pressure.

The high intake of saturated fats such as lard and suet can increase the cholesterol level in some individuals and so increase the risk of heart disease. Adults and children over 5 years of age are advised to avoid taking in more than one-third of their total energy or calorie requirement in the form of fat. When people put on weight, they do so gradually and usually do not notice it happening. The strain of carrying that extra weight around affects your heart, muscles and back.

Unhealthy diets (those which tend to include too much salt, sugar and fatty foods) are linked to heart disease, stroke and tooth decay. About a third of all cancers are caused by a poor diet.

Poor-quality diet

Suppose you have less than £50 a week to feed five of you. Your main purpose in buying food would be to stop people from feeling hungry rather than meeting all their nutritional needs (see Figure 8.11). The easiest, fastest way to stop hunger is to eat high-fat carbohydrate foods, such as chips and tinned spaghetti on toast. Advice from the experts about eating five helpings of fruit and vegetables a day is less easy to follow when you are living on a limited income. Poverty can spiral people into ill-health (see Figure 8.12)

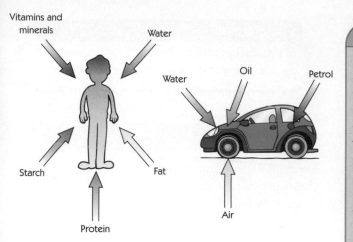

Figure 8.11 Just as a car needs petrol, we all need the correct food to keep our bodies in working order

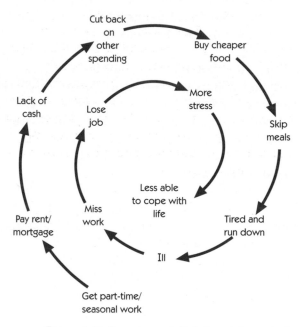

Figure 8.12 Poverty and diet: the vicious circle

Short-term effects	Long-term effects
Feeling cold	Sleeplessness
Being less sensitive to pain	High blood pressure
	Irritability
Being more sensitive to touch	Loss of appetite
	Heart disease
Tense muscles	Indigestion
Faster breathing	Ulcers
Dry mouth	Poor circulation
Flared nostrils	Nerves
Wide eyes	Aching muscles
Pale face	Body tension
Hair on end	Headaches and migraines
Faster heart beat	Short temperedness
Butterflies	Poor sex life
Urge to pass water	Unhappiness
Sweaty hands	Anxiety
Diarrhoea	Eczema
	Asthma
	Angina – heart muscle pain
	Accidents
	Breakdown of relationships
	Mental illness
	Violent or suicidal tendencies
	Become withdrawn

Figure 8.13 The short and long-term effects of stress

Stress

Stress occurs when a person has to respond to demands made upon him or her, be they physical or mental. Most people suffer from stress at some time in their lives, and a small amount of stress can be good for us, making our bodies respond more vigorously to meet the challenges of life. It is the grind of continual stress that is so harmful to us (see Figure 8.13). Stress causes the body to secrete the hormone adrenaline (see Figure 8.14).

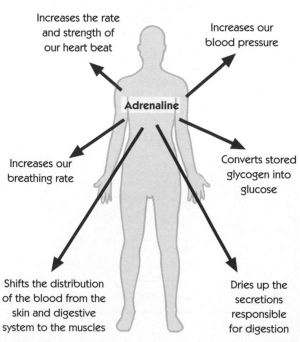

Figure 8.14 The effects of adrenaline

Causes of stress

Stress is a very individual matter but it is generally acknowledged that major life changes are stressful. These include the death of someone close, divorce, illness, loss of a job and many more.

Lack of personal hygiene

Poor personal hygiene isn't just unpleasant, it can affect our health in a negative way. Human beings are an ideal medium for bacteria to grow in. We are the right sort of temperature, we produce moisture in the form of sweat and we produce food for bacteria in the form of dead skin cells, and in the chemicals in our sweat. Bacteria can be passed from one person to another (see Figure 8.15) and also in food, so it's important to try to reduce the number of bacteria that are using us as host (see Figure 8.16).

Health and social care workers have to have excellent hygiene routines as they have to

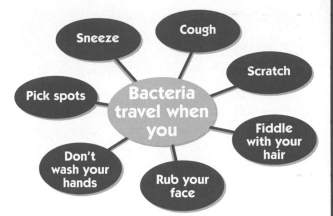

Figure 8.15 How we pass on bacteria

work closely with other people, often in a confined space. Young babies or older people are less resistant to diseases and can suffer more damage from bacteria passed on by unwashed hands preparing their milk or food. Besides maintaining their own personal hygiene, workers have to help clients with their personal hygiene routines. For example, older people with mobility problems need to be kept clean and well groomed for their own self-esteem, so personal hygiene is important for a client's well-being.

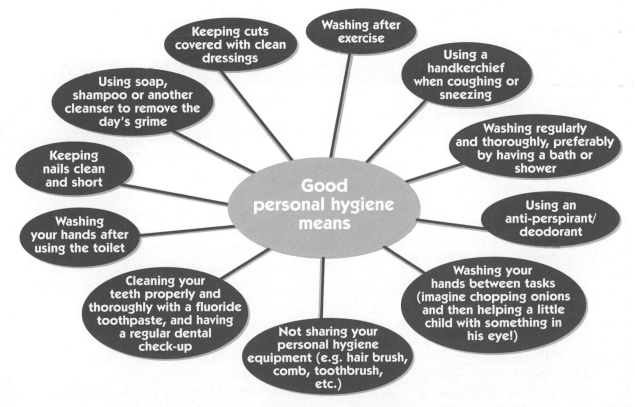

Figure 8.16 Good personal hygiene is essential

Lack of regular physical exercise

A lack of physical exercise has many effects on our bodies (see Figure 8.17) Our lungs are never fully inflated and deposits collect at their bases. The bowel is sluggish and this leads to constipation. Our weight is not under control and, frequently, as middle age sets in, our body weight increases steadily. If, as a care worker, you are encouraging people to exercise, you need to think about the sort of physical activities they are able to do, taking into account their health, age and their ability to exercise.

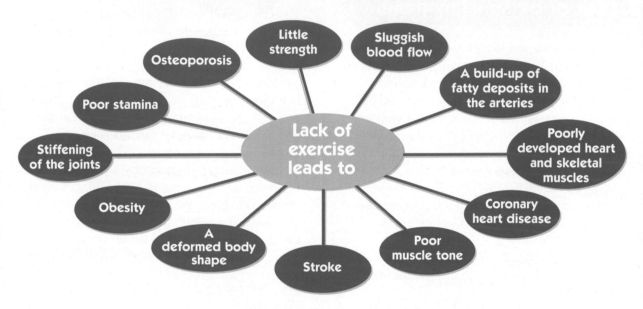

Figure 8.17 Some of the effects of a lack of physical exercise

Case study

Adam

Adam is 5 years old and lives on a nice estate tucked away on the edge of the open countryside. Occasionally, the odd driver comes round the bend in the road too quickly but it is usually pretty quiet and safe. Adam loves to play football outside the house with his other little friend. Sadly he was knocked over in the road outside his house three months ago by a youth who had just started driving. Both his legs were broken and he has been in a wheelchair since he came out of hospital. He is now learning to walk again.

1 What will have happened to Adam's muscles while he has had both his legs in plaster?

2 What do you think will have happened to the rest of his body?

3 What activities do you think his care workers might suggest to help him develop the strength to walk again? List at least five.

1 What problems do you think Adam's parents will face with him during the time he is learning to walk again?

2 His parents are likely to say he cannot play in front of the house again but he will be upset because his friends still do so. Suggest some practical ideas for:
- his parents
- his friends
- the other residents on the estate to stop this situation arising again. You must say how you would persuade each group to act on your suggestions.

Unprotected sex

Sex is a natural part of human life – the continuation of the human race depends upon males and females having sex. Because people are actively engaging in sex at a younger age, they are often not aware of the consequences of unwanted pregnancies and of the possibilities of contracting diseases that are transmitted through the act of sexual intercourse. Sex can occur between males and females or between two people of the same gender. The latter cannot result in pregnancy but still carries a serious risk of disease. The greater the number of sexual partners a person has, the greater the risk of being infected with disease, and the greater the risk of passing it on.

Most hospitals have special clinics, called genito-urinary medicine (GUM) clinics, dealing with sexual diseases (see Figure 8.18). They give advice and treatment. Doctors and nurses will not pass on details of results or treatments to a client's own doctor.

HIV (human immuno-deficiency virus) and AIDS (acquired immune deficiency syndrome)

AIDS is caused by HIV and, although only first reported as recently as 1981, AIDS is now a major worldwide epidemic. AIDS is the term used to describe the condition people who have advanced HIV infection suffer from. The virus, a simple living organism, gets into the bloodstream and attacks and destroys the body's natural defence mechanisms so that the person's body is unable to fight off certain infections and cancers (see Figure 8.19).

Sexual condition	Signs	Symptoms
Gonorrhoea	Discharge from the penis or vagina	Burning feeling when passing water
Syphillis	A small hard 'sore' called a chancre. This disappears after a few weeks. Rash and swollen glands	Years later heart, brain and nervous system become infected leading to death
HIV/AIDS	No signs	No symptoms until years later when death is the result
Non-specific urethritis	Discharge from the urethra (the tube through which urine passes)	Burning feeling when passing water
Genital herpes	Blisters around the genital area	Pain and fever. There is no cure for this. The blisters and pain go away with treatment but can return at any time
Lice	Crab lice living in the genital area of the body. They can spread to other parts of the body as well	Severe itching and skin irratation
Chlamydia	There may be none or women might have vaginal bleeding	Women may have abdominal pain or pain during sex. Men might have stinging sensation when passing water

Figure 8.18 Signs and symptoms of some sexually transmitted diseases

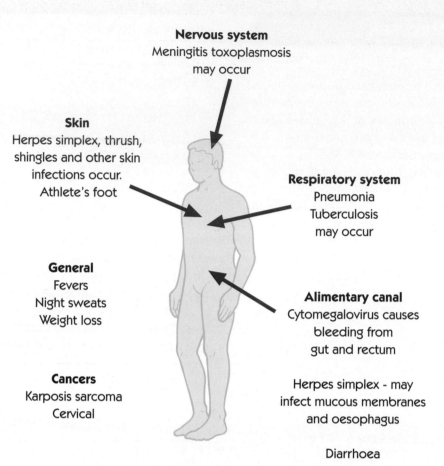

Nervous system
Meningitis toxoplasmosis
may occur

Skin
Herpes simplex, thrush,
shingles and other skin
infections occur.
Athlete's foot

Respiratory system
Pneumonia
Tuberculosis
may occur

General
Fevers
Night sweats
Weight loss

Alimentary canal
Cytomegalovirus causes
bleeding from
gut and rectum

Cancers
Karposis sarcoma
Cervical

Herpes simplex - may
infect mucous membranes
and oesophagus

Diarrhoea

Figure 8.19 AIDS-related illnesses

Generally the AIDS patient is prone to **opportunistic infections** and cancers that do not usually cause illnesses in healthy people. There is still no cure for AIDS, although several therapies are now known to prolong the life expectancy of AIDS sufferers. Therefore the only way to avoid HIV infection is to avoid behaviours that put a person at risk, such as having unprotected sex or drug users not sharing needles.

Checkpoint

An **opportunist infection** is one that takes advantage of a weakness in the immune system. Examples are thrush (a fungal infection of the mouth, throat or vagina) and viruses that cause cold sores and genital herpes.

Transmission of HIV

The main ways in which the virus is passed on to others are as follows:

- Unprotected sexual contact with an infected partner.
- The sharing of blood-contaminated needles or syringes between drug-injecting users when one user is infected.
- An infected mother to her baby during pregnancy or at birth.
- Contact with infected blood (rare because blood donations are now screened).
- Accidental jabs or cuts with needles, etc., when passed between an infected client and care worker (also rare).

Scientists have found no evidence of transmission through saliva, tears, urine, faeces, towels, bedding, toilet seats, swimming pools, telephones, food utensils or biting insects.

Activity

- Examine Figure 8.20, which shows AIDS cases by country and by year of report of diagnosis. Draw a bar chart showing how the total number of cases of AIDS in the UK has changed each year. Try to explain the pattern you see.

- Calculate the percentage increase or decrease in cases of AIDS in each country in the UK between the years 1986 and 1987 and again between 1999 and 2000.

Example of a calculation

The increase in cases of AIDS between 1989 and 1990 is 1145 − 979 = 166 for England. This is a percentage increase of:

$$\frac{166 \times 100}{979} = 17\%$$

- Comment on each country's apparent success in the promotion of health in relation to AIDS as suggested by these figures. Write a short report that identifies the main trends of AIDS infection. Include graphs or pie charts to illustrate the data.

| Year of diagnosis | Country | | | | |
	England	Wales	N.Ireland	Scotland	Total
1985 or earlier	389	7	2	10	408
1986	452	9	1	12	474
1987	641	6	1	32	680
1988	844	22	7	32	905
1989	979	16	8	78	1081
1990	1145	18	6	75	1244
1991	1267	16	6	98	1387
1992	1475	15	8	80	1578
1993	1625	28	9	122	1784
1994	1698	30	12	111	1851
1995	1596	30	13	125	1764
1996	1320	20	1	83	1424
1997	981	11	2	70	1064
1998	716	13	2	36	767
1999	645	13	7	50	715
2000	667	6	5	40	718
2001*	134	2	1	5	142
Total	**16574**	**262**	**91**	**1059**	**17986**

* Reported in the first two quarters of year

Figure 8.20 AIDS cases by country and by year of report of diagnosis

Protection from HIV infection in the workplace

Figure 8.21 shows measures that can be taken to reduce the risk of contracting HIV in the health and social care workplace.

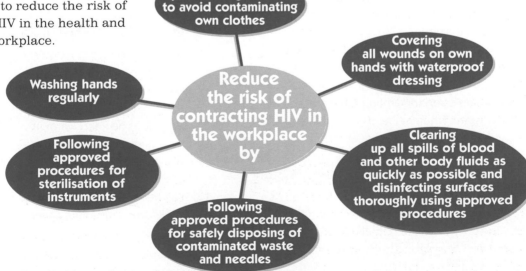

Figure 8.21 How to reduce the risk of contracting HIV in the workplace

Social isolation

So far we have looked at health risks to people who mainly have their health under their own control, who make their own choices as to whether to smoke, diet, exercise, drink alcohol, etc. However, some people have little choice about what they eat or what care they take of themselves and this includes the homeless.

Homeless people do not have regular access to resources that meet their basic needs. Many people in the UK today live on the streets. Most of these people have no choice about the situation, having little money. Their main concerns are for basic food and shelter, and the inadequacies in these mean they have an increased risk of illness. They are also at risk from diseases caused by a shortage of particular nutrients in their diet.

Case study

Michael

Michael lives in Manchester. He does not have a home and spends most of his time on the streets trying to keep warm and dry. When he wakes in the morning he is so stiff from being cold all night that it takes him ages before he can walk without pain in his joints. It is not often he has enough money to buy food as well as coffee to get warm. There are not many cafès open at six o'clock in the morning but he knows where the nearest one is.

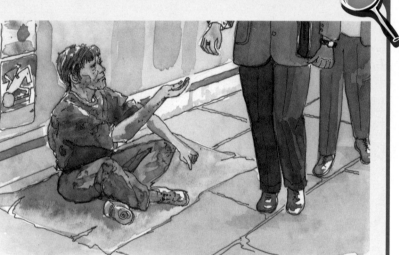

Having a wash and shower is usually out of the question unless he is staying at one of the hostels for the homeless. He enjoys staying in the hostel because he always gets warm food and a comfortable bed for the night. However, he is only allowed to stay there for a maximum of three nights in one month. He would love to have a house of his own but while he has no address he cannot claim benefits or even register with a doctor. He usually calls upon the emergency service at the local hospital when he needs medical help.

What Michael hates most about being homeless is the names people call him. When he is begging for money, he already feels very guilty but he feels there is nothing else he can do to survive. The last thing he needs is people telling him to get a job and get off the streets.

As a class, discuss the following questions about Michael:

1 Where does he get his food from?
2 What sort of food might he get?
3 How does he know whether the food is safe to eat?
4 What would he do if he got a stomach bug?
5 How does he wash himself?
6 How does he exercise?
7 Where does he get water to drink?
8 Where does he sleep?
9 How does he keep warm in winter?
10 How does he get any privacy?
11 Will he be treated with respect by members of society?
12 Will he know how to get information about health and community services?
13 What other needs does he have?

Think about PIES to make sure you have covered all aspects of his health needs.

Other people who are socially isolated include some elderly people who are physically or mentally unable to look after themselves and who do not get the round-the-clock care they need. Also, many elderly people live alone or with their partner and many never see any relatives or friends for long periods of a time. They might lack company and become depressed. Lack of conversation can lead to mental deterioration and loneliness. Loss of status and role in life, loss of company, loss of income, loss of bodily functions and health are all examples of how the health and well-being of elderly people can be affected.

For most people contact with others is important to promote social and emotional development during all the different life stages. People can become socially isolated by illness, social exclusion, language or cultural difficulties. They can also become isolated because of having to live in high-rise tower blocks or bedsits. Their isolation reduces opportunities to develop supportive relationships and so reduces their self-esteem and well-being.

Poverty

Another area over which many people have no choice is their level of income. Some people live in *absolute poverty*. This means that despite welfare benefits being available, they do not receive sufficient money to be able to afford enough food, clothing or housing. Other people live in *relative poverty*. This means that, although they have enough money for the essentials to live, they have less than other people and so are unable to afford to take part fully in the community in which they live. People who live in poverty are more likely to suffer ill-health and have their opportunities for personal development restricted. We have already seen how poverty affects diet earlier in this chapter.

About one fifth of the people of the UK live below the official poverty line, which is defined by the amount of money paid to people receiving income support. The key groups of people who mostly live below the poverty line include:

- elderly people;
- unskilled couples with only one person working;
- people who are unemployed; and
- people who sick or disabled.

The number of people who live in poverty continues to increase.

People who are poor may have enough money for food, for some clothes and for heating, but poverty means there is little money for purchases that make for exciting lifestyles, giving limited life choices. Even jogging for exercise isn't possible if you feel your neighbourhood isn't safe to go out in. Children living in poverty may have limited life chances to develop their full social, emotional and intellectual potential.

Inadequate housing

Our income affects where we are able to live and how we can afford to live there. Our housing is where we spend much of our time. If a home is overcrowded, damp and cold it is likely to be the cause of ill-health.

Cold and damp housing can aggravate conditions such as:

- rheumatism
- arthritis
- asthma
- bronchitis
- tuberculosis.

Overcrowding can:

- encourage the spread of infections and diseases;
- lead to accidents;
- cause sleeplessness; and
- cause stress.

People living in high-rise apartments can suffer from social isolation and so depression. Children have nowhere safe to play. The government is now phasing out such buildings and not building new housing blocks that extend beyond four floors.

Unemployment

To have no job at all is extremely stressful. Unemployment means very little money coming in and a restricted lifestyle. In some areas of the UK, unemployment figures are so high it is very difficult for people to get jobs. Unemployment has a profound effect on self-esteem and motivation. Gaining qualifications may seem pointless if there are no jobs to apply for.

Unemployment affects the way we treat other people. We may think we cannot, or have no right to, approach others for help. It also affects the treatment we receive from others, the services we are entitled to and our attitudes to life. People who are unemployed are often sick and very depressed.

Case study

Alan

Alan lost his job three years ago and has been unable to get another one. His house has been repossessed by the building society and he now lives in council accommodation with his wife and three young children. His wife cannot work because they cannot afford to pay anyone to look after the children and they have no family nearby. He works off and on as a casual labourer and in between jobs he sometimes begs on a bridge going over a road into a busy shopping centre, unless he is moved on by the police. He hates having to do this but is too proud to claim benefits, as he feels he should be earning money to support his family.

▶ 1 How do you think Alan will feel about himself?
2 How do you think his wife will feel about him?
3 How will the way his wife feels about him affect him?
4 How do you think he will feel when people throw him money without even saying anything?

▶ 1 How do you think Alan will behave at home, given his money problems?
2 Why do you think it is important to Alan to support his own family?
3 What will be the effect on the children of the situation Alan and his wife find themselves in?

Environmental pollution

The environment in which we live has a major impact on our health and well-being. We all need clean air and water, and proper waste disposal facilities. However, we cannot, in many cases, do anything as individuals to clean up the air we breathe, although such changes can sometimes be brought about by groups of committed individuals. A healthy environment and clean surroundings can enhance your outlook on life and the way you feel about yourself.

Certain illnesses can affect groups of people who live in the same area. For example, the increased amount of ozone in the air in a city during the summer can increase respiratory conditions such as asthma. Those who live in the city will also be affected by motor vehicle fumes, emissions from factories, and noise and light pollution.

Types of pollution

The environment we live in contains many different organisms which depend on each other and on their environment to stay alive. Human activities can disturb the environment in many different ways causing damage to living organisms, including humans. This damage is called pollution.

Carbon monoxide poisoning is the most common cause of poison-related deaths in the USA. It is a tasteless, colourless, odourless gas produced by the incomplete burning of fuel containing carbon. Car exhaust, coal gas and furnace gas are all sources of carbon monoxide. When carbon monoxide and soot particles from exhaust gases mix with the air, sunlight sets off reactions that make ozone. The result is a lethal concoction of gases that makes asthma worse and even kills people with severe breathing problems.

Dust from quarries, mines and factories can cause lung disease, while lead poisoning affects the nervous system, the blood and the digestive system. This can come about by contamination from lead paints, dust, contaminated soil and car exhaust gases, although the latter is being tackled by the use of more and more lead-free petrol.

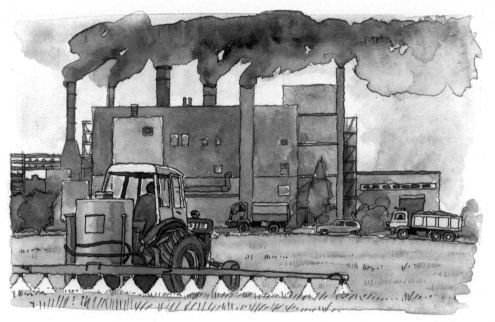

Our environment has become damaged by pollution

Mercury and cadmium are poisonous pollutants and are produced by industrial sources. They can get in your lungs and gradually build up until they reach poisonous levels.

Other sources of environmental pollution are pesticides and herbicides, often taken into the body through their accidental contact with food. Toxic substances around the home, such as detergents, bleaches and rat poison, can also poison children who accidentally swallow them.

If an accident happens, radioactive waste from a nuclear power station can contaminate the air, sea and soil.

Noisy aircraft, drills, etc., can damage hearing.

Sulphur dioxide is another poisonous gas formed by factories.

Activity

Look at the two graphs in Figure 8.22.

1   Can you see any connection between the deaths from bronchitis and the distance from a city centre?

2   What is unusual about the number of bronchitis deaths 8 miles from the centre of the city? Can you suggest a reason for this? (Remember – what goes up, must come down!)

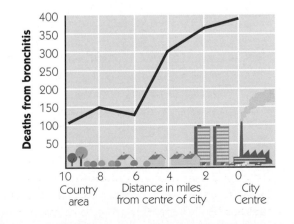

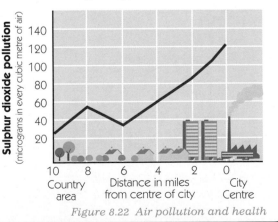

Figure 8.22 Air pollution and health

1. What word is used to describe the condition caused by too little food over a long period of time?
2. Why is overeating bad for your health?
3. Name three types of food an unhealthy diet might contain.
4. How does poverty affect health?
5. What is adrenaline?
6. Name three effects of adrenaline.
7. Name three effects of stress you have experienced in, for example, a race at sports day or in an exam.
8. Give three reasons why good personal hygiene is essential.
9. Name three effects of a lack of exercise.
10. What are two of the main risks from having unprotected sex?
11. What is meant by the term 'social isolation'?
12. Name three groups of people who are at risk of social isolation.
13. What is the difference between absolute and relative poverty?
14. Name three effects of having inadequate housing.
15. How can a healthy environment and clean surroundings affect your health and well-being?

Case study

Nigel

Nigel is 27 years old and has no family. He suffers from a mental illness that is kept under control by drugs, which he is meant to take regularly but he occasionally forgets. When he doesn't take his pills he gets stressed very easily by little things and can become aggressive. He doesn't have many friends and has a poorly paid, boring job. His diet consists of meals such as egg and chips and he drinks beer regularly, sometimes to excess. He also smokes because he doesn't get much exercise and he finds that smoking keeps his weight down. One of the reasons he doesn't have many friends is because he is rather lazy about personal hygiene so has body odour.

Nigel lives in a rather cold flat on the third floor of a building in a run-down area of a big town. The woman from the flat below sometimes keeps him company because she also has no family and very few friends. They sometimes have unprotected sex, usually when they have had too much to drink.

1. Write a list of all the factors that are likely to affect Nigel's health and well-being.
2. Write down how each of these factors put Nigel's health at risk.
3. Suggest ways in which Nigel could reduce the risks to his health and well-being and live a more healthy lifestyle.

Chapter 9 — Indicators of physical health

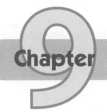

Key issue

How can an individual's physical health be measured?

In this chapter you will learn that some indicators of physical health can be measured. You need to know how the measures listed below can be taken and how they are used to assess the state of an individual's physical health:

- blood pressure;
- peak flow;
- body mass index; and
- resting pulse and recovery after exercise.

You will find out that a person's age, sex and lifestyle have to be taken into account when interpreting the measurement that is recorded.

Indicators of good physical health

In the previous two chapters we have looked at factors that promote good health and at risks to health but we have not said how good health can actually be measured. When you are trying to improve your health and well-being, you need some kind of measure on which to set some targets for yourself and to monitor your progress against.

The kind of health targets people set for themselves, or have set for them by a health professional, could include any of those shown in Figure 9.1. Using measures of progress can strongly motivate people, particularly if they show how well a person is doing. The hardest part of making any change in our lifestyles is sticking to it!

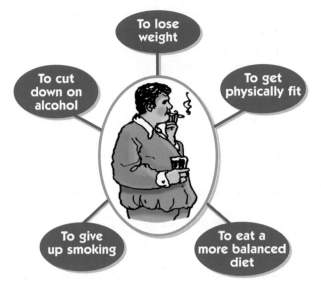

Figure 9.1 Examples of health targets

Activity

Can you think of any other targets people might set for themselves? You can include things that will improve other aspects of their health, such as visiting relatives more.

There are, in fact, many different ways of measuring health and the one we are probably most familiar with is height and weight charts.

Height and weight charts

As soon as babies are born they are weighed and measured, and centile charts are used regularly to assess the growth rates of babies and young children. Babies are weighed and measured regularly because weight gain shows they are being fed properly. They are usually weighed every week for the first two months of their lives, then once a month for the next ten months and, every six months after the age of 1 year old.

On average a healthy baby triples its birth weight by the age of 1 year, whilst increasing its height by about 50%. If a baby does not grow either as quickly or slowly as predicted by standard charts (described in more detail in Chapter 11), health care workers will keep an even closer eye on the baby to make sure there is not anything wrong with the way in which it is developing. It might be a child is too fat because it is overeating and not getting enough exercise – a simple change in diet and trips out can put the problem right. It is important to bear in mind, however, that these charts are only a guide. Those charts used in the UK are based on the white British population and do not include babies of other ethnic minorities. African and Caribbean babies and children tend to be taller and heavier than white British babies and children, while Asian babies and children are usually smaller and lighter.

As children reach a certain height they are then measured on the height and weight charts for adults, which you have probably come across in magazines. These show ideal height and weight ratios – that is, they show whether a person is the correct weight for his or her height. They are found in three main forms, the first being in the form of a graph. An example is shown in Figure 9.2. It is important to be realistic about these charts. They are only a guide. Someone who is small but does a lot of

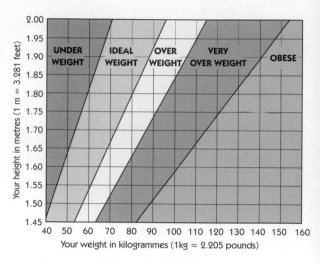

Figure 9.2 An example of a height/weight graph

exercise might be heavier than someone who is fat, because muscle weighs more than fat.

The other two forms of these charts are tables, as in Figures 9.3 and 9.4. These tables take into account the person's frame size and gender. Frame size is a person's bone size and build. Most people know whether standard clothing and shoe sizes fit them.

If someone falls into the severely overweight range, he or she is at risk of cardiovascular diseases, high blood pressure, diabetes, arthritis and other conditions. They people should be advised to seek help from their family doctor, as should anyone who is

Height (in shoes)		Small frame				Medium frame				Large frame			
m	ft in	kg kg	st lb	st lb		kg kg	st lb	st lb		kg kg	st lb	st lb	
1.575	5 2	50.8 – 54.4	8 0 –	8 8		53.5 – 58.5	8 6 –	9 3		57.2 – 64.0	9 0 –	10 1	
1.6	5 3	52.8 – 55.8	8 3 –	8 11		54.9 – 60.3	8 9 –	9 7		58.5 – 65.3	9 3 –	10 4	
1.626	5 4	53.5 – 57.2	8 6 –	9 0		56.2 – 64.7	8 12 –	9 10		59.9 – 67.1	9 6 –	10 8	
1.651	5 5	54.9 – 58.5	8 9 –	9 3		57.6 – 63.0	9 1 –	9 13		61.2 – 68.9	9 9 –	1012	
1.676	5 6	56.2 – 60.3	9 12 –	9 7		59.0 – 64.9	9 4 –	10 3		62.6 – 70.8	1012 –	11 2	
1.702	5 7	58.1 – 62.1	9 2 –	9 11		60.8 – 66.7	9 8 –	10 7		64.4 – 73.0	10 2 –	11 7	
1.727	5 8	59.9 – 64.0	9 6 –	10 1		62.6 – 68.9	9 12 –	1012		66.7 – 75.3	10 7 –	1112	
1.753	5 9	61.7 – 65.8	9 10 –	10 5		64.4 – 70.8	10 2 –	11 2		68.5 – 77.1	1011 –	12 2	
1.778	5 10	63.5 – 68.0	10 0 –	1010		66.2 – 72.6	10 6 –	11 6		70.3 – 78.9	11 1 –	12 6	
1.803	5 11	65.2 – 69.9	10 4 –	11 0		68.0 – 74.8	1010 –	1111		72.1 – 81.2	11 5 –	1211	
1.829	6 0	67.1 – 71.7	10 8 –	11 4		69.9 – 77.1	11 0 –	12 2		74.4 – 83.5	1110 –	13 2	
1.854	6 1	68.9 – 73.5	1012 –	11 8		71.7 – 79.4	11 4 –	12 7		76.2 – 85.7	12 0 –	13 7	
1.88	6 2	70.8 – 75.7	11 0 –	1113		73.5 – 81.6	11 8 –	1212		78.5 – 88.0	12 5 –	1312	
1.905	6 3	72.6 – 77.6	11 4 –	12 3		75.7 – 83.5	1113 –	13 3		80.7 – 90.3	1210 –	14 3	
1.93	6 4	74.4 – 79.4	11 8 –	12 7		78.1 – 86.2	12 4 –	13 8		82.7 – 92.5	13 0 –	14 8	

Figure 9.3 A weight/height chart for men

Height (in shoes)		Small frame			Medium frame			Large frame		
m	ft in	kg kg	st lb	st lb	kg kg	st lb	st lb	kg kg	st lb	st lb
1.473	4 10	41.7 – 44.5	6 8 –	7 0	43.5 – 48.5	6 12 –	7 9	47.2 – 54.0	7 6 –	8 7
1.499	4 11	42.6 – 45.8	6 10 –	7 3	44.5 – 49.9	7 0 –	7 12	48.1 – 55.3	7 8 –	8 10
1.524	5 0	43.5 – 47.2	6 12 –	7 6	45.8 – 51.3	7 3 –	8 1	49.4 – 56.7	7 11 –	8 13
1.549	5 1	44.9 – 48.5	7 1 –	7 9	47.2 – 52.5	7 6 –	8 4	50.8 – 58.1	8 0 –	9 2
1.575	5 2	46.3 – 49.9	7 4 –	7 12	48.5 – 54.0	7 9 –	8 7	52.2 – 59.4	8 3 –	9 5
1.6	5 3	47.6 – 61.5	7 7 –	8 1	49.9 – 55.3	7 12 –	8 10	53.5 – 60.8	8 6 –	9 8
1.626	5 4	49.0 – 52.5	7 10 –	8 4	51.3 – 57.2	8 1 –	9 0	54.9 – 62.6	8 10 –	9 12
1.651	5 5	50.3 – 54.0	7 13 –	8 7	52.7 – 59.0	8 4 –	9 4	56.8 – 64.4	8 13 –	10 2
1.676	5 6	51.7 – 55.8	8 2 –	8 11	54.4 – 61.2	8 8 –	9 9	58.5 – 66.2	9 3 –	10 6
1.702	5 7	53.5 – 57.6	8 6 –	9 1	56.2 – 63.0	8 12 –	9 13	60.3 – 68.0	9 7 –	10 10
1.727	5 8	55.3 – 59.4	8 10 –	9 5	58.1 – 64.9	9 2 –	10 3	62.1 – 69.9	9 11 –	11 0
1.753	5 9	57.2 – 61.2	9 0 –	9 9	59.9 – 66.7	9 6 –	10 7	64.0 – 71.7	10 1 –	11 4
1.778	5 10	59.0 – 63.5	9 4 –	10 0	61.7 – 68.5	9 10 –	10 11	65.8 – 73.9	10 5 –	11 9
1.803	5 11	60.8 – 65.3	9 8 –	10 4	63.5 – 70.3	10 0 –	11 1	67.6 – 76.2	10 9 –	12 0
1.829	6 0	62.6 – 67.1	9 12 –	10 8	65.3 – 72.1	10 4 –	11 5	69.4 – 78.5	10 13 –	12 5

Figure 9.4 A weight/height chart for women

moderately overweight. However, it is important that people do not become so obsessed with their weight that they develop serious eating disorders such as anorexia nervosa or bulimia nervosa.

Being slightly overweight is not a problem but being very underweight *is* a problem. If someone has recently started to lose weight for no reason, he or she may have an undiagnosed illness. Such people should be advised to consult a medical practitioner. Some people are very sensitive about others knowing their weight. When working with people, you will need to anticipate such sensitivity. Do not tell other people about someone's weight without first asking for his or her permission.

Activity

▶ Look at Figure 9.2 showing heights and weights of adults.
Put a ruler against your weight and another across from your height. Look at the point where the two rulers meet. Make a note of which section of the chart you fall into. You will need this information for the 'Me Now' activity at the end of this chapter.
Do you need to do anything about your weight?

▶ Look at either Figure 9.3 or 9.4, depending on whether you are male or female. Decide what kind of frame you have and work out your ideal weight.

Blood pressure

Your blood provides all the organs of your body with the materials to stay alive and healthy. The circulatory system is a network of blood vessels through which the blood flows and is pumped round this system continuously by your heart. Blood pressure is the pressure blood exerts against the walls of the arteries in which it is contained. The arteries are flexible, thick-walled vessels that carry blood away from your heart to the rest of your body. The amount of blood depends upon the strength and rate of the heart's contraction, the volume of blood in the circulatory system and the elasticity of the arteries.

Normal blood pressure varies from person to person, but usually normal blood pressure at rest is anything up to 140/90. It is lower in children. *Systolic pressure*, the top number, represents the maximum pressure in the arteries as the heart contracts and ejects blood into the circulation. *Diastolic pressure*, the bottom number, represents the minimum blood pressure as the heart relaxes following a contraction. Together, the diastolic and systolic pressure give the measure known as blood pressure.

Blood pressure is measured using an instrument called a *sphygmomanometer*. It is made up of a rubber bag that is placed around the arm and inflated by means of a rubber tube from the inside of the rubber bag to a mercury pressure gauge or, increasingly more usual, a digital pressure gauge.

When the pressure in the bag is the same as the pressure in the artery, the artery is gently compressed and the blood flowing through it is temporarily stopped, causing the person's pulse to disappear. A stethoscope attached to the ear of the person taking the blood pressure is placed over the brachial artery in the bend of the elbow. Each beat of the heart increases the pressure and the height to which the mercury in the pressure gauge is forced is the systolic pressure. The rubber tube is then gently deflated and the heart beat gradually disappears. The last beat is the diastolic pressure.

A single blood pressure reading, unless it is very high or very low, should not be considered abnormal. Usually, several readings are taken on different days and the results are then compared. It is important to remember that blood pressure varies with age.

High blood pressure is called *hypertension* and is a major problem that needs treatment as soon as possible. The heart pumps blood too forcefully around the body. It can damage the wall of the body's arteries. In the early stages the artery wall becomes thickened. Later, fatty patches form in the wall and further reduce the flow of blood through the artery. If left untreated it can damage the heart, blood vessels and kidneys and lead to conditions such as strokes and heart disease. It can also cause an artery to rupture and bleed. If this happens in the brain it may cause a haemorrhage.

Checkpoint

Haemorrhage is the technical name for bleeding.

Hypertension can also cause eye damage and even blindness. The arteries of the retina may narrow (see Figure 9.5), small haemorrhages can occur and areas of damaged retina appear.

Low blood pressure is called *hypotension* and is often just normal for a particular person.

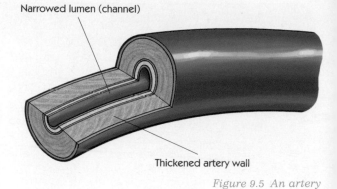

Narrowed lumen (channel)

Thickened artery wall

Figure 9.5 An artery

It may even indicate a prolonged life expectancy. It often has no symptoms and is diagnosed during a routine visit to the doctor for some other reason. Sometimes, though, the sufferer might go to the doctor complaining of feeling dizzy, especially when standing up quickly (called postural hypotension). Most cases get better without treatment. However, it can also be the result of some underlying problem, such as Parkinson's disease.

Peak flow

Another way of checking on your health is by using a peak flow meter. A peak flow meter is the name of a special kind of *spirometer*, an instrument that measures the breathing rate and the volume of air taken in by a person during each breath. These have many different uses but basically they are used to see how effective a person's lungs are. A peak flow meter usually measures the maximum rate at which air is expelled from the lungs when a person breathes out as hard as he or she can. This is called *forced vital capacity*. This is an example of a *pulmonary function test*, because it monitors an aspect of respiratory function.

This measurement is used to assess the width of the air passages (bronchi). The most common use of peak flow measurements is to monitor the degree of bronchospasm (narrowing of the air passages) in people who suffer from asthma, and their response to the drugs they take for the condition. It is also a useful measurement in people who have respiratory problems, such as intermittent

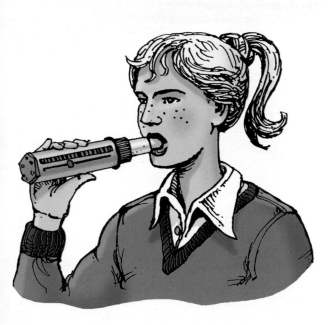

Figure 9.6 A peak flow meter

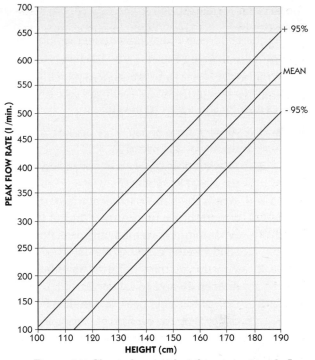

Figure 9.7 Chart showing height against peak flow
reading for children aged 5–18 years

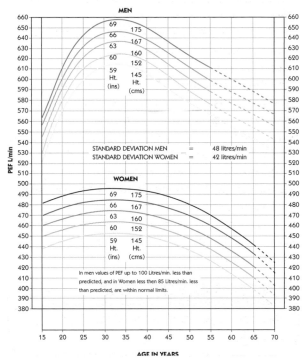

Figure 9.8 Chart showing age against peak flow
reading for adults aged 15–70 years of age

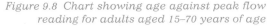

coughing or difficulty with breathing. It can help to assess whether they have developed asthma (see Figure 9.6).

To use a peak flow meter the person has to blow as hard as he or she can into a tube. This than moves a pointer to a certain point, at which you can read off the number it has reached. The best score out of three blows is usually used. Regular physical exercise can make a difference to the score you reach on a peak flow meter. Exercise makes the lungs more powerful and improves their ability to take in oxygen. Fitness suites in gyms and sports centres often employ peak flow measuring equipment (see Figures 9.7 and 9.8).

The peak flow meter can be used to diagnose whether someone has a problem with his or her lungs by comparing his or her score with that on a chart of expected scores. Readings are generally higher in males than in females. Readings are lower in obstructive lung diseases such as bronchitis or asthma. Other conditions that can cause shortness of breath include blood clots in the lungs, lung cancer, heart failure, cystic fibrosis, emphysema and chronic bronchitis.

Monitoring peak flow helps an asthma sufferer monitor changes and adjust the medication dose accordingly. Each person with asthma who uses a peak flow meter has a personal-best peak flow reading and a peak flow reading of less than 80% of that personal best indicates the need for action.

This chart shows the peak flow meter readings for Elizabeth, aged 48 years old, who has had asthma since the age of 16. She is not very good at remembering to use her peak flow meter three times a day and only uses it when she is feeling unwell.

▶ **1** At what time of day is her peak flow reading usually at its lowest?

2 At what time of day is her peak flow reading usually at its highest?

3 Why is the pattern lower at the start of the period shown on the chart than at the end?

▶ **1** What might have made the peak flow reading so low in the evening on 7 January?

2 Why do you think her peak flows fall off a little on 15 and 16 January?

3 Do you think her peak flow reading will go up or down on the evening of 17 January? Why?

4 Why do you think the readings stopped on 16 January?

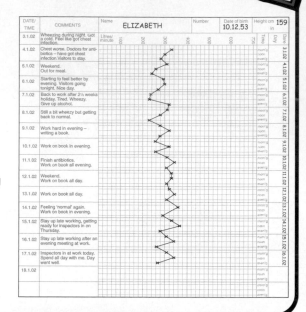

Body mass index

This is an indicator of good health that measures the amount of fat in a person's body in relation to his or her height. It is not the same as a height/weight chart. The body mass index (BMI) uses weight in kilograms and height in metres to assess a person's general state of health. A person's weight should be in proportion to his or her height. A person is considered to be obese when his or her weight is more than 20% above the average weight for people of the same height and similar other characteristics. BMI is worked out using the following calculation:

$$\frac{\text{weight (kg)}}{\text{height (m)}^2} = \text{BMI}$$

For example, if your height is 1.82 m, you will divide your weight by 1.82 × 1.82. If your weight is 70.5 kg then:

$$\frac{70.5}{1.82 \times 1.82} = 21.3$$

People with BMIs between 19 and 22 appear to live the longest; death rates seem to be highest in people with BMIs of 25 and over. BMIs are different for males and females (see Figure 9.9).

Female	Significance	Male	Significance
Less than 18	Underweight	Less than 18	Underweight
18–20	Lean	18–20	Lean
21–22	Average	21–23	Average
23–28	Plump	24–32	Plump
29–36	Moderately obese	32–40	Moderately obese
37+	Severely obese	40+	Severely obese

Figure 9.9 Body mass indexes

▶ Copy out the table shown in Figure 9.10. Calculate the BMI for the people given in the table. Decide what area of the chart they fall into.

Name	Age	Weight in kilograms	Height in metres	Body mass index
Rachel	28	54	1.62	
Mike	28	94	1.85	
Siobhan	15	60	1.60	
Robert	15	80	1.84	
Alana	15	49	1.62	
Ben	15	60	1.68	
Linzi	15	70	1.72	
Sarah	16	52	1.59	

Figure 9.10 Chart for calculating BMI

Resting pulse and recovery after exercise

Each time the heart beats it forces a quantity of blood under pressure into our circulatory system. These beats cause a pulse, or shock wave, that travels along the walls of the arteries. This pulse can be felt in several parts of the body by placing the finger over an artery. Arteries at which the pulse can normally be felt easily are the *carotid arteries* in the neck and the *radial arteries* in the wrist.

The pulse rate is normally measured by feeling the radial pulse, using two fingers (**not** the thumb), found near the thumb side of the front surface of the wrist. The number of pulse beats counted in 10 seconds is multiplied by 6 to work out the rate in beats per minute. The pulse is usually felt for longer to check for an irregular pulse rate and the strength or weakness of the pulse is also usually noted. The pulse rate shows how fast the heart is beating. To take a person's resting pulse, make sure he or she is calm and has been sitting quietly for 5–10 minutes. Take at least three readings and calculate the average pulse rate (add all the readings together and divide by the number of readings you have taken).

Example

Zola had the following counts for her resting pulse rate:

65, 68, 72, 74, 68, 65

$$\text{The average} = \frac{65 + 68 + 72 + 74 + 68 + 65}{6}$$
$$= 69 \text{ beats per minute}$$

The pulse rate in a healthy adult at rest is typically about 60–80 beats per minute. Athletes may have slower heart rates, while babies and children have faster pulse rates. A young baby has a pulse rate of about 140 beats per minute. The pulse rate increases during exercise to increase the output of blood from the heart. The rate is also raised by excitement, emotion, infection, blood or fluid loss, shock or heart and respiratory disease.

Usually, the lower the pulse rate, the fitter a person is. The pulse rate increases during exercise and then it quickly returns to normal. The shorter the recovery time the fitter the person. If you ever watch athletes running on television you will know they are often able to be interviewed almost straight after the race. However, in an unfit person, exercise makes the pulse rate go very high and it returns to normal only slowly. Measuring the pulse rate before and after exercise and seeing how long it takes for the pulse rate to return to normal is therefore another good way of measuring the physical health of a person.

Activity

Measure the resting pulse rate of yourself or your partner. Suggest some form of mild exercise for you or your partner, such as running on the spot for 30 seconds or stepping up and down a step for a short length of time. The exercise should be enough to get you or your partner out of breath but not painfully so. Bear in mind your own, and your partner's, state of fitness! Measure the pulse rate immediately after the exercise and again every minute until the pulse rate returns to the resting rate.

▶ 1   Draw a graph of pulse rate against time to display your findings and mark the time at which the pulse rate returned to the resting rate.

2   Repeat this activity but this time make sure the other one of you does the exercise. Keep the information about yourself. You will need it for the 'Me Now' activity at the end of this chapter.

▶ 1   Look at the table given in Figure 9.11, which shows the effects of regular exercise on the body. Write down the other effects regular exercise has on your body, besides slowing down your pulse rate.

	Before months of regular exercise	After months of regular exercise
Pulse rate (beats per minute)	76	65
Breathing rate (breaths per minute	16	14
Heart volume (cm³)	125	138
Volume of blood pumped out of the heart during each beat (cm³)	60	75

Figure 9.11 The effects of regular exercise on the body

Use of measures of health

It is important to remember that as no two people are exactly alike, the measures of good health we have been looking at are only a general guide. When measuring a person's physical health it is necessary to take into account his or her age, gender, culture and any physical disability. Once such measures have been made, advice can be given and targets set to improve a person's health, if necessary or possible.

Check your knowledge

1 Give three examples of the kind of health targets people might set themselves.
2 What do we mean by 'an indicator of good health'?
3 Name two indicators of good health.
4 What is meant by the term 'blood pressure'?
5 What does the amount of blood pumping round your body depend on?
6 What does the top number of a blood pressure reading represent?
7 What is another name for high blood pressure?
8 Why is high blood pressure a problem?
9 What does a peak flow meter measure?
10 Why is it useful to measure peak flow?
11 Why is your BMI useful to your doctor?
12 Calculate the BMI for the people given in Figure 9.12.
13 What causes a pulse?
14 Do fit people (such as athletes) have a low or a high resting pulse rate?
15 Why is it important to remember that all these measures are only a guide?

Name	Age	Weight in kilograms	Height in metres	Body mass index
Emma	15	60	1.67	
Andrew	16	80	1.78	
Michaela	15	46	1.59	
Robin	15	78	1.76	
Catherine	15	58	1.64	
Chris	15	89	1.80	
Jenna	15	55	1.57	
Joe	12	44	1.56	
Jemma	15	54	1.61	
Christopher	12	37	1.46	
Aimie	15	56	1.69	
Sanjeev	46	71	1.69	
Kirsty	15	52	1.57	
Hannah	15	64	1.61	
Nathan	12	36	1.39	

Figure 9.12 Calculating BMI

Practice activity

Me Now

In this chapter you have already checked your own health by looking at:

- a height and weight chart;
- a body mass index chart;
- your resting pulse rate; and
- your recovery after exercise.

Have you had your blood pressure measured recently? Is there a peak flow meter available in school for you to measure your personal-best peak flow reading?

Draw up a table like the one shown here. Complete the 'Me now' and think carefully about what you would like your 'Me in the future' column to say. You do not have to show this piece of work to anyone else.

1 What do you need to change in your life?
2 What are you willing to change in your life?
3 Is there anything you cannot change in your life? If so, why not?

	Me now	Me in the future
Section of height weight chart (for example, obese, underweight, normal weight)		
Section of body mass index chart		
Resting pulse rate		
Recovery time after exercise		
Blood pressure if known		
Peak flow if known		

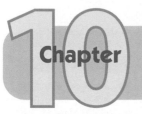

Chapter 10

Health promotion and improvement methods

By the end of this chapter, you will have learnt why physical health assessment and target-setting should happen before a health improvement plan is produced for an individual. You will learn how realistic health improvement targets are established for others. You will find out how different health behaviours can help people achieve their targets.

You will also learn about the different types of health promotion materials that are used to inform, motivate and support people to improve their health and well-being.

Health promotion and the medical profession

The NHS was set up in 1948. Before then, people had to pay for health care. Many poor people, especially women and children, didn't receive the medical treatment they needed. When the NHS was established, it was thought at first that demand for the service would eventually fall, as people got healthier. We now know that the opposite has happened. Demand grows year by year and there is never enough money or staff available to meet the public's needs.

At the same time, it is believed that people have become too dependent on the medical profession. There is a huge demand for medical treatment for relatively minor ailments such as colds, as well as common conditions such as headaches, period pains and the effects of ageing.

This expectation has had the effect of taking responsibility for a person's health away from the individual and passing it on to the medical profession. People expect more from

the health services and some *health professionals* believe people could do more to help themselves.

Health promotion aims to help people take responsibility for their own health. It does this by:

- providing information;
- giving advice; and
- providing support.

Health promotion information is available in many forms. These include leaflets, videos, TV campaigns, posters and slide shows. There are many different types of health promotion materials available to inform and motivate people. Each is suitable for different groups of people and for use in different settings. All materials must be easy to understand, accurate and contain the information the group or

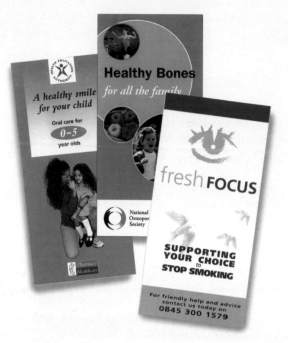

Examples of health promotion leaflets

individual needs to know. It is helpful if the information is presented in an attractive or entertaining way, as this will increase the chance of holding the users' attention. It will make it more likely that the information will be absorbed and remembered.

Health promotion aims to give people the confidence to feel able to look after themselves instead of expecting health professionals to look after them. In the long term, encouraging self-help in people will benefit those individuals more than improving medical treatment. Smoking provides a clear example of this point. More people will improve their own health by giving up smoking than will ever be helped by the medical profession once they have become ill with a smoking-related disorder such as lung cancer, emphysema or pneumonia.

Activity

List all the things you do that are *good* or *bad* for your health. Think about what you eat, whether you smoke or drink alcohol and how much sleep you get. You will have other ideas to include as well. When you have finished, look at your lists. Which is longest? Describe how much you are prepared to do to make the second list shorter.

Physical health assessments and target-setting before devising a health improvement plan

Checkpoint

A **health improvement plan** is developed by a health professional such as a GP or practice nurse. The plan could be for someone to lose weight, stop smoking and eat a more healthy diet, or anything that would improve the client's health in the long term. It should include targets to aim for and a timetable to reach the target. The plan could be devised as a result of a suggestion by the doctor or because the client asked for help from the health professionals.

Before a person can be persuaded to improve his or her own health, he or she has to be *motivated*. This means people want to make the necessary changes and improvements to their lifestyle enough to put up with short-term difficulties. This can be surprisingly hard for people to do. For example, many people want to lose weight and know their health would benefit if they were to do so. However, they still lack the motivation to stick to a diet that would enable them to lose the excess pounds.

Bearing all this in mind, before people are given a health improvement plan they must be:

1 persuaded it will do them good. This is generally not difficult as people usually know they should do some exercise, stop smoking, etc.; and
2 motivated to carry out the plan for long enough to allow the plan to have a positive effect.

Problems usually occur with the second of these. A psychologist called Albert Bandura has done research into motivation and behaviour. He said that behaviour could be predicted and explained by three factors. These factors are as follows:

1 **Incentives:** People may try to lose weight if

they believe it will make them look and feel better.

2 **Outcomes:** A person is more likely to stick to a diet if he or she believes it will work eventually. The plan must not be too difficult to achieve.

3 **Ability:** A person has to believe he or she is capable of making the necessary changes and sticking to them. The plan must be realistic.

It is important that health professionals remember this research when setting targets for an individual.

A physical health assessment is necessary to decide exactly what targets need to be set for an individual. If a woman wants to lose weight then, first of all, she should be weighed and measured to see how much weight she needs to lose. A height/weight chart or a BMI calculation can be used to do this (see Chapter 9). A peak flow or resting pulse and recovery after exercise will give the health professional more information about the effect of excess weight upon the general fitness of the person. It may also provide additional evidence to persuade the client of the need to lose weight.

Activity

▶ Look at the list you wrote earlier of things that are not good for your health. For each item on the list, state what you need to do to change the behaviour. For example, a smoker would need to cut down smoking or stop completely.

▶ Now use Bandura's explanation of motivation to explain why you have not made the necessary changes to improve your health. Explain which of the three factors he identified is preventing you from changing your behaviour.

Check your knowledge

1 When was the NHS first set up?
2 What happened to poor, ill people before the NHS existed?
3 What is the aim of health promotion?
4 Suggest different types of health promotion materials.
5 What is a health professional?
6 What is a health improvement plan?
7 Why can it be difficult for people to improve their own health?
8 How does Bandura's research on human behaviour and motivation help health professionals to set targets for others?
9 Why is a physical health assessment necessary before targets are set?

Case study

Alan

Alan is 18 years old. He has been overweight since he was a small child. His mum is a keen cook and he enjoys eating what she has made. However, he has now decided to try to lose weight. The final straw had come earlier in the spring when he had got stuck in a turnstile as he tried to get into a theme park. He is going to university in the autumn and wants to be thinner when he begins his new life away from home.

His cousin has been going to Weight Watchers for two months and he can see that she looks thinner, although she still has some weight to lose before she reaches her target. He has seen her diet books and thinks they look varied enough to make sticking to a diet a possibility this time. He has decided to go to the next meeting with her and, this time, really to give it a go.

▶ Use Bandura's theory about motivation and behaviour to explain why Alan has a good chance of losing weight this time.

▶ How will his weight loss affect Alan emotionally and socially?

Setting realistic health improvement targets

The role of the health professional

The health professional is needed to give information, help set realistic targets and provide support. Before setting targets and making a plan, the health professional has to be aware that people are not always ready to change their lifestyle enough to make real differences to their health. Certain features about a person's life may mean he or she will not stick to a health improvement plan, even when he or she knows he or she would benefit from it. Such factors could include:

- People don't always believe 'experts'. Different warnings, given by scientists about food scares such as eating eggs and beef, mean people are aware that experts are sometimes wrong.
- People have different values. A doctor knows that smoking is harmful but a teenager who smokes is also concerned about the opinions of her friends. She will probably be more concerned about fitting in with them, if they smoke, than pleasing a doctor.
- Adults do not like being told what to do. That is why targets must be agreed jointly.

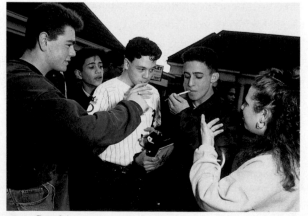

Smoking can earn the approval of the peer group

- Individuals do not have total freedom of choice. Shift work makes regular meal times more difficult. Lack of money means cheap, processed foods are chosen rather than fruit and vegetables. Targets must be realistic and fit in with the client's lifestyle.

Factors affecting the success of the plan

When devising a health plan, it has to be recognised that various factors will affect the person's ability to carry it out. It would be silly to devise an exercise plan and think it could be used for both an overweight teenager and a middle-aged businessman. The two people are very different and so their health improvement plans must differ too. Different factors affect the chances of the plan being a success. These factors often *interrelate* (come together) and should be considered before a plan is drawn up. The following factors need to be considered:

1. **Levels of stress**. Harmful behaviour that reduces stress (e.g. smoking and drinking alcohol) can be difficult to give up unless an alternative activity can be suggested to have the same result.
2. **Occupation**. Some jobs are positively harmful to the worker but people still have to carry on doing them (e.g. people in manual jobs are more likely to be physically injured at work).
3. **Age and gender**. Women tend to be more concerned about their health than men. Older people may see less point in changing their behaviour because 'they have less time left'.
4. **Peer group and social pressure**. This is extremely important especially to young people who seek the approval of the peer group. Social pressure can slowly cause a change in behaviour. This can be seen by the fall in numbers of people who drink and drive.
5. **Social class**. People who belong to higher social classes tend to be more health conscious than people in lower social classes. As a result, they are more likely to change their behaviour.

6   **Self-concept**. This is the person's view of him or herself. A positive self-concept means the person will be more optimistic about his or her ability to change his or her behaviour. (You will learn more about self-concept in Chapter 14.)

Health professionals have to try to consider all these factors when devising a plan for an individual.

Case study

Richard and Debbie

Richard and Debbie are married. Debbie is a social worker. She works with a group of mentally handicapped men, helping them to live in the community. The work is very stressful as some of the patients can be violent and abusive to the staff and each other. She has to work shifts at weekends and bank holidays. Richard is a director of his own company that provides specialised computer systems. The company is successful, but Richard works long hours and travels a lot round the country, meeting new customers. If Debbie is not in, he doesn't bother to cook for himself but, instead, uses the local Indian and Chinese takeaways. When they are both off together, they often go out to eat as a form of relaxation. Both of them smoke, as they often feel stressed. Debbie has been for a check at the Well Woman clinic at her GP's surgery and has been told her blood pressure is too high. She needs to stop smoking and lose some weight. Richard will not go to the Well Man clinic that is held at the same surgery although Debbie suspects he would be told the same thing, if he were to go.

▶ Imagine you were a practice nurse who is trying to advise Debbie on her health problems. Which features of Debbie and Richard's life will make changes for the sake of their health difficult?

▶ Suggest reasons why Debbie is more likely to make changes to improve her health than Richard is.

Involving the individual in devising a health improvement plan

As we have said, health promotion would be easy if people simply did as they were told (i.e. stopped smoking, lost weight, ate a more healthy diet, etc.). However, although people often know what they should do, they very often do the opposite. Health professionals cannot therefore simply tell people to do things. The person has to be involved in the process of developing the targets so that the chances of success are greater. Sometimes this is described as giving the person *ownership* of the targets. This means the person has a feeling of responsibility because he or she has been actively involved in devising the targets with the health professional. Target-setting will require five stages:

1   Identifying the health need (e.g. drinking less, eating a better diet).
2   Discussion of the need. This is necessary to build trust and understanding between the person and the health professional who is working with him or her.
3   Discussion of different options (e.g. whether to join a gym, start swimming or exercise with a friend to become more fit).
4   Decide which of the options that have been discussed to follow.
5   Development of the plan. This will need the knowledge of the health professional, plus his or her understanding of the person involved.

It is vital the health professional and the person decide targets jointly if there is to be any chance of success.

Activity

You are to devise a role play to demonstrate how a health professional should carry out a discussion with a person who needs to be persuaded to drink less. Working in pairs, one person is to play the professional and the other is to play the person who drinks. When devising the role-play, think about the points made above.

Communication between health professional and client

When communicating the plan, the health professional should remember the **KISS** rule. This stands for **K**eep **I**t **S**imple and **S**traightforward. Information should be clear. Medical and technical words that can be confusing should be used as little as possible. Such language is off-putting to the person listening. There are many reasons why communication between the two people is poor:

- The person is not interested in the subject.
- The information is not clear.
- The two people involved don't like each other.
- The person is frightened of what is going to be said so doesn't listen properly.
- The person is bored or confused.
- The health professional doesn't fully understand the subject so questions cannot be answered satisfactorily.
- The health professional tries to 'boss' the person or to impress him or her with his or her greater knowledge.

The meeting should be held in a quiet room, where there are unlikely to be interruptions.

The meeting should not be held in a place where there are likely to be interruptions

Devising the plan

When actually devising the plan with a person the following guidelines help to clarify the process.
The **SMART** rule:

S – The plan should be **specific** (e.g. give up smoking, eat more healthily, etc.).

M – The plan should be **measurable** (i.e. the amount of weight lost, the fall in numbers of cigarettes smoked).

A – The person must feel he or she can **achieve** the goal (remember Bandura's theory?).
A weight loss of one kilogram in two weeks is reasonable; a loss of three kilograms a month is not.

R – The plan must be **realistic**. An elderly woman is unlikely to take up weight lifting.

T – There should be a **timetable** set so both the health professional and the individual have a goal to work towards.

If all these points are considered, there is a good chance of the plan being carried out.

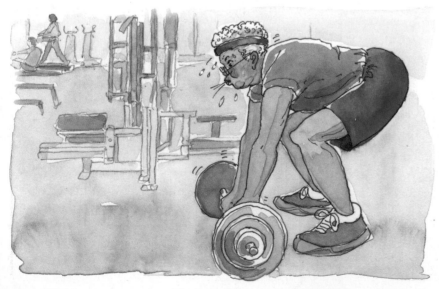

The health improvement plan must be realistic

How different health behaviours can help people achieve their targets

You should realise by now that developing and carrying out a health improvement plan is a complicated process. You are asking others to change behaviour they have seen as pleasant and acceptable. They are being asked to do something they are likely to find difficult and unpleasant, especially at first. You must not be surprised if people don't manage the change easily or quickly. Studies have been done on people who are attempting to change their behaviour in this way. Their behaviour can be described as in Figure 10.1.

At each stage the following happens:

- **Pre-contemplation:** People don't feel any need or interest in changing their behaviour.
- **Contemplation:** People are thinking about change.
- **Commitment:** The person has made the decision to change his or her behaviour.
- **Action:** The person is actively changing (e.g. he or she has stopped smoking or has gone on a diet).
- **Maintenance:** People have carried out the change but may be finding it hard to keep going. If they are successful, they could be said to have left the cycle as they carry on with their healthy lifestyle.

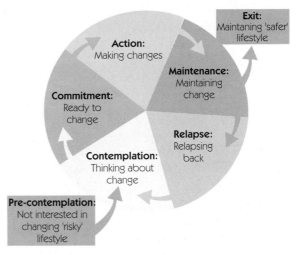

Figure 10.1 Stages in changing health behaviour (adapted from Neesham, C., 1993 and Prochaska, J. & DiClemente, C., 1984)

- **Relapse:** The person abandons the plan (e.g. abandons the diet).

The diagram is shown in a circle because many people go through these stages several times before eventually succeeding in making the change to their lifestyle permanent. Most smokers go around the cycle three times before stopping smoking entirely.

When people are in the action and maintenance stages they will often need help to keep going. The following strategies can help people to remain motivated enough to continue with the plan:

1 **Self-monitoring**. The person keeps a diary of his behaviour (i.e. how often he wants a drink, etc.). By looking at the pattern of his

Case study

Vicky

Vicky has smoked since she was a teenager. She is now 33 years old and is considering giving up smoking. Recently, she has started to cough first thing in the morning and she knows that this is probably linked to her smoking habit. Her partner is also a heavy smoker and she is trying to persuade him to stop as well. They work for the same company, where they are allowed to smoke in a particular area, away from the non-smokers. They have always wanted to go on a safari holiday and Vicky has worked out

that they could afford the holiday next year, if they were to stop smoking and save the money.

1 Using Figure 10.1, identify what stage Vicky is at now.

2 What stage is her partner at?

3 What strategies is she already using to try to support her desire to give up smoking?

1 If she manages to stop, what strategies could she use to try to remain a non-smoker?

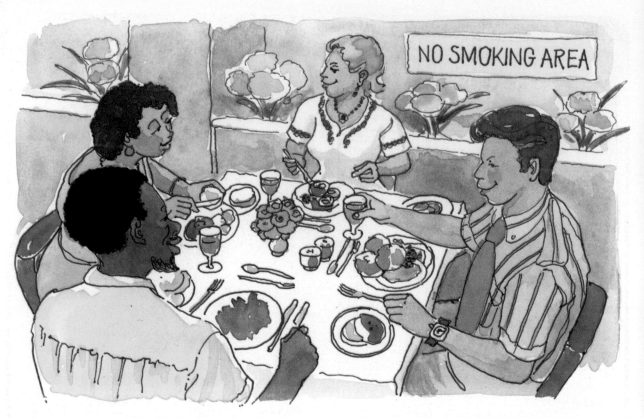

Using no-smoking areas can be a useful strategy for a person who is trying to give up

behaviour, a person can learn something about his or her own actions and learn to recognise when he might be in danger of losing motivation.

2 **Giving rewards**. Rewards for following a health improvement plan tend to be long term (e.g. better health, a slimmer figure, etc.). If possible, it helps if there can be rewards in the short-term as well.

3 **Devising coping strategies**. These are ways of helping people get through the first few days or weeks when it may seem difficult to keep going. Strategies for a smoker could include using Nicorette gum or sitting in non-smoking areas.

4 **Reviewing targets**. The targets set should be realistic but, if they are not being met, they need to be reviewed to see if different ones will improve the chance of success.

Check your knowledge

1 What is the role of the health professional?

2 Why do people sometimes not follow a health improvement plan?

3 What factors affect the chances of a health improvement plan being a success?

4 Why is it important to involve the individual when setting targets for a health improvement plan?

5 Describe possible barriers to communication between the individual and the health professional devising the plan.

6 Why do health improvement plans fail?

7 Why are the stages of health behaviour drawn in a circle?

8 What strategies can be used to help motivate people who are following a health improvement plan?

▶ There is now a great deal of information available on all aspects of health promotion (see Figure 10.2). Use the Internet to research an aspect of the subject that interests you (e.g. drug abuse, losing weight, the benefits of regular exercise). Use a search engine such as Google. Collect information on your chosen subject and then present it in a way that should appeal to students in your age group. Include an image to improve the quality of your work.

▶ Use the information you have found to devise a health improvement plan for a person with a particular need (e.g. a teenager who needs to eat a healthier diet). Consider the points listed above when drawing up the plan.

Type of health promotion material	Examples	Uses	Advantages	Disadvantages
Leaflets and handouts	Information on diet, hygiene, overuse of anti-biotics	For the individual to read in his or her own time. Supports other health promotion activities	Can be read at home, at a time and place to suit the reader. Easy and cheap to produce. Can be used to summarise information previously given in a talk	Information may be too general to be of real value to the individual. Requires the reader to have good reading skills. Usually only produced in English so non-English speakers will be unable to read them. Easily lost.
Posters and wall charts	Posters on dental health, HIV and AIDS. Found in GPs and dental surgeries, family planning clinics	Raises awareness of a subject. Conveys basic information to large numbers of people	Can provide basic information with addresses, phone numbers and website addresses for more detailed information. Cheap to produce. Seen by large numbers of people	Can become tatty and untidy. They need changing regularly or people no longer notice them. High-quality posters can be expensive
Videos	Exercise programmes. Hygiene information. The menopause	Can be used to show real-life situations such as childbirth. Can start discussions and pose problems for the viewer to discuss	Can be started and stopped, watched again to allow for discussion. Useful for people with poor reading skills. Can be used with large numbers of people	Requires reliable, specialist equipment. The films need to be up to date as old-fashioned clothes, etc., are off-putting to the viewer
Slides	Pictures of foods to help understanding of diet. Pictures of hazards in the home.	Provides stimulation for discussion. Adds interest to lectures. Graphs and charts can easily be seen. Can be used with large groups.	Can be used again. Can be added to and the order rearranged to suit the audience. Holds attention by adding interest	Needs specialist equipment
Audio cassette tapes	Relaxation tapes. Children's stories related to health issues	To reinforce information. Can be taken home and used when needed. Can accompany written information	Small and easy to carry. Cheap to obtain and use. Useful for the visually impaired	Attention may wander because there is nothing to look at
Computer programs	Diet analysis. Information on drugs	Problem-solving. To give information. To question the user about his or her health behaviour	People often enjoy using the program. Can be used again	Requires access to computer equipment. User needs computer skills to follow the program
OHP transparencies	Used to highlight important points. Diagrams of parts of the body	To improve presentation of facts and ideas. To show diagrams, graphs and charts	Holds attention of the audience. Can be used with large numbers of people. Diagrams help understanding of difficult ideas. Can be later produced on paper so that the audience can take the information away with them	Needs specialist equipment. Must be prepared in advance if they are to be of a good quality
Flipcharts	Brainstorming to get discussion going. Summarising of points at the end of a discussion	Draw quick diagrams to clarify points that need more explanation. Recording information to be used later in the talk. Used to start and end talks and lectures. Suitable for small and medium-sized groups	Can give immediate response to comments from the audience. Inexpensive and easily available	Can look messy while in use. Teacher has to turn away from the audience
Toys and models	Food models used to explain basic nutrition. Teddy bear used to explain an operation to a child	Teaches skills. Enables people to be actively involved in their own learning	Can be used repeatedly. Can be used to explain difficult ideas more simply	May get broken or damaged
Blackboards and whiteboards	Writing key words. Drawing diagrams	Draws attention to important points. Clarifies ideas that are proving to be difficult for the audience. Suitable for small and medium-sized groups	Immediate response to comments from the audience. Easy to use. Can be wiped clean and reused easily	Need chalk and special pens. Needs practice to write clearly. Teacher has to turn his or her back on the audience

Figure 10.2 The types of health promotion materials used to inform, motivate and support people

Assignment

You need to produce a health plan for improving or maintaining the physical health and well-being of one individual for your portfolio. Your plan must:

(a) include an explanation of what is meant by health and well-being;

(b) identify factors which have both a good and bad effect on an individual's health and well-being, and explain the effect these factors have;

(c) identify appropriate information to set targets and measures of health for the individual;

(d) include an assessment of how the plan may affect the individual, together with an evaluation of the difficulties which might be met in following and achieving the plan, and how these difficulties may be overcome.

The individual could be you, one of your friends or a member of your family. Ideally the individual you choose should have several factors which affect her/his health and well-being in a negative way, for example, smoking and obesity, to give you the chance to gain as many marks as possible. The case study is provided to help you practise for the assignment for this unit.

N.B. When you produce your actual assignment you can follow the instructions in the grid, but remember to use the name of your selected individual instead of Jemma!

Practice assignment

Case study

Jemma is 28 years old and for the last 10 years she has spent the holiday season working on a popular holiday island in the Mediterranean. She spends a lot of the day in the sun, has healthy skin and tans easily so doesn't bother with creams or moisturisers. The job involves her getting plenty of exercise and she eats lots of salads during the day, as she is determined to eat as healthily as possible. She never takes drugs although she is offered them regularly. Her nights are spent in the clubs with the holiday makers; she drinks at least 2 pints of lager and a couple of spirits every night, smokes 20 cigarettes a day and has had a succession of brief relationships, sometimes sexual. She left school with 5 good passes at GCSE and 1 A-level. She rarely reads a book but does read an English tabloid newspaper each day.

In the winter Jemma returns to England and lives with her parents. They are always pleased to see her but worry that she does not look after herself well enough during the summer. They cook her 3 meals a day and she goes out with ex-school friends to clubs and pubs when she is not working. She still drinks and smokes. She works part time in a pub. Each winter she puts on weight and goes on a crash diet before returning to her island in the sun at the start of the next summer season.

Jemma is 1.72m tall and weighs 62.2kg. She is a medium frame. Her blood pressure is 130/80 and her usual peak flow reading is 350 litres per minute. Her resting pulse rate is 80 beats per minute and it takes about 4 minutes for her pulse rate to return to normal after mild exercise.

Use the case study to practise for the real assignment. To achieve the highest possible mark you need to include everything from all three mark bands for areas A to D.

Total marks available	Mark Band 1 Average Grade FF	Mark Band 2 Average Grade CC	Mark Band 3 Average Grade AA
(a) 10 marks available	1 – 4 marks	5 – 7 marks	8 – 10 marks
	You need to **describe** what is meant by health and well-being. Give at least two definitions and make it clear that you understand the difference between positive and negative descriptions. You need to show how at least one definition has changed over time.	You need to give an **accurate and precise description** of three or four different definitions of health and well-being, with reference to influences such as the World Health Organisation and with examples to explain each one. You must show how these definitions have changed with time. You need to make some reference to physical, social, emotional or intellectual influences.	You must give a **clear, precise and accurate description** of three or four different definitions of health and well-being and give examples which clearly show that you understand how these have changed over time.
(b) 16 marks available	1 – 6 marks	7 – 11 marks	12 – 16 marks
	You need to **state** at least five or six factors that have an effect on Jemma's health and well-being. Some should be positive, for example, 'Jemma eats a balanced diet which means that her body receives the right balance of the nutrients she needs.' You need to say what a healthy diet is made up of. You also need to give some negative factors, for example 'Jemma smokes 20 cigarettes a day,' and explain what effect the cigarettes will have on her.	You need to state **and explain in detail** at least five or six factors that have an effect on Jemma's health and well-being, including both positive and negative factors. You need to include quite a lot of detail when you explain the effects on Jemma, for example, 'Jemma gets plenty of exercise so will be physically tired so will sleep better. This will mean she wakes up more refreshed and alert and will be more likely to be in a positive and optimistic mood.' You need to get your information from a wide range of sources and list those sources.	You need to **state and explain in detail** at least five or six factors that have **the most** effect on Jemma's health and well-being. Your explanations need to be detailed, for example, 'Jemma eats healthily. She knows that smoking is bad for her health but does not want to give up as she is afraid her appetite will increase and she will put on weight.' You need to go on to describe in detail all the effects, for example, smoking could have on Jemma's health and well-being. All the factors that you describe need to be in as much detail. You need to select relevant information from a wide range of sources without any help from others. You need to list your sources of information.

Total marks available	Mark Band 1 Average Grade FF	Mark Band 2 Average Grade CC	Mark Band 3 Average Grade AA
(c) 16 marks available	1 – 3 marks	4 – 6 marks	7 – 16 marks
	You need to **list** the details about Jemma which will make it possible to suggest targets to improve her health, for example, her weight and height. You need to suggest how these details are measured and suggest **simple targets** to help her improve on them, for example, 'Her lung capacity can be measured with a peak flow meter. She can improve this by stopping smoking.'	You need to list the information about Jemma that will be needed to set targets and explain **in detail** how the information has been gathered, for example, explain how a peak flow meter reading is taken. You also need to suggest **targets**, for example, cut down her cigarettes by 10 in the first six months.	You need to list all the **relevant** information available about Jemma that will be needed to set targets and explain **in detail** how **each** piece of information will be gathered. You also need to suggest **short and long-term targets**, which are appropriate and realistic, for example, cut down her cigarettes by 5 in the first month, by 10 in six months and stop smoking altogether after a year.
(d) 15 marks available	1 – 6 marks	7 – 10 marks	11 – 15 marks
	Write your plan out in a form which will be useful and easy for Jemma to read, for example, in the form of a table. Say **how you think the plan will affect** Jemma, **listing any difficulties** you think she might have in trying to stick to it. Say how she **might overcome these difficulties**. Giving up smoking, for example, will help her breathing but she might find it hard to give up smoking because she spends so much time in clubs and will be tempted to smoke. She could try to overcome this problem by chewing gum.	Your plan should include more ways in which Jemma can be motivated to improve her health. You need to identify **some of the most significant effects** that your plan will have on Jemma. You need to say why you think some of these are most significant. For example, a significant physical effect is that she will be less at risk from respiratory problems so be less likely to develop diseases such as lung cancer, which is life threatening, if she gives up smoking. You need to **clearly identify any difficulties** she might encounter at each stage of the plan, for example she might find it harder to give up all together after a year than she did to cut down at first. You also need to **compare the effects of each target**, for example, she might find it harder to stop smoking than to eat healthily all the time. You should also suggest **some ways to overcome the difficulties**.	Your plan should be **very detailed, with clear and** accurate arguments to support the points you make. You need to identify **all the most significant effects** that your plan will have on Jemma. You need to suggest the **relative impacts of the different effects** and say **how** these will have different effects at different stages of the plan. You need to show very clearly that you understand what you are trying to get Jemma to achieve by following your plan. You also need to suggest **alternative approaches** in your plan when you anticipate Jemma having difficulties, for example, going out for a special meal for her birthday might tempt her to smoke so you could suggest that she picks a totally non-smoking restaurant.

Understanding personal development and relationships

Introduction to Unit 3

Health, social care and early years workers need to know about the different ways that people grow and develop during their lives. This unit will help you to find out about the process of human growth and development, and the different factors that can affect an individual's experience.

What you will learn

In this unit you will learn about:

- the stages and pattern of human growth and development;
- the different factors that can affect human growth and development;
- the development of self-concept and personal relationships;
- major life changes and how people deal with them; and
- the role of relationships in personal development.

Why do you need to learn this?

People who work in the caring professions are helping people of all age groups, ethnicity and social backgrounds. However, the factors that affect the healthy growth and development of individuals are similar for all people, regardless of their apparent differences. You therefore need to know what factors promote the satisfactory development of people, throughout their lives. If people are experiencing difficulties in their lives, you will be more able to help them if you have some understanding of how factors can cause development that is less than satisfactory.

At the end of this unit you will be looking at the types of support that are available for people who need help in times of difficulty. There are many leaflets available to explain what help can be obtained. Such help could include information about benefits or advice for carers of the elderly or small children. You can find information leaflets of this type in the library, at the doctor's surgery or at the town hall, among other places. Try to get hold of some leaflets of this type while you are studying this unit.

Assessment

This unit is assessed through a set examination. Your overall result for this unit will be a grade from G to A*.

Key issue

How do individuals grow and develop during each life stage?

By the end of this chapter you will have learnt that growth refers to an increase in physical size (mass and weight) and that development is concerned with the emergence and increase in the sophistication of skills, abilities and emotions. You will be able to describe the expected patterns of physical growth and change, and the physical, social, intellectual and emotional developments that typically take place during each of the five main life stages. These are (in years):

* infancy (0–3)
* childhood (4–10)
* adolescence (11–18)
* adulthood (19–65)
* later adulthood (65+).

Introduction to human growth and development

The term *growth* means an increase in mass and height. This happens because:

* the total number of body cells increases;
* each cell gets larger as it carries more information; and
* the body cells become more specialised in the jobs they do.

Development refers to the gradual change and increase in abilities, emotions and skills as people get older. Both growth and development occur most rapidly until the person is about 19 years of age. After this, people continue to change and develop, but at a slower rate than before. One way of looking at the human life span is to study the way we develop *physically, intellectually, emotionally* and *socially*. The

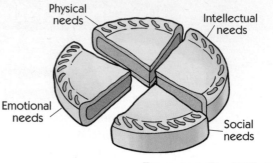

Figure 11.1 The PIES circle

first letters of these words spell PIES. Unit 2 explains that PIES is a way of thinking about human development (see Figure 11.1).

Checkpoint

Growth means an increase in physical size.
Development means an increase in skills, abilities and emotions.

Physical development

Physical development describes the way the body increases in weight and height during the lifetime of the individual. It is our *hormones* that control our growth. Hormones are chemicals made in the *endocrine glands* of the body. They are transported around the body by the blood system. The thyroid gland in the neck produces growth hormone or *thyroxin*.

Physical development can also be called *ageing*. This describes the way in which the body gradually changes as a person gets older. Physical development in children can be measured on *centile* charts (see Figure 11.2). A child's weight and height are measured and are compared with the chart. The chart shows the normal range of height and weight you would expect for children between the ages of 0 and 5 years. By plotting the individual's measurement in the chart, it is possible to see if the child is growing at a satisfactory rate. There are different charts for boys and girls.

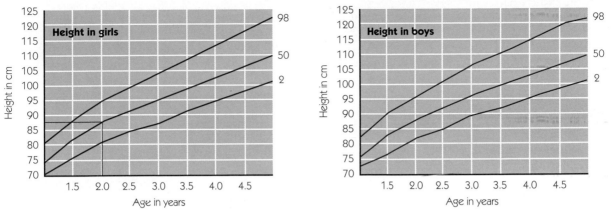

Figure 11.2 Centile charts allow health professionals such as nurses to check that a child is growing at a healthy rate

Intellectual development

This describes the way in which the individual acquires the ability to use language, to develop concepts and to think. It is sometimes called *cognitive development*. Again, development is rapid in the first years of life.

A psychologist called Jean Piaget described the way in which children develop mentally. Figure 11.3 shows the different stages in Piaget's theory of child development. Children progress gradually through each stage as they get older. Intellectual development occurs most rapidly before the child is 18 years old but development can continue into middle or even old age.

Emotional development

As we get older we learn to understand our feelings and those of other people. We also learn to take other people's feelings into account. This is *emotional development*. Emotional development starts through a successful *attachment relationship* or *bonding* between the child and the main carer. This must occur during the first few years of the child's life or he or she may have difficulty forming successful relationships with people throughout his or her life.

Sound emotional development leads to a satisfactory *self-concept*. Our self-concept describes the sum total of the ways in which we think about ourselves.

Stage of development	Age	Key issue
Sensori-motor	0–18 months/2 years	Children do not understand how objects exist
Pre-operational (pre-logical)	2–6/7 years	Children do not think in a logical way
Concrete operational	7–11 years	Children can understand logic if they can see or handle objects. Children do not fully understand logical arguments in words
Formal operational	11 years onwards	People can understand logical arguments and think in an abstract way

Figure 11.3 Piaget's stages of child development

As we become older, emotional development is maintained through our relationships with family, friends and then with a long-term sexual partner. Like physical development, emotional development continues throughout our lives.

Social development

As children become older, they gradually learn how to get on with other people. Children learn to *socialise*. A child's first relationship is with his or her parents or main carers. If they bond successfully with them, children will feel able to make other relationships as they grow older.

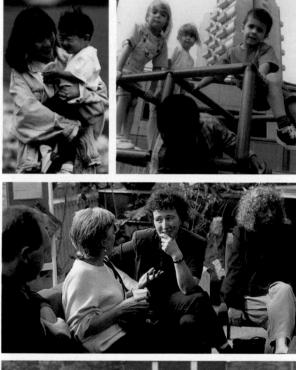

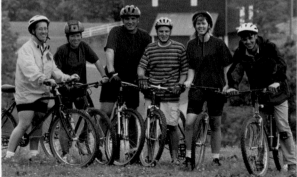

A child's first relationship is (a) with his or her carer; (b) social development continues through friendships with children of the same age; (c) people form friendships at work; (d) shared interests help social development

These will be less intense relationships, but they are still important. These are relationships with siblings (sisters and brothers), the extended family and other children. Adults will make relationships with colleagues, neighbours and the other adults they meet through shared interests.

Social development contributes to our self-concept. Human beings are social beings. We all need the support, comfort and company of other people to feel confident and secure. Satisfactory social development will help to bring this about.

Nature versus nurture

Every individual (except identical twins) is unique. He or she is biologically different from every other human being. People both look and behave differently from each other. These differences can be described as our *characteristics*.

> **Checkpoint**
>
> A person's **characteristics** are features of the person that determine the way he or she looks, behaves, feels and thinks.

Doctors and psychologists (people who study human behaviour) have debated for a long time the factors that decide how we look and behave. This argument is known as the nature versus nurture debate. Some people believe that all the characteristics of a person are inherited from his or her parents. For example, we can see quite clearly when we have inherited features such as hair or eye colour from our parents. This is the nature argument.

Other people believe that our characteristics are decided by the way in which the child is brought up. They believe that certain types of behaviour and attitudes are learnt from the parents. A child who is taken to football matches may become very keen on the sport as he or she grows older. This is the nurture argument. Others believe that the two features cannot be easily separated. They believe some aspects of an individual are formed from inherited characteristics, whereas other aspects are learnt.

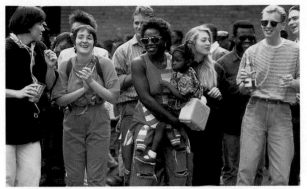

Every person is biologically unique. Scientists disagree about what causes the differences between people

Infancy (0 – 3 years)

In the first three years of life, a baby is called an 'infant'. Once he or she starts crawling, pulling him or herself up and walking, the baby is often called a 'toddler'. During this stage, development is very fast, with the body changing and growing quickly. During the first years of life the human infant is completely dependent on his or her carers. All the infant's basic needs have to be met by someone else if he or she is to survive.

Physical development

Babies develop very rapidly during the first three years of life. They are born with a number of physical *reflexes*.

> **Checkpoint**
>
> A **reflex** is an automatic, uncontrollable response to a physical change (e.g. moving your hand away from a hot plate).

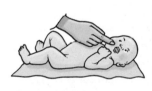

Rooting reflex
The baby turns its head in the direction of the touch, enabling it to find the nipple of its mother's breast to obtain food.

Moro reflex
When startled, a baby throws out its arms and legs, then pulls them back with fingers curved.

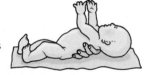

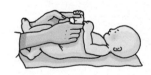

Grasp reflex
A baby will grasp an object placed in its hand.

Walking reflex
When a baby is held with its feet touching the ground its legs make forward movements, as if walking.

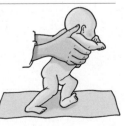

Figure 11.4 The primitive reflexes of a newborn baby

Activity

▶ What makes you different from other people? Make a list of your own characteristics. Start with physical characteristics such as hair and eye colour. Then think about aspects of your personality. Are you impatient, hard working, laid back, etc.? Put your description in your file.

▶ Working with another person, decide which category (physical, social, emotional and intellectual) the characteristics in your list above should go into. For example, is being kind a social or a physical characteristic? Finish the activity and put your conclusions in your file. Then decide if you have acquired the characteristic through nature, nurture or a combination of the two.

Check your knowledge

1   What is meant by growth and development?
2   What role do hormones play in human development?
3   What is a centile chart and how is it used?
4   What is cognitive development?
5   What is emotional development?
6   What is necessary for our successful emotional development?
7   How do adults maintain emotional development throughout their lives?
8   Why is satisfactory social development necessary?
9   How do we acquire our characteristics?

Age	Gross motor skills	Fine motor skills
New born	Primitive reflexes (see Figure 11.4)	
1 month	Lifts up chin, some control of head	
3 months	Reaches towards objects. Lifts head when laid on the stomach	Holds rattle for a few seconds. Moves hands towards a bottle
4/5 months	Sits supported	
6 months	Sits unsupported. Rolls over, can kick strongly. Lifts head and chest when lying on the stomach	Can move objects from one hand to another. Picks up dropped toys if they are in sight
9 months	Stands alone, holding on to something. Tries to crawl. Active movement of all limbs. Can lean forward without falling over	Begins to have 'pincer' movement between finger and thumb. Stretches out for held toy. Can release toy by dropping it
12 months	Pulls to stand. May walk alone or holding on to furniture. May crawl upstairs. Sits upright well	Good pincer movement. Bangs things together. Throws toys deliberately
15 months	Can walk without help	
18 months	Runs	Holds small objects. Can hold a pencil to 'draw'
2 years old	Picks things up without falling over. Kicks a ball	Eats competently with a spoon. Can build a tower of six bricks
2/3 years old	Stands on toes, jumps off a step. Can ride a tricycle	Can use crayons competently

Figure 11.5 Gross and fine motor skills in children aged 0–4 years

Some early reflexes are shown in Figure 11.4. These early reflexes fade away as the baby gets older and are replaced by others. At first, babies have little control over their bodies. During the first three years they gradually learn to control their muscles and movements. The control of large muscles, such as in the arms and legs, is called the *gross motor skills*. The control of smaller muscles and movements, such as those in the fingers, is called *fine motor skills*. Fine motor skills are more difficult to acquire (see Figure 11.5).

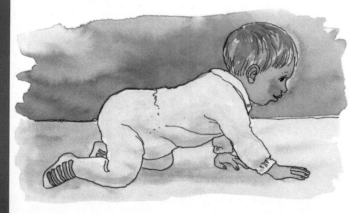

Children gain more complicated gross motor skills as they get older

Intellectual development

Perhaps the most important intellectual development a child makes is the ability to use and understand language. Babies understand simple words such as 'bye-bye' at 6–9 months old and will have a vocabulary of about three words at 1 year old. At around 2 years of age, most children have started to speak, using two-word phrases such as 'Zoe sleep' (meaning Zoe wants to go to sleep). As children grow they start to use their own type of language pattern to communicate, such as 'I want a drink' and 'the cat goed' (the cat has gone out). Young children of 2 or 3 years of age do not use adult language and it is probably best not to correct what they say. Children may go through stages of language development such as the examples listed below:

Two-word statements ('Cat goed').

Short phrases ('I want drink').

Being able to ask questions ('What that?' 'Where is cat?').

Using sentences ('Jill come in and the doggy come in').

Adult sentences ('I would like a drink and a piece of cake').

By the age of 5 or 6 years, children can use adult speech and have a reasonable knowledge of words. However, children continue to develop their knowledge of words and their ability to understand and use speech throughout childhood.

Intellectual development is helped by play. Children investigate objects by putting them into their mouths, which is the most sensitive area of the body. They learn by handling things, listening to things and by looking at things that are pointed out to them. The role of the carer is vital here as he or she teaches the child simple facts such as parts of the body and names of animals. Children can look at picture books with an adult or older child to help stimulate them and to increase their ability to recognise everyday objects. At this stage, children will copy many actions.

Emotional and social development

Emotional development only occurs satisfactorily in the older child if a secure *attachment relationship* has been made in the first years of life. As well as forming a secure relationship with their main carer, children now begin to form relationships with siblings and other members of the extended family they meet regularly. Children will recognise these people and will be at ease with them.

As the child gets a little older, he or she will begin to be interested in other children. By the age of 2 years, he or she will play alone next to another child. This is called *parallel play*. A child is about 4 before he or she can play properly with another child. The child can now be involved in *co-operative play*.

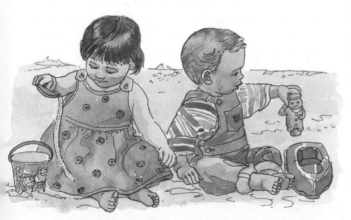

Children under 3 years of age play near each other, but not with each other. This is called parallel play

Bonding

During the first 18 months of life, infants develop an emotional bond with their carers. This bonding process ties the infant emotionally to familiar carers. Some theorists think it is very important that children are not separated at any time from their mothers during infancy so that this emotional bond can develop. Other theorists argue that an infant's main emotional attachment is not always with the mother – fathers and other carers are also important. Some theorists say it is the quality of the love and care that matters most, and not whether carers ever leave their child (for example, to go to work). There is agreement, however, that infants need to experience a loving attachment with a carer and, if this does not happen, that a children's social and emotional development will be damaged.

Case study

Ahmed

Ahmed is 9 months old. He is his parent's first child and is very much loved. After his mother has fed him, she holds him till he goes to sleep. If he doesn't fall asleep quickly, she talks to him, pointing out things that might take his interest. At the weekend, his parents try at take him out so that he sees things outside his home. Ahmed's mother is doing an Access course at college two afternoons a week. On those days, his grandparents, who live nearby, look after Ahmed. As he has spent a lot of time with them since he was born, he is at ease when he is at their house.

> 1   Whom is Ahmed likely to bond with?
> 2   Use examples from the case study to explain how Ahmed is likely to form satisfactory emotional attachments.

> 1   Describe the person/people you formed an attachment relationship with when you were a young child.

Young children (4–10 years)

Physical development

The physical appearance of children begins to change as they get older. He or she loses his or her baby shape and begins to look like a small adult. The infant's fast rate of growth begins to slow down during childhood. Physical, intellectual, emotional and social development is still taking place but the child is now beginning to learn some very complicated skills. As the child grows and develops, their balance becomes very good. This means they can run, climb and jump (and, of course, get into all sorts of danger as a result!).

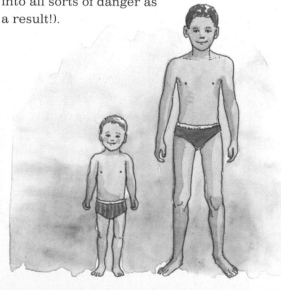

Intellectual development

The development of the brain and the mind is all part of childhood intellectual development. (The features of intellectual development are shown in Figure 11.6.) Children are interested in everything. It is by asking questions (and getting answers) that the child will learn about his or her environment and the culture (customs and practices) of the society in which he or she lives.

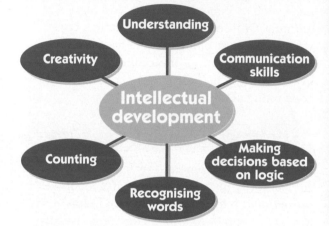

Figure 11.6 The features of intellectual development

As the child's intellectual development continues, he or she can begin to carry out a range of more complex activities, such as:

- reading and sums;
- making and keeping relationships;
- table manners;
- writing his or her own name; and
- understanding the rules of team games.

The child begins to mix different skills to complete a complicated task. For example, playing a team game like football requires a child to understand the rules (intellectual development), to be able to kick the ball in the right direction (physical development) and to talk to his or her team-mates about the strategy to follow. They also have to cope with negative (or positive) feelings when the game has been won or lost (emotional development).

Children learn how to do things by watching others. This is called *modelling*. It is often amusing to see a small child copying something his or her parents have said or done. On the other hand, as they get older, some children learn from poor behaviour which can lead to difficulties.

Emotional development

Children have to cope with their own feelings and the feelings of others in the same way they have to learn a new skill, such as table manners. Children learn to cope with their emotions through playing with other children. Some emotional characteristics are shown in Figure 11.7.

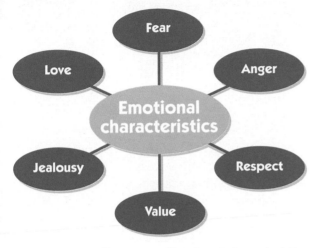

Figure 11.7 Emotional characteristics

Infants may be prone to temper tantrums. However, as infants get older these become less frequent. By the time the infant is 5 years old, he or she usually wants to be in the company of other children. At this age infants are able to play together and to join in team games. By the time a child is 10 years old, he or she has begun to learn how to cope with his or her feelings. Infants will have discovered jealousy and anger and appropriate ways of coping. Children are very sensitive to criticism and do not react well to 'a telling off', especially in front of other people.

Social development

Developing good relationships with other people is a skill we begin to learn from birth onwards. The way we learn and the kind of skills we learn will depend on the culture we are born into. For example, a person from a culture that does not approve of males and females mixing together outside the home may choose to become friendly with someone of his or her own sex. On the other hand, some societies allow mixing between all age groups and between both sexes.

Some children are good at developing lots of social relationships; others are better at keeping a few special friends for a short time. We are all different! During childhood, a child learns to make friends with others. He or she learns the importance of good relationships in a variety of settings. For example:

- in the home;
- at school;
- in clubs and groups (sports, drama, music, etc.);
- where he or she lives; and
- in religious settings.

The importance of play

Play (see Figure 11.8) is necessary to ensure children learn. The way children play changes as the child grows older. Play activities at any age can help the child to develop:

- practical skills and abilities (e.g. making things from kits);
- social skills and good relationships with others (e.g. playing co-operatively with a toy or with a game); and
- intellectually (e.g. by looking at picture books with an adult or older sibling).

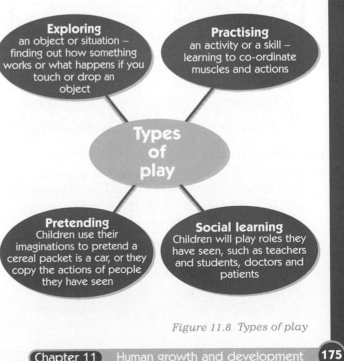

Figure 11.8 Types of play

Activity

▶ Use magazines to find pictures of babies and children aged 0–10 years old. Stick the pictures into your notes. By the side of the picture, state the child's age (you will have to guess this). Use the information from the section above to describe the child's physical, intellectual, emotional and social development at this age. Try to find enough pictures to cover the age range of this section.

▶ Use catalogues to find examples of children's toys. Take each toy in turn and suggest how the toy is designed to help the child's physical, intellectual, emotional or social development. For example, a toy sewing machine is designed to develop the child's fine motor skills, a type of physical development. Put the picture of the toy and the explanation of its value by the side of the child's picture.

Check your knowledge

1 How does the physical appearance of children change between 4–10 years old?
2 Why do children ask questions?
3 What is 'modelling'?
4 How do children learn to cope with their emotions?
5 Where do children learn the importance of social relationships?
6 Why is play important?

Adolescence (11–18 years)

Individuals enter this stage of their lives as young children and emerge as young adults. Next time the whole school is gathered together, look at the Year 7 students and compare them with Year 11. The difference in body size, knowledge, experience and ability is huge! Yet these changes are made in a relatively short time, in about only four or five years.

During this stage of life, new roles and responsibilities are developed. Young people are:

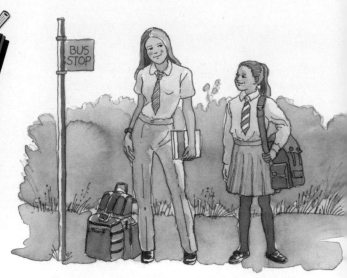

There is great physical, intellectual, emotional and social development during the teenage years

- developing relationships with people of all ages and of both sexes;
- learning skills, ready for work;
- achieving independence;
- developing a set of values and morals;
- developing socially responsible behaviour; and
- preparing for a lasting relationship.

Activity

▶ You have developed a great deal since you were in Year 7. Under the headings 'Physical development', 'Intellectual development', 'Emotional development' and 'Social development', make lists of the ways you have developed. For example, you are taller, which is *physical* development. You can cope with more complicated ideas and concepts, which is *intellectual* development. Put your ideas in your file.

▶ Think of a person (or persons) who is older than you and whom you know well. What sort of skills or abilities does he or she have that you feel you have not yet acquired? For example, the person may have more confidence when speaking to strangers. Make a list of his or her skills. Now decide whether each skill or ability is a physical, intellectual, emotional or social skill. Categorise each skill in this way.

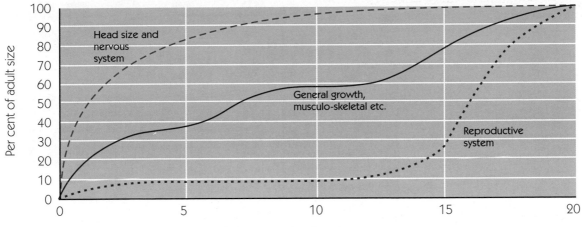

Figure 11.9 *Some body systems have different growth rates*

Physical development

Physical changes start to occur at any time from the age of 8 years onwards, and some body systems have different growth rates from others (Figure 11.9). The changes happen in girls sooner than boys (see Figures 11.10 and 11.11).

The hormones secreted by the pituitary gland cause these changes. These glands stimulate the production of *oestrogen* in girls and *testosterone* in boys. During puberty, the boys catch up and overtake the girls' head start in growth. Boys therefore end up heavier and taller than girls, although there is a wide variation in mature heights and weights in both sexes.

Intellectual development

Adolescents are able to imagine and think about things they have never seen or done before: they can imagine their future and how they might achieve things in the future. Children are not able to plan and think ahead in this way. Adolescents can solve problems in the same manner as adults.

Piaget called this stage of development *formal operational* (or formal logical). Formal logic helps people solve problems at work and in daily life. Whereas children often make guesses when they have to solve problems, adolescents can often work things out logically. Although adolescents can reason in an adult

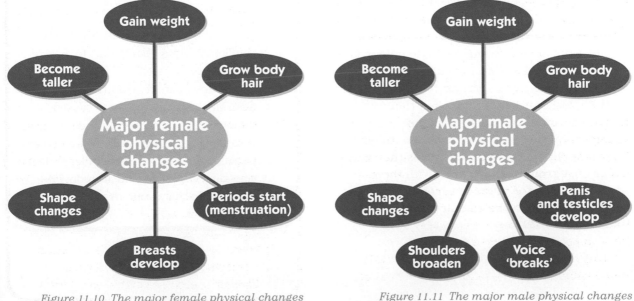

Figure 11.10 *The major female physical changes*

Figure 11.11 *The major male physical changes*

way, they may often not know enough to make the right decisions. Decision-making skills are something we acquire throughout our adult lives.

Emotional development

Emotions are often very important during the teenage years. Hormones may be out of balance and, in some cases, this can lead to mood swings or aggressive behaviour. These kinds of emotions usually settle down as the teenager becomes older. However, while moods swings last, they can make caring for someone in this age group very difficult. During this time of development and change, it is important for the adolescent to be able to talk to someone who can help him or her understand the variety of feelings and strong emotions he or she is having.

Lack of confidence and low self-esteem are problems faced by many teenagers. Some teenagers will even become very depressed about their lives. It is not always easy for them to talk to their parents or carers about these problems. They may need to talk to understanding friends and relatives instead.

Social development

Adolescents become increasingly independent of their families. Instead, they become much more dependent on their friends or *peer group* to provide support and advice. This is explored in more detail in Chapter 13. This phase of development is called *secondary socialisation*. Adolescents have a strong desire to belong to a group, and this is shown through their clothing and interests. Between 12 and 18 years of age, most adolescents begin to explore their sexuality, which includes testing out relationships and sexual behaviour with others. As young people take on adult roles they may experience trouble and conflict with their parents. This is the stage at which adolescents are trying to assert their adult independence (see Figure 11.12).

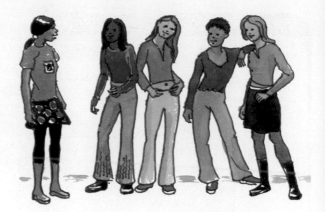

Figure 11.12 During adolescence, friendship groups become more important than the family in the development of social skills

Activity

▶ The people we mix with affects our decision-making. The things we see in the media (i.e. on TV and in magazines) also affect us. Make a list of all the things you make a decision about. The list could include your hairstyle, clothes, TV programmes you watch and the music you listen to. (You could think of many other items to add to the list.) By the side of each item you have listed, identify the person or factor that influences you when you make your choice. By looking at your completed lists, summarise who or what seems to be having the most effect on the decisions you make.

▶ Parents and teenagers often experience conflict as young people start to make their own decisions instead of 'doing as they are told' by their parents. Using the list above, describe the issues that have caused disagreement between you and the adults who care for you. Do you now feel you are beginning to become more independent of your carers' opinions and attitudes? Be prepared to share your ideas with the rest of the group.

Adulthood (19–65 years)

Adulthood is the longest stage of our development and is often a time of 'stability' (we begin to settle down). Many new skills and a great deal of knowledge have been learnt. We never stop learning, but the speed at which we learn can slow down. Problem-solving becomes a major part of life. We have to solve problems about:

- where to live;
- whom to live with;
- what job to do;
- how to find the money we need to live; and
- how to keep fit and healthy.

Physical development

People in their 20s and 30s are at the height of their physical powers and at their reproductive peak. As people enter their 40s, there are gradual physical changes in the body. These changes include the following:

- Men may start to lose their hair.
- Both sexes may find their eyesight deteriorating so they need glasses.
- The skin loses elasticity so wrinkles appear.
- Women continue to have periods till about 45 years old, when the *menopause* will start. Their fertility declines.
- Sperm production in men lessens, although they continue to be able to father children into their 80s.

Intellectual development

Intellectual skills and abilities may increase during adulthood if these skills and abilities are exercised. Older adults may be slightly slower when it comes to working out logical problems, but increased knowledge may compensate for slower reactions. Many older people are thought to have wisdom. Wisdom comes from many years of experience of life and so age may help people to make better decisions.

Emotional development

During adulthood most people look for steady and satisfying relationships. Some form couples in order to satisfy the need for love, security and companionship. Often couples have children, which arouses feelings of protectiveness, love and togetherness. In contrast, some adults may choose to live their lives alone. Adult relationships can also involve a variety of other emotions, such as anger, resentment and jealousy.

Coping with emotional changes can be difficult at times, so it is important adults learn to communicate with each other openly and honestly. Sometimes relationships fail and this can result in anxiety, stress and bitterness. As adults reach their older years, they may find their own parents need help and support as they become elderly and frail. This can cause emotional difficulties as the adult 'child' has to take on the role of carer to the parent.

Social development

Many things can bring about a change in the social life of adults, such as having children. For example, it may not be possible to go out to have a meal with friends in a restaurant if children have to be cared for. Instead, many adults maintain their social relationships with friends in their own homes.

Many people experience stress when trying to cope with the demands of being a parent, partner and worker. Going to work while maintaining a family home can create social and emotional problems. Adult life often involves trying to balance the need for money with the needs of partners and other family members.

Later adulthood (65+ years)

Many people think that becoming older is a negative thing to happen, but there are some advantages, such as being able to retire from work and to do more of the things they want to do. The ageing process involves some changes to the body and lifestyle, such as:

- Adjusting to having less physical strength.
- Getting used to retirement.
- Accepting the loss of friends and partners.
- Changing accommodation to supported housing or residential care.
- Teaching grandchildren.
- Adjusting to poor-quality eyesight or hearing.
- Enjoying more leisure time.

Physical development

The ageing process is subtle and the changes it brings are so slow and tiny we tend not to notice them. However, once we reach our mid-60s, we begin to notice some changes:

- Skin becomes thinner and less elastic so wrinkles appear.
- Bones become more brittle and more likely to break, particularly in women.
- Joints become stiffer and may become painful as the cartilage on the bone-ends becomes worn away and the ligaments that reinforce our joints become more loose.
- Height is reduced as the vertebrae in the spine get closer together; the spine may also become more rounded.
- Muscles become weaker.

- Sense of balance becomes impaired.
- Sense of taste and smell deteriorates.
- Hearing and sight deteriorate; vision can be further impaired because the lens of the eye starts to block light. This can be the forerunner of cataracts.
- There is a general reduction in the skin's sensitivity so that we are susceptible to burns and hypothermia. Hypothermia is when the body temperature falls too low. Some older people do not realise they are cold and this can be life-threatening.
- Breathing is less efficient because muscles around the lungs are weaker.
- Blood pressure increases because the walls of the arteries have become hard and less elastic. This can lead to a higher risk of strokes and brain haemorrhages.
- Insufficient insulin (a hormone) may be produced, leading to the start of diabetes, particularly in the overweight.
- The glands that provide hormones (endocrine glands) do not function as well as they used to. The rate of metabolism the chemical reactions in the body cells is reduced due to a reduction in thyroxine (a hormone needed to regulate metabolism). Lack of effective insulin from the pancreas frequently leads to diabetes, particularly in elderly people who are overweight.

Although the elderly may suffer from more than one of these problems, elderly people can live healthy and fulfilling lives. People now live much longer than they used to and with the right support and help, their quality of life can be good.

Intellectual development

People do not become less intelligent as they become older! However, older people might need support when gaining new abilities, especially if it is a long time since they acquired new skills and knowledge. Support will increase their confidence and improve their chances of success.

On the other hand, people who enjoy good health and who exercise their minds often retain their mental abilities and continue to develop their store of knowledge. Even if thinking slows down, the opportunity to acquire wisdom may increase with older age.

Emotional development

People's concepts of themselves continue to develop as life progresses. Changes such as retirement can affect self-concept as the person no longer has a clear idea of who he or she is now he or she no longer has a job. Older people may not only develop health problems but they can also be stereotyped by other people who assume they are less able than they are. This also affects the person's view of himself or herself. Some older people may be at risk of losing their self-confidence and self-esteem because of the way others treat them. The death of friends or partners can leave elderly people feeling emotionally isolated.

Social development

Older people can lead very varied lives. Many retired people have a greater opportunity for meeting and making friends than when they were working and bringing up a family. A network of friends and family can provide vital practical and emotional support. Alternatively, health problems and impairments can sometimes create difficulties that result in social isolation. For example, an elderly person may have difficulty in visiting friends if he or she has to use a wheelchair.

Moral development

Moral development changes throughout the stages of our lives. As children get older their understanding of moral issues becomes more sophisticated. When young, they know they should not do something because they could get punished. They believe that everyone should be treated the same, with no allowance for individual differences. As they get older, they begin to consider the opinions of others because they have more understanding about the feelings of those around them. Adolescents gradually recognise that the whole of society has to be considered when decisions are made that affect people. An adult eventually forms principles and values that will affect the way he or she chooses to live his or her life.

Check your knowledge

1 Describe the physical changes that occur in later adulthood.
2 Why do some older people need support in their learning?
3 How does stereotyping affect the self-confidence and self-esteem of the elderly?
4 How can health problems affect social development in this age group?
5 How do views about morals change as the individual gets older?

Case study

Alfred

Alfred is 73 years old. He used to have a stressful job as a doctor in the casualty department of the local hospital. He was glad to retire as he found the job exhausting in his last few years. Since he retired he has enjoyed doing the garden and doing improvements on his home. In the winter, he and his wife have taken French lessons as they enjoy taking their mobile home to Europe each summer. He never had time for these types of activities before. However, Alfred has just had some bad news. He has an incurable eye condition, which means he will eventually have to stop driving. His wife doesn't drive.

▶ 1 Why would Alfred have welcomed his retirement?
2 How is Alfred ensuring that his intellectual and physical development continue now he has retired?

▷ 1 What are the implications for the personal development of Alfred and his wife when he is no longer able to drive? When answering this question, think in terms of the PIES.

Chapter 12

Factors that affect growth and development

Key issue

What factors affect growth and development and how do these factors influence a person's health, well-being and opportunities in life?

At the end of this chapter you will have learned about the factors that cause individual differences in patterns of growth and development. These include the following:

1. **Physical factors:** Genetic inheritance, diet, amount and type of physical exercise, experience of illness or disease, etc.

2. **Social and emotional factors:** Gender, family relationships, friendships, educational experiences, employment/unemployment, ethnicity and religion, and various life experiences such as birth, marriage and death, etc.

3. **Economic factors:** Income and material possessions.

4. **Environmental factors:** Housing conditions, pollution, access to health and welfare services, etc.

You will understand how these factors inter-relate and affect a person's:

- self-esteem;
- physical and mental health;
- employment prospects; and
- level of education.

Physical factors

A physical factor is something that affects the growth and development of the body (e.g. a good diet or a clean home). We cannot control some of the factors but others we can change if we wish to.

Genetic inheritance

Our genetic inheritance is the collection of *genes* we have inherited from our parents (see Chapter 8). They determine our characteristics. These characteristics include our hair colour, eye colour, whether we are short or tall, or the likelihood we have an ability like our parents.

Diet

Our diet has a great effect on the condition of our bodies. As you read in Chapters 7 and 8, not eating enough food or eating the wrong type of food can prevent the body from developing properly.

Physical exercise

Obesity is defined as someone being more than 20% above his or her ideal body weight. Currently, 20% of 4-year-olds are overweight and, of adults, 20% of women and 17% of men are obese. The cause of this dramatic increase is due, in some part, to a lack of physical exercise. Read Chapter 8 again to remind yourself about the dangers to health and well-being of a lack of physical exercise.

Experience of illness or disease

A person is said to have an illness or disease when he or she suffers a variety of symptoms that mean the person is unwell. It is not difficult to appreciate that experience of long-term illness and disease will inevitably affect the sufferer. It is not easy for any individual to achieve his or her full potential in life if he or she suffers from a serious illness and is in pain.

For the individual affected by an illness or disease, there is an increased likelihood he or she will be affected financially by his or her problems. Some 34% of people with disabilities and illnesses are living in poverty, and the average income for an adult of working age with a disability is only 72% of the income of non-disabled people.

However, it should not be forgotten that individuals who live with those who are very ill could also be seriously affected. A small but significant number of children are the only (or major) carers for their disabled or ill parents. Such children will find it more difficult than others to give their full attention to schoolwork. They will not have the time to develop social activities for themselves.

Check your knowledge

1. Why do we often look like our parents?
2. What is the main cause for the rise in obesity in Britain?
3. If a person suffers from ill-health, what effect can this have on other members of the family?
4. What problems will a child carer have (a) at school and (b) at home?

Social and emotional factors

Checkpoint

Social and *emotional* factors are those things that influence our feelings about something or someone.

Gender

The term *sex* is concerned with the biological differences between males and females. The term *gender* refers to the behaviour society expects of men and women. For example, society still expects that at times of tragedy women will cry, whereas men are commended for their ability to hide their feelings.

Until recently, women were seen as a 'second sex' as they left school earlier than boys and earned less money than men. This happened even when they were doing the same job. However, girls and women have been making great gains and the gap is narrowing. Similar numbers of men and women are employed in the workforce (although women are still only paid, on average, 80% of men's wages). Girls now achieve better results in public examinations. Nowadays, a major issue in education is to find ways of closing the gap so boys do not get left behind.

Gender strongly influences a person's chances in life. Things are changing rapidly in society so there is some evidence that women are now seen as having more opportunities than men. This is most clearly seen in the world of work where there has been a massive decrease in traditionally male jobs in mines, steel works and heavy industry. At the same time, there has been an increase in such jobs as retailing, insurance and banking. These are seen as being more suited to women.

Case study

Dave

Dave is 47 years old and, until two months ago, worked in the local steel works. He started working there when he was 17 years old. He was the foreman and used to enjoy his job. Since the steel works closed down he has been very fed up. His wife has asked him to go to the job centre to see what jobs are available. Dave was horrified when he went – he was offered work at the local supermarket on the checkout or a job in the office of a local company. He was also told his chances of getting a job would be better if he could use a computer. Dave has told his wife that 'these sorts of jobs are not for him'.

▶ 1. What does Dave mean when he says these jobs are not for him?
2. Do you agree with Dave?
3. What would you say if you were married to Dave?
4. What do you think Dave should do to get a job again?

▶ 1. How is Dave demonstrating traditional ideas concerning the issue of gender?

Family relationships

A family is a social group made up of people who are 'related' to each other. This means that other people (society) recognise that this group is related. In British society, 'family' is the word used to describe groups where adults act as parents or guardians to children. Belonging to a family can have many advantages – family relationships can provide a safe, caring setting for children. Family groups can guide and teach children, and they can provide a source of social and emotional support for adults and older family members (see Figure 12.1).

There are four different types of family.

The extended family

This type of family consists of three (or even four) generations of one family (i.e. grandparents, parents and children). They may live together or very near to each other and maintain very regular contact. This type of family is less common in today's society. The extended family provides a strong support network so that individuals are less likely to require help from outside agencies such as social services or Meals on Wheels. Grandparents may look after children while parents work. In return, children may run errands for a sick or elderly relative. Such families are more common in some ethnic communities in Britain.

The nuclear family

This family includes two parents (who may be married or cohabiting) and their children. In developed countries such as Britain, this type of family is more common than the extended family. When watching the television it seems as though the majority of people live in families like these: in fact, the nuclear family represents only 23% of households. These days it is common for both parents (or neither) to work. Although the nuclear family may not live near other generations of the family, members of the family still stay in good contact – by phone, visits and e-mail.

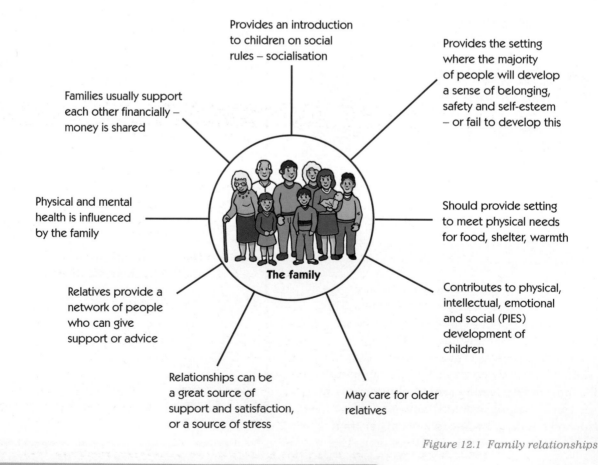

Provides an introduction to children on social rules – socialisation

Provides the setting where the majority of people will develop a sense of belonging, safety and self-esteem – or fail to develop this

Families usually support each other financially – money is shared

Physical and mental health is influenced by the family

The family

Should provide setting to meet physical needs for food, shelter, warmth

Relatives provide a network of people who can give support or advice

Contributes to physical, intellectual, emotional and social (PIES) development of children

Relationships can be a great source of support and satisfaction, or a source of stress

May care for older relatives

Figure 12.1 Family relationships

The lone-parent family

This consists of one parent (90% are female) and their children. There are three causes of one-parent families:

- The parent has been widowed.
- The parent is divorced or separated.
- The parent has never been married to the parent of her children.

In 2000 there were over 1.5 million one-parent families in Britain, involving 2.8 million children under 16 years of age. These families are more likely to live in poverty because it can be more difficult for a lone parent to work and earn money (see Figure 12.2).

The reconstituted family

In this type of family, individuals with children form a relationship with a person who may or may not have children from a previous relationship. As a consequence, the family has at least one step-parent. The adults may go on to have a child or children together. About 6 million people live in reconstituted families in Britain.

However, families do not remain the same and children may live in more than one type of family in their childhood. A child may live in a nuclear family until his or her parents divorce, live in a one-parent family with his or her father and then in a reconstituted family if his or her father remarries.

> ### Activity
>
> ▶ Select one of the types of family described above. It might be easier to choose the one you are most familiar with. List the advantages and disadvantages of the type of family you have chosen (e.g. in an extended family there can be a number of adults to give advice).
>
> ▷ Now get together in small groups. Discuss the advantages and disadvantages of each type of family. Select one person who is prepared to share the group's views on each type of family with the rest of the class.

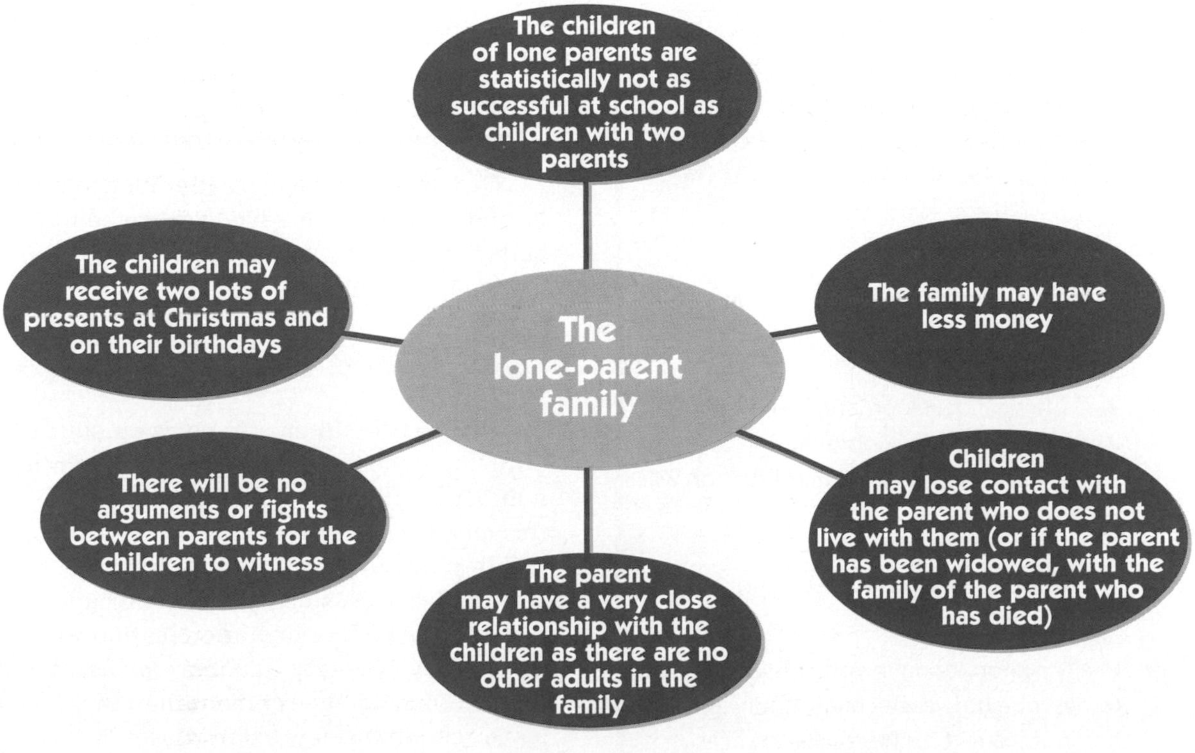

Figure 12.2 The lone-parent family

Case study

Anil

Anil is 8 years old and was born into a family where his parents had good jobs and enough money for lots of toys, books and computers. Anil learned to play on his father's computer when he was only 3 years old. This has helped him to learn. Anil always has someone to talk to at home because he lives with his sister and grandparents in a large house. The family is happy and Anil can go out on his cycle and play with friends in the local park. Anil's family are not afraid of crime in their neighbourhood. Anil is doing very well at school. He has many friends and enjoys school. Anil does not miss school very often.

Rick

Rick is 8 years old and was born into a family where both his parents had difficulty in finding work. Because Rick's parents cannot get jobs, there is not much money for toys, books or computers. Rick lives in a crowded block of flats on a housing estate. Rick's mother does not let him out to play because she is afraid of the crime and drug-taking that take place on the estate.

Rick's mother has periods of depression when she does not talk to Rick. Rick is often unhappy because he has few friends and he gets bored indoors. Rick often gets colds and misses a lot of school. Rick is like one third of children who grow up in low-income households. He does not have the same chance of a happy and wealthy life as Anil.

▶ Use the ideas you looked at in Chapter 11 to explain how Anil's home situation will affect his:
  1   physical development; and
  2   intellectual development.
  Now explain how Rick's home situation will affect his:
  1   physical development;
  2   intellectual development; and
  3   social development.

▶ Use the information in your answers above to describe how each child's family and home will affect his future life chances.

Friendships

Friendships play an important role in our lives as they provide us with social and emotional support. We tend to become friends with people whom we think are like ourselves, with similar values and attitudes. Female and male friendships are rather different. Female friendships tend to be emotionally closer, sharing feelings and opinions and acting as emotional support in times of trouble. Male friendships tend to be based around shared interests or activities, such as going fishing together or playing on the same football team.

Activity

▶ Get into small groups. Each group should, if possible, include at least one member of the opposite sex. Discuss how friendships between boys and girls differ. Be prepared to share your ideas with the rest of the class.

▶ As they get older, students are more likely to have friends (not girl or boyfriends) of the opposite sex. Try to explain what each sex gains from its friendships with members of the opposite sex. Does it change the way you view the world? Is it important to have friends of the opposite sex? Put your conclusions in your file.

Our friends have a great influence on us. Friends improve our social life, make us feel better about ourselves and provide practical help and advice.

Educational experiences

By law, every child must receive an education until he or she is 16 years old. Except for a tiny number of children who are educated at home, this means children attend school. Although all children must receive an education, not all will be equally successful. As a generalisation, those who go on to further education will earn more. They will work in a more pleasant and secure working environment than those who leave school with few exam passes (see Figure 12.3).

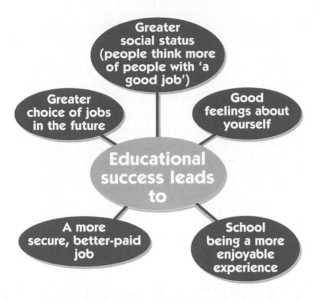

Figure 12.3 *The benefits of educational success*

The reasons why some students succeed in school and others do not are varied and complicated. Poverty, parental attitude and cultural difference between home and school can all have an effect.

Once in school, the child's success will be affected by the quality of teaching. Schools in affluent areas tend to attract good teachers. Pupils who attend schools in less affluent areas may have teachers who are less interested or less able to keep good discipline. This is likely to affect the pupils' success in school.

Educational experiences have a great effect on an individual's chances in life. However, there is now a greater understanding of the problems some children have in school so there are more chances for adults to return to education and acquire qualifications they did not gain in school.

Employment/unemployment

Checkpoint

Employment means to have a job (usually outside the home) for which you are paid. **Self-employed** people work for themselves and earn money from this work.

To be in work or to be self-employed provides people with the following benefits. People:

* receive an income. The larger this is, the more expensive the home, car, holidays, etc., people and their families can afford;
* gain social status in the eyes of others. We tend to be impressed by people who have 'a good job' (e.g. a solicitor);
* gain positive feelings about themselves because they feel they are contributing to society; and
* have a busy life (although this may leave them with less time for leisure activities).

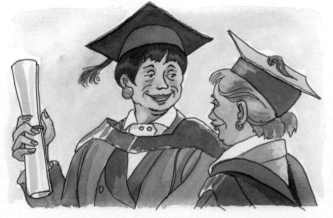

Nowadays it is never too late to gain educational qualifications

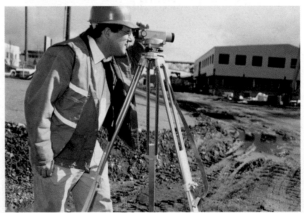

Work gives people social status and money for material possessions

People who are in regular employment, therefore, gain many benefits from having a job. In contrast, those who are unemployed suffer in the following ways:

- They have less money for their home and to spend on leisure activities. This can have an effect on diet, quality of housing and treats for the children and the family.
- The unemployed lose their status in society, as we tend to regard anyone in a job (no matter how low paid) as of higher status than those without a job.
- Unemployed people can lose their positive feelings about themselves. They feel that society does not need them because they are not joining in the world of work.

Within all types employment, those with more qualifications tend to earn more than those with fewer qualifications. Men on average earn more than women and white people tend to earn more than members of ethnic groups.

Ethnicity and religion

Checkpoint

Ethnicity is used to describe a group of people who share the same way of life and culture. A **religion** is a set of beliefs, often focused on one individual being (e.g. God, Allah), that might guide a person's behaviour.

An individual's life and way of behaving are often influenced by his or her religious beliefs. Very often, one of the things a group of people will have in common is their religion. For instance, many members of the Asian communities are Muslims, Hindus or Sikhs. Many members of white Caucasian communities are Christians. It is therefore reasonable to link ethnicity and religion together to see if these factors affect a person's life chances.

Checkpoint

Ethnic means belonging to a certain race or culture. An **ethnic minority** is a group of people who belong to a different race or who share a different culture from the majority of the people in the society in which they live.

Research has shown that ethnicity and religion have a major effect on a person's opportunities. People who belong to ethnic minorities tend to have poorer housing than the general population. When they go to school, overall, members of ethnic groups tend to do less well than the white population. In Britain, about 40% of Asians and 25% of those of African-Caribbean origin get five or more C grade GCSEs, compared to 45% of white students. However, Indian girls tend to do considerably better than other Asian groups (both girls and boys). Girls of African-Caribbean origin are much more successful than boys of African-Caribbean origin.

Life experiences

Birth

As we have already seen, the family a child is born into has a great effect on the life chances of that child. A child born into a loving home will have the following advantages:

- The child's parents will love and care for him or her. The child will have a good diet and warm clothes. He or she will make sure he or she goes to bed at a sensible time so he or she has enough sleep.
- The child will have toys and things to play with and to stimulate him or her.
- The child's parents will encourage him or her to play with other children so that he or she learns how to get on with people.

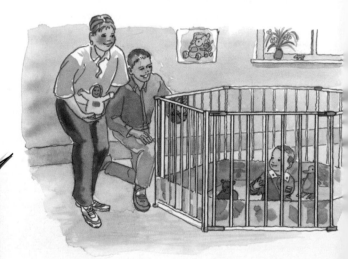

A loving home gives a child the best possible start in life

- When the child goes to school, his or her parents will be interested in his or her progress.
- They will make sure the child does not watch unsuitable TV programs and videos when he or she is young as they may scare or upset him or her.
- The child's parents will not hit him or her if he or she does something naughty but, instead, will find some other way of showing him or her that he or she has done wrong.

All these actions will help the child to have the best possible start in life. This will enable the child to make the most of his or her opportunities and be a successful, happy adult.

Activity

▶ Take the list above. Explain how each of these advantages will help the child to grow into a happy and successful adult. You could list each factor under the headings PIES.

▶ Use each of the advantages listed above to identify features of a poor home in which to raise a child. Explain how these features would affect the child's development. Again, this could be done in terms of the PIES.

Marriage

Although there is an increasing number of people who cohabit (live with a member of the opposite sex in a monogamous, sexual relationship), most of the population – between 75% and 80% – will marry at some point in their lives. The reasons why people marry are shown in Figure 12.4.

Even today, marriage seems to favour men rather than women. Married men live to a greater old age than single men. Single women live longer than married women.

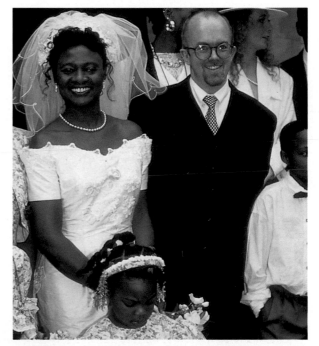

Some 60% of marriages in Britain last 'until death do us part'

To make a public statement about the feelings they have for each other

To have a big party (perhaps not the best reason!)

To gain legal protection and benefits (important if the relationship breaks down)

The reasons why people get married

To ensure their children are legitimate (this is much less important than it was but still matters when money is inherited, for example)

Because of their religious beliefs

To please their parents and family and to gain approval from society

Figure 12.4 The reasons why people get married

Divorce

In Britain, the divorce rate has doubled in the last 30 years. In 2000, a total of 142,500 children under 16 years of age old were in families whose parents had divorced. Some 25% of these children were under 5 years of age. Only the death of a close relative is ranked higher as a cause of stress for an individual. The reasons for the increase in the divorce rate include the following:

- Women have greater independence and better jobs than they used to. They do not need a man to provide a home for them like they did 50 years ago.
- Women are less tolerant of men who do not treat them well (in 1997, approximately 52% of women gave their husband's unreasonable behaviour as a reason for the divorce).
- Changes in the law have made it easier to get a divorce.
- There is less social disapproval of people who get divorced. People who divorced used to try to keep it a secret.
- People travel more so there is greater chance of them marrying someone of a different culture, which increases the chances of the marriage not lasting.

Children of parents who divorce are likely to live with their mother, and a large number of them will lose contact with their father after only two years. For the adults themselves, both men and women are likely to have less money after the divorce. This is because each now has to pay for a home instead of sharing the expense of one house.

Children of divorced parents are twice as likely to do badly in school or to have mental health problems when older. They are more likely to drink and smoke heavily and to take drugs. They are also more likely to be divorced themselves. However, some people believe these problems can be caused by the arguments that lead to divorce as well as the divorce itself. They say that an unhappy couple staying together 'for the sake of the children' is as harmful to them as simply separating and divorcing.

Death

During the last 200 years, there has been a dramatic decrease in the *death rate*. This is due to:

- better housing;
- cleaner water;
- better diet;
- the care we receive from the NHS;
- the introduction of vaccination programmes; and
- improved medicines and operations.

> ### Checkpoint
> The **death rate** is the number of deaths per 1,000 people in the population. Wealthy countries such as Britain have a lower death rate than poorer, less developed countries.

Death of a child

This is likely to be painful for all family members. For a long time the parents may feel unable to enjoy life, to laugh or to have fun because they still feel so saddened by the loss of the child. These feelings may last months or even years.

Death of a parent of young children

When a parent of children still living at home dies, the children will experience sad feelings at the loss. If their parents lived together in a nuclear family, suddenly the children are part of a lone-parent family. Eventually, the lone parent may meet a new partner so the children could become part of a reconstituted family.

Death of a partner

In a happy, stable relationship, the death of a partner is bound to be traumatic for the person who remains. For an elderly couple, who have been married for many years, it is difficult to make a new life as a single person again. The situation may bring practical problems as elderly couples are often able to manage in their own home if there are two of them but feel unable to cope alone.

Check your knowledge

1 What are the benefits (other than money) of having a job?
2 Which groups of people in society are most likely to earn low wages?
3 What does 'ethnicity' mean?
4 How does ethnicity affect a person's life chances?
5 Give five advantages of a loving home for a child.
6 Why do people get married?
7 Why has the divorce rate increased?
8 What problems can arise for the children of divorced parents?
9 How would the death of a parent affect a young child?
10 Describe the problems that can occur when a partner dies.

Economic factors

People do not all have an equal chance to develop their skills and abilities: some are born into a life that holds fewer opportunities than the lives of others.

In 1999, the DSS (now the Department for Work and Pensions) published a report called *Opportunity for All*. In this report the government states: 'Our aim is to end the injustice which holds people back and prevents them from making the most of themselves.' The government says its goal is 'that everyone should have the opportunity to achieve their potential. But too many people are denied that opportunity. It is wrong and economically inefficient to waste the talents of even one single person'.

Checkpoint

When we discuss **economic factors**, we are always discussing money or the cost of things to buy or make.

Income and material possessions

Checkpoint

Income is the money people receive from their work, their savings, their pension or from benefits from the state.
Material possessions are objects people can go to the shops to buy that are not usually essential (such as videos and designer-label clothing).

Everyone has to pay for essentials such as housing, food and clothing. Wealthy people are likely to have a far wider range of material possessions than the poor as, once essentials have been paid for, money left over can be spent on the things people want (not to be confused with need, though we often do). The people who are most likely to be poor are the very young, the elderly, people who are unemployed and members of the ethnic communities. Women are more likely to be poor than men.

Wealth includes:

● savings in bank accounts or building societies;
● the value of your home if you own it;
● shares, life assurances and pension rights; and
● any other property that belongs to you.

Wealth is not shared out evenly in the UK. The poorest half of the population only own 8% of the country's wealth and property. The top 1% of the richest people own 19% of the UK's wealth. The richest 10% of the population own 50% of the wealth.

Activity

The government recently sent some British soldiers to help keep the peace in a country in Africa. One soldier was killed. At the time, his long-term girlfriend was pregnant and she has now had a baby girl. The girlfriend wants the army to pay her a widow's pension. She would have received this automatically if she had been married to the soldier when he died.

Do you think the army should give her a pension? Discuss her situation with members of the class. Make a list of the reasons for and against giving her a pension.

Check your knowledge

1 What is income?
2 What are material possessions?
3 Which groups of people in society are more likely to have low incomes?

Environmental factors

Checkpoint ✓

Our **environment** is the place around us. This can simply mean our home. Alternatively, it can mean a larger geographical area such as the neighbourhood in which we live or the town our neighbourhood is apart of.

Housing conditions

You have already looked at how poor housing can affect people. Figures 12.5 and 12.6 show how a poor neighbourhood and poor housing can affect an individual.

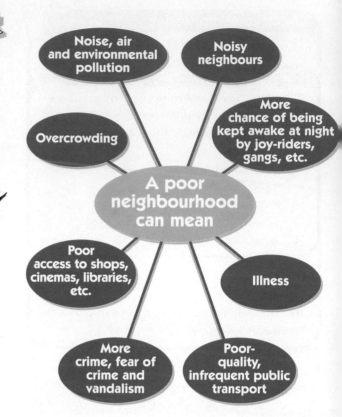

A poor neighbourhood can mean

- Noise, air and environmental pollution
- Noisy neighbours
- More chance of being kept awake at night by joy-riders, gangs, etc.
- Overcrowding
- Illness
- Poor access to shops, cinemas, libraries, etc.
- More crime, fear of crime and vandalism
- Poor-quality, infrequent public transport

Figure 12.5 A poor neighbourhood can affect the quality of a person's life

Door hinged outward to create space (safety hazard)

Windows kept shut to conserve warmth – resulting in poor ventilation

Overcrowded bedroom – helps spread airborne infection when combined with poor ventilation

Portable electric fire (Safety hazard)

Poor maintenance of building – increased accident risk

Damp patch on wall from broken gutters outside – risk of infection from fungal spores

Poor lighting

Poor hygiene maintenance of bathroom facilities (lack of cleaning agents) – increased risk of skin and other contagious diseases, especially if facilities are shared

Overcrowding may increase interpersonal stress and, coupled with other stressors, may lead to poor mental health

Figure 12.6 Poor housing can affect the quality of a person's life

Pollution

Checkpoint

Pollution is a general term used to describe the spoiling of our environment (e.g. carbon monoxide from cars is responsible for polluting the air).

Pollutants are anything that causes pollution. Many of these pollutants can affect a person's health. Some pollutants cause harmful physical effects (e.g. lead particles in the air can affect the development of babies' brains).

Access to health and welfare services

Some people have poor health and well-being because their access to health and welfare services is not as good as it should be. Such services include GPs surgeries, social services and benefit offices. The reasons for this are varied:

- People who are poor may lack confidence when dealing with the professional staff (doctors, nurses, social workers, etc.) who work in the service.
- Some people may be embarrassed at their low reading age. As a result, they may avoid using the services in case they are asked to read leaflets or fill in forms.
- If English is not their first language, people can find it difficult to describe their worries or problems when asking for help. They will also have difficulty in reading information leaflets and in filling in forms.
- They may have to use public transport, which means that simply getting to a health centre or benefit office can be difficult.
- Women in certain ethnic groups may not feel comfortable dealing with male members of staff and so may be reluctant to approach the staff to gain assistance.

All these reasons mean that some people do not gain the help they need from health and welfare services that could improve their quality of life.

Check your knowledge

1 What do we mean by the 'environment'?
2 Give five problems of living in low-income housing.
3 How does living in a poor neighbourhood affect people?
4 What is pollution?
5 Give four reasons to explain why the poor have more difficulty in gaining access to health and welfare services.

How factors interrelate to affect an individual

You have now looked at the different factors that affect a person's growth and development. All these factors *interrelate* (combine together) to affect your growth and development. Because we all have a different mix of these factors, we all develop differences in how we react to things and how we behave.

The next section of this chapter looks at how these factors affect the following aspects of our lives:

- Self esteem.
- Physical and mental health.
- Employment prospects.
- Level of education.

Self-esteem

Checkpoint

Self-esteem means how you value yourself. We all have an opinion of ourselves (e.g. 'I've got nice hair', 'I'm good at PE', 'I'm not good at meeting new people'). We may never share this view of ourselves with other people. If the view is realistic and generally positive then we will have high self-esteem.

Self-esteem is important because it helps us cope with the problems we all experience in our everyday lives (e.g. failing exams, being made redundant, breaking up with a boy or girlfriend). Parents are very important in the

Young people with high self-esteem	Young people with low self-esteem
Parents are interested in them	Parents are less interested in them
Parents expect them to do well	Parents are less strict with them
Parents are reasonably strict and make it clear to their children how they should behave	Parents do not know the names of their children's friends
Children set themselves high targets to achieve	Children set themselves lower targets
Children often meet their high targets	Children are generally less successful
Children are confident in expressing their opinions	Children don't give their opinions in case others disagree with them
Children are generally successful	Children are more likely to be ill, especially with headaches and stomach upsets

Reprduced with permission from Hayes, N. (1993) *The Principles of Social Psychology,* Hove: Psychology Press

Figure 12.7 The effects of high and low self-esteem in young people

development of high self-esteem in their children (see Figure 12.7).

Physical factors that contribute to self-esteem

- People who are good looking are often thought to be more intelligent or interesting than plain people.
- A fit body looks and feels good.
- Being a member of a sports team increases the chance of friendship and improves social life.
- A healthy family gets maximum enjoyment and benefits from life.

Social and emotional factors that contribute to self-esteem

- Parents should regard both boys and girls as equally important.

- When family relationships are strong, people care for each other. Parents take an interest in all aspects of their children's lives.
- Close friendships make us feel good about ourselves and help us if things go wrong.
- Religion provides a support and set of beliefs to live by, which is especially useful if things are going wrong.
- Being a member of a religious community provides more opportunity for friendship as people are drawn together by shared beliefs.
- Our ethnic background gives us support (as long as we don't suffer prejudice or discrimination).
- In a strong relationship, the couple look after each other and provide support for each other.

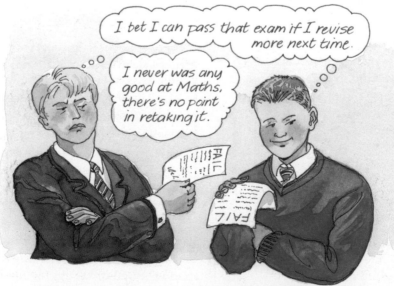

The different effects of self-esteem on an individual

Economic factors that contribute to self-esteem

- Buying children educational toys and games increases their chances of educational success.
- Taking children on visits to interesting places and holidays gives children new experiences.
- Having enough money to buy what our friends have helps us to feel we fit in.

Environmental factors that contribute to self-esteem

- A clean, comfortable home helps us to have good health. We sleep better and recover from illnesses more quickly.
- An unpolluted environment is more pleasant to live in and helps promote good health.
- Good health and welfare services provide assistance if things go wrong so that problems are solved more easily.
- We are pleased to bring friends back to a nice home, which helps to build close friendships.

Few people are lucky enough to gain all the advantages shown above. What affects our self-esteem is the balance between good and less good factors in our lives. Sometimes one or two positive factors can outweigh many other negative aspects of our lives so that we can achieve success despite a difficult background.

Check your knowledge

1 What is self-esteem?
2 How does high self-esteem benefit children?
3 How does low self-esteem disadvantage children?
4 Describe three physical factors that affect self-esteem.
5 Describe five social and emotional factors that affect self-esteem.
6 Describe three economic and social factors that affect self-esteem.
7 Describe three environmental factors that affect self-esteem.

Physical and mental health

Illnesses can be divided into groups by looking at how serious they are.

Physical illnesses

Physical illnesses can be grouped in the following way:

1 Short-term infectious illnesses such as colds, 'flu', stomach upsets and measles.
2 Longer-term illnesses that may disrupt school attendance, including glandular fever, TB and pleurisy.
3 Chronic illnesses the patient has to 'learn to live with' (e.g. asthma, arthritis, psoriasis and angina). These illnesses can be helped with drugs and other treatments such as physiotherapy.
4 The diseases that often end in the death of the sufferer, such as cancers, heart and circulatory problems and kidney failure.

Mental illnesses

These illnesses can be grouped in different ways, but the simplest way is to classify them depending upon their severity (i.e. those illnesses that still allow the patient to take part in everyday life and those illnesses that do not). In these more serious illnesses, the patient cannot hold down a job or college place, cannot maintain a relationship or, at worst, cannot even look after him or herself.

For example, depression can be successfully treated with drugs so that the patient can still go to work and carry out his or her daily routine. However, at its worst, a patient with depression may need hospital treatment. Many mental illnesses respond well to long-term drug treatments that, along with various therapies such as counselling, can keep these illnesses at a manageable level.

Physical factors that affect physical and mental health

- It is believed that we can inherit the chances of getting some illnesses (e.g. the chances of getting breast cancer increase if a close relative has suffered from it).
- A poor diet affects the body in a variety of different ways (see the section on diet).
- Children in large families are more likely to catch infections from each other.
- Caring for a sick person at home can cause the carer to become ill due to lack of sleep,

lifting the patient, etc.

- If a member of the family is suffering from illness, relatives can become distressed and anxious.

Social and emotional factors that affect physical and mental health

- Women are more health conscious than men. There are more 'well woman' clinics and they are better used than 'well man' clinics. However, women are more likely to suffer mental health problems.
- Men drink more than women. More teenage girls smoke than teenage boys.
- Some jobs carry physical risks (e.g. miners often suffer from lung diseases).
- Some illnesses are linked to certain ethnic groups (e.g. African-Caribbean people can suffer from sickle cell anaemia).
- Intermarriage between family members is more common in some ethnic groups. This increases the chance of inherited diseases in their children.
- Some jobs (such as the police, teaching and the prison service) are recognised to be more stressful than others.
- Members of ethnic groups may suffer discrimination or racial abuse. This can lead to depression.
- Children of divorced parents are more likely to suffer mental illness in later life.
- The loss of a partner, relative or close friend can cause unhappiness, which may develop into depression.

Economic factors that affect physical and mental health

- A greater income means that people live in a warmer, more comfortable home, which promotes good health.
- More money means a family can have regular holidays.
- Lack of money causes stress and anxiety as people struggle to pay for essential items.

Environmental factors that affect physical and mental health

- Damp, poorly maintained homes increase the chance of physical illnesses such as colds and chest infections.
- Overcrowding increases the chances of infectious illnesses spreading.

- Children in tower blocks have limited access to play areas, which makes them irritable and depressed.
- Noise and other types of pollution can cause physical and mental ill-health.
- Greater access to health and welfare services increases the chance of better care for all types of illnesses.

Case study

Amy

Amy lives in a small terraced house with her baby sister, older brother and her parents. The house is near a factory and the workers often wake her up as they pass at the beginning and end of the night shift. Amy has to share a room with her sister, which means she must do her homework downstairs as her sister is put to bed earlier than she is. The house is very old and gets cold in the winter because there is no insulation. The family does not have a garden, only a small backyard. Amy has been to the homes of some of her friends but is not keen to invite them to her own home. This is because she is embarrassed about its size and condition.

▶ 1 How will Amy's housing affect her success at school?
  2 What effect could the home have on the health and well-being of the rest of the family?

▶ 1 How could the house affect her physical and mental health?
  2 How will Amy's home affect her emotionally and socially?

Check your knowledge

1 Describe how physical factors affect our physical and mental health.
2 Read the list of social and economic factors that affect health. Choose the five factors you consider to be most important. Describe each of them and try to explain why you think they are the most important.
3 Describe how economic factors can affect physical and mental health.

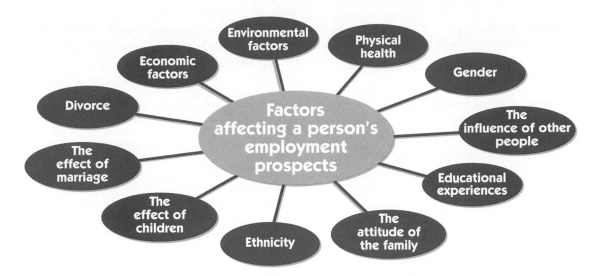

Figure 12.8 Factors that affect a person's employment prospects

Employment prospects

A person's *employment prospects* are the chances a person has of getting a good, well paid job that interests him or her, and the chances of that person keeping the job, once he or she has started it (see Figure 12.8).

Physical health

If you are to have and hold down a good job it is important you are as healthy as possible. Employers need reliable employees who do not take time off regularly. People who take a lot of time off get a reputation for unreliability and are less likely to get a good reference if they apply for a new job.

Gender

In the world of work, women are disadvantaged in relation to men. They earn, on average, 80% of male wages and are more likely to work part time. As we will see, girls achieve much better results in school exams but they do not carry this advantage through the workplace. There are many reasons for this:

- Women may take a career break to look after small children. This means they fall behind on the promotion ladder.
- There seems to be a *glass ceiling* in many workplaces. This means that many women work their way up in their company or workplace until they reach a certain point and then, for some reason, they don't get any further.
- Part-time employees are less likely to be promoted. As more women work part time than men, this penalises women.
- Men may simply prefer to work with other men. They therefore find reasons not to promote women. This is illegal, but in view of the small numbers of women in senior positions at work, it seems likely this does go on.

However, there have been great improvements in women's opportunities in the workplace as there has been an increase in jobs in shops, banking, sales and insurance. Women are believed to be more suited to these types of jobs.

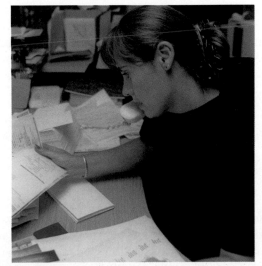

There has been an increase in job opportunities for women

The influence of other people

We are all greatly affected by the people we come into contact with. If all your friends can use a computer confidently, it is likely you will want to be able to do so also. If our friends take their work seriously, it is more likely we will do too. This helps a person's employment prospects.

Many people find work through friends, relatives and contacts. An older member of the family may offer to look out for any vacancies at his or her workplace. A family connection of this type gives a person the 'edge' over another.

Educational experiences

There are many examples of people being very successful in their careers in spite of a lack of qualifications. However, generally speaking, good results from school that lead on to a university degree or further qualifications are a great help when trying to get a good job. These days it is expected that employees should be keen to improve their skills. People have to be prepared to gain new skills if their job demands it.

The attitude of the family

Young people whose parents have a strong *work ethic* (belief in the value of work) are most likely to find a job. There are some families where no one has worked for many years and young people from such families are less likely to find work. In such families, unemployment is a way of life and there is less pressure put on the younger members of the family to find a job.

Ethnicity

Members of ethnic groups are more likely to have fewer well paid jobs, to work shifts and to be unemployed. As we have seen, these are generalisations and do not apply to both sexes and to all ethnic groups. For example, African-Caribbean boys are less likely to be in higher-status jobs than African-Caribbean girls. These girls also outperform boys in school. People of Indian origin are more likely to be in high-status jobs than Bangladeshi people.

Life experiences

The effect of children

After the birth of a child, many women take a break from work. The woman may miss out on new initiatives, training or promotion.

The effect of marriage

In contrast to childbirth, marriage is likely to benefit employment prospects as married people are seen as having responsibilities that will cause them to take their work more seriously.

Divorce

Divorce is an extremely upsetting experience. However, once the initial trauma is over, the divorced person may feel free to devote more time and effort to his or her career. This will increase his or her chances of promotion or of gaining a better position somewhere else.

Economic factors

There is evidence to suggest that those people who have more money are likely to have better job prospects than those who are poor. People who live in *poverty* (have very little money) are more likely to have feelings of hopelessness, which means they believe there is no possibility of changing their difficult circumstances. As a result, they may be less likely to try to find work.

At a simple level, having more money and some material possessions can improve the chances of finding a job, for the following reasons:

- A person with a car can travel longer distances to find work.
- Access to the Internet means a person has another place to look for vacancies.
- Word-processed job applications look better than hand-written letters.
- Poorer people may have fewer smart clothes to wear at interviews.

Environmental factors

In every large town there are areas or estates known for their high numbers of social problems (e.g. vandalism and high crime rates). Local employers can be prejudiced against people who live in such well-known areas. For people from these areas trying to find work, their postcode may a problem they have to overcome.

People who live in the country or any area that has poor public transport will encounter difficulties in finding work, in comparison with those people in towns or who own a car. They have to travel longer distances to get to work. They may not have easy access to an FE college so that gaining qualifications or re-training are very difficult for them.

Check your knowledge

1 What do we mean by 'employment prospects'?
2 Why is employment important?
3 Why are women disadvantaged at work in relation to men?
4 How do your friends affect your attitude to work?
5 How can your friends and family help you get a job?
6 How do family attitudes to work affect the individual?
7 How does ethnicity affect employment prospects?
8 How do children affect a mother's employment prospects?
9 How does divorce affect the person's employment prospects?
10 How can living in poverty make it harder to get a job?

Level of education

'Level of education' refers to the point at which people leave education and the examination results and qualifications they have when they leave. A person can leave school in the summer after his or her sixteenth birthday. In reality, most will either return to school or the local college in the autumn or go into training and education supported by the government or an employer.

Nowadays, employees of all ages are encouraged to go on courses to update their knowledge and skills. Education is seen as an ongoing process all adults of working age should take part in. The government calls this 'lifelong learning'. Because of this, to talk of 'level of education' is rather misleading because many adults may raise their level of educational achievement in their 40s or 50s, after having achieved little in school when they were young.

Physical factors that affect the level of education

- Some people believe that intelligent parents will have intelligent children (remember the nature and nurture argument?).
- A balanced diet and physical exercise contribute to good health. This means students have less time off school so they don't fall behind.
- If there is a sick member of the family, attention may be focused upon them. Children will lose interest in school if no one is interested in their progress.

Social and emotional factors that affect the level of education

- Girls develop earlier so have the maturity to cope with the demands of school. They are more likely to see a purpose to passing exams and work harder for them.
- Many boys long to be seen by others as 'hard'. This means boys tend to *underachieve* (i.e. do less well than their actual ability).
- Some parents allow their children to miss school to help them at home or to provide company for themselves. Missing school regularly leaves the child confused when he or she returns, making more absences likely.
- Young people are much influenced by their friends. If someone's friends are anti-school, it is difficult for a person to work hard because he or she risks being left out of the group.
- A good school, with firm discipline and enthusiastic, committed teachers, will

ensure all children achieve as much as they can.

- If the child lives in an area of high unemployment, he or she may make less effort because the child knows his or her efforts will give him or her little advantage in difficult economic circumstances.
- Girls under the school-leaving age who become pregnant are unlikely to be able to complete their education. As they have a baby to care for, it is very difficult for them to return to education after the baby's birth.
- Statistically, children of divorced parents do not do as well at school as the children of parents who stay together.

Economic factors that affect the level of education

- When each child has a room of his or her own, children are able to get on with homework without interruption from the TV or other family members.
- Wealthier parents may send their children (under school age) to a nursery. This can give them a good start when they go to infant school.
- Parents in higher income families are able to buy their children educational toys when they are young and computers when they are older.
- Children of parents with good, well paid jobs will probably want to have the same standard of living for themselves when they are adults. They are therefore more likely to work hard to achieve it. However, poverty may provide children with a drive to escape their poor background.
- Some able children from poorer families do not go to university because they don't want to run up large debts they will have to pay off when they start work. Better off parents can help their children financially when they are at university. These children are therefore more likely to attend university.

Environmental factors that affect the level of education

- Overcrowding can lead to tensions in the home, which can make schoolwork seem very unimportant. Children will therefore not do as well in school as they should.

- Noise from neighbours can disrupt sleep, leaving the child too tired to concentrate in school the next day.

Case study

Shahiid

Shahiid lives with his parents and younger brother in a large detached house, about two miles from a large town. The house is on an estate where there are several other families with children, so he has several friends nearby. His home has a garden and he has his own bedroom. He and his brother use the spare bedroom as a 'playroom' (as his mother calls it) where they have a computer between them. His parents got fed up of sharing theirs with the boys! His parents both work in their business and so the family has a cleaning lady who comes twice a week. The family enjoy their regular summer holiday and now the boys are older they have started going on shorter holidays at half-term to visit foreign cities.

1. List the factors that indicate Shahiid is likely to achieve educational success.
2. Take each factor you have identified in turn. Explain how each factor would increase the chances of Shahiid's educational success.

1. How will educational success affect Shahiid's self-esteem?
2. How will educational success affect Shahiid's employment prospects?

Check your knowledge

1. What do you think the government means by 'lifelong learning'?
2. Suggest some reasons why girls do better in school than boys.
3. How can schools increase the chance of exam success for their students?
4. Describe the ways in which parents with more money can help their children achieve educational success.
5. Why are poorer children less likely to go to university?
6. Describe the environmental factors that affect a child's chance of educational success.

Effects of relationships on personal development

By the end of this chapter, you will have learnt that, throughout their lives, people have many different types of relationship. These include:

- family relationships (with parents, siblings and as parents);
- friendships;
- intimate personal and sexual relationships; and
- working relationships (including teacher/student, employer/employee, peers, colleagues).

You will find out which relationships play a key part in an individual's social and emotional development during each life stage. You will be able to identify how these relationships can have a positive or negative effect on personal development. You will also be able to identify what effect abuse, neglect and lack of support can have on personal development.

Throughout our lives, we are strongly affected by the relationships we have with others. The nature of these relationships changes as we grow older. For babies, for example, the relationship with one main carer is very important. For teenagers, relationships with friends become increasingly important. For adults, intimate personal and sexual relationships are significant. Let's look at the changing nature of relationships through the different life stages.

Relationships in infancy (0–3 years)

Babies at birth are totally helpless and need someone to provide them with food, warmth, shelter and safety. As a result of being cared for, the child begins to form his or her first relationships. Babies are born with certain simple abilities that enable them to begin to form relationships with others (see Figure 13.1).

The adult carer is encouraged by the reactions of the child to spend time with him or her, talking, cuddling and reassuring the child. As a result, the baby and his or her parents start to build their relationship.

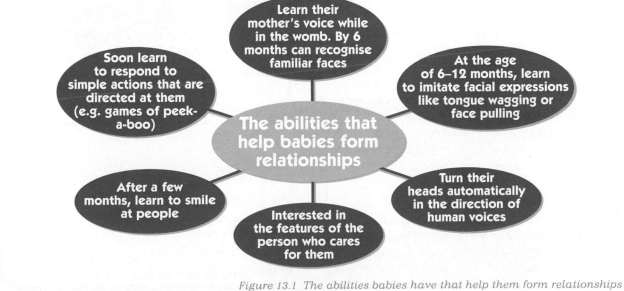

Figure 13.1 The abilities babies have that help them form relationships

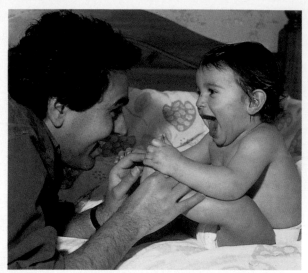

Babies have abilities that enable them to build relationships

Babies and family relationships

It is essential for the healthy development of the child that he or she forms a *bond* with at least one adult figure (usually the parents) who cares for him or her. The relationship between parent and child (or parent substitute) is the most important one the child will ever have. This is because it will determine the child's ability to form relationships with the other people with whom he or she comes into contact.

Parents and attachment relationships

The psychologist, John Bowlby, carried out many experiments with babies and their parents which enabled him to describe what he called an *attachment relationship*.

Checkpoint

An **attachment relationship** is formed between the child and one or two people who are the child's main carers. The relationship develops as the adult interacts with the child (i.e. talks, cuddles and looks at the child). An adult who simply feeds her or changes her nappy is not important enough to the child to be the person with whom the child will establish this key relationship.

The importance of attachment relationships

This type of relationship is very important to ensure the child develops into an emotionally secure adult. A good relationship between parent and child should result in the following positive effects on the child:

- The child will feel secure as his or her needs for food, warmth and safety have been met.
- He or she will begin to love and trust others.
- He or she will gain self-confidence when making the first moves towards independence (e.g. when starting to walk or beginning to feed him or herself).
- As he or she gets older, the child will have self-confidence at nursery school.
- He or she will settle into school happily and there will be fewer behaviour problems.

Grandparents

Research shows that it can be beneficial to the child to have more than one attachment relationship. It is possible that the child will form such a relationship with a grandparent if he or she sees him or her regularly. This is particularly good for the child if he or she is brought up in a one-parent family, as a grandparent can provide a *role model* to help replace an absent parent.

Checkpoint

A **role model** is someone a person can copy. There can be good and bad role models. Children learn how to behave as a boy or girl through copying adult behaviour. Parents and other adults act as role models for their children.

Siblings

The baby's relationships with his or her siblings (sisters and brothers) will vary, depending on the age gap between them and the degree of jealousy that exists. Research shows that small children learn how to tease and annoy their elder siblings at a very early age (around 12–15 months old). The relationship with siblings is the first the child has with a near equal. It provides an early opportunity for the child to begin to understand and influence other people in his or her own age group.

Friendships

Babies gradually develop a sense of themselves as individuals. It takes up to two years for the child to develop an understanding of him or herself and others. This is called having a *sense of self*. Until the child has acquired this ability, the child cannot begin to form relationships with other children. However, research with children aged between 12 and 18 months shows that children of this age are interested in others of the same age. This can be seen by the way they will look towards them, smile at them or make a noise to attract their attention.

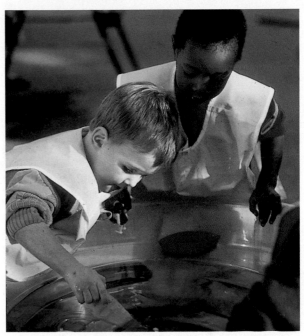

A child's 'peer group' are those children of a similar age

Checkpoint

A **peer group** is the people of the same age as the individual (e.g. a child's peer group could be the other children in his or her class).

When relationships go wrong

If the attachment relationship between parents and child is not adequate, problems may occur (see Figure 13.2). If the child encounters these problems there is a possibility he or she will start to show signs of emotional disturbance through his or her behaviour.

The signs of emotional disturbance include the following:

- The child is very anti-social: he or she hits, bites and is unpleasant to others.
- The child is very shy and is reluctant to leave the adult he or she is most familiar with.
- Intellectual development can be slowed down by a childhood that is very seriously deprived (see the section on abuse on page 216).
- The child develops physical behaviours, such as bed wetting (after previously being dry at night), rocking, head banging or pulling out his or her own hair.

Causes of emotional problems in babies

- Has many carers so unable to make an attachment with anyone
- Jealousy of a new baby, sibling or favouritism of one child above another by the parents
- Separation from the parent at a young age, when they have no understanding of the reason or of time
- New situations they are not ready for and cannot cope with (e.g. starting nursery school, being sent to stay with people with whom they are not familiar)
- If the parents are very young, they may not be able to provide the emotional security needed because they still have needs as children themselves

Figure 13.2 The causes of emotional problems in babies

Emotional behaviours such as these may stop as the child gets older, but if the problems are not resolved they may reappear in a different form (e.g. the child may start to steal or bully others when he or she gets to school).

Case study

Mandy

Mandy is 18 months old. She lives with her parents, Steph and Joe. After she had Mandy, Steph changed her job so she could work part time. Both she and Joe believe it would be better for Mandy if she was cared for mainly by Steph.

Mandy has been walking for about four months. She understands a lot of what is said to her and she is beginning to say her first words. Joe spends time with her when he gets home from work and takes her out on a Sunday morning so Steph can have a little time for herself. Steph takes Mandy to a mother and baby group on a Thursday morning. Steph enjoys meeting other young mums while Mandy plays alongside her.

▶ 1   Who is Mandy likely to form an attachment relationship with?
  2   Use the information from the case study to explain how this is likely to happen.
  3   Why does Mandy only 'play alongside' her mother?

▷ How will Mandy's upbringing help to increase her self-esteem?

Check your knowledge

Describe the abilities babies have which mean they can begin to form relationships.
1   What is an attachment relationship?
2   Whom do babies form attachment relationships with?
3   Why are attachment relationships important?
4   What is a role model?
5   What is a sense of self?
6   Describe five causes of emotional problems in babies.
7   Describe the behaviour of emotionally disturbed children.

Relationships in childhood (4–10 years)

As children get older, relationships with school friends and other adults will begin to be of importance.

Family

As the child gets older, the parents will begin to pass on more complex values and ways of behaving that will help the child become a well balanced, happy, useful member of society. During childhood the parents' role is to:

- be a good role model for the child and teach the child the difference between right and wrong;
- provide comfort when the child is worried or frightened of something;
- teach the child good manners and how to behave when meeting strangers or when in new situations;
- pass on the values of the society and group in which the child lives;
- help the child deal with strong and sometimes unpleasant feelings of hate, jealousy and dislike;
- give the child clear moral values about honesty, the way to treat others, telling the truth, etc.
- provide encouragement and help for the child so he or she feels able to tackle new challenges and cope with change satisfactorily (e.g. starting school, moving house, etc.); and
- continue to help the child develop self-esteem and self-worth through loving and caring for the child.

Friendships

By the time the child is 4 years old, he or she will be able to make friends with other children. Girls tend to become friendly with one or two others and the friendship can be intense. Boys tend to make more friends that link together in looser groups so that a boy is not so dependent on the company of a particular individual.

Friendships among younger children tend to be based upon common activities between children who simply live near each other. Children between the ages of 4 and 9 years have to learn that if friends do something for them, it is reasonable they should do something in return. At this age children fall out regularly. This is because they are not yet able fully to understand another child's point of view. It is only by the age of 12 that children understand fully that friendship is a two-way relationship.

Friendship helps to build self-esteem in the child. The feeling of being wanted and important to another person, and also feeling socially accepted by his or her peers, all help the child to feel good about him or herself.

Activity

▶ Think about the person with whom you were friendly at primary school. (You may still be friends with this person.) List the types of things you did together when you were 6 or 7 years old. Try to describe your friendship then.

▶ If you are still friends with the same person, try to describe how your friendship has changed over the years. If you are no longer friendly, describe why you drifted apart. Describe how your friendship has altered as you have got older, linking the changes to your intellectual and social development.

Friendships and a child's future

There has been found to be a clear link between high peer-group approval and low numbers of mental health problems in the child when he or she is older. Those children with few friends at a young age are far more likely to drop out of school when they get older. The ability to make friends, therefore, has an effect on the child's future opportunities.

Siblings

Many children are about 3 or 4 four years old when their parents decide to have another child. For the child who has been used to having all the parental attention up until now,

this can be a rather unpleasant change in his or her life. Some children will adapt well, as they may not resent the presence of the new baby, but others may be greatly upset by the new arrival and may show signs of jealousy.

If the introduction of a new baby to the house is not done with care and sensitivity, the feelings of jealousy will remain with the older child throughout his or her life. However, if managed carefully, the older child should gradually accept the baby without problems and begin to form a good relationship with him or her.

Teachers

In Britain, children start school around the age of 5 years. They will spend each year in primary school with, mainly, one teacher. As they spend so long in the company of one person, the relationship the child builds with that teacher is very significant. If the relationship is not one of trust and respect, the progress, achievement and happiness of the child will be badly affected throughout the whole of the year.

If the relationship is good, it will increase the child's positive feelings about him or herself and improve his or her self-esteem. A child with good self-esteem will have a strong sense of his or her own ability and value.

When relationships go wrong

Young children are not good at expressing their feelings so often their unhappiness will be shown through their behaviour. A child will become very unhappy if:

- he or she is being bullied by siblings or by other children;
- he or she feels unwanted or unloved;
- the parents separate or divorce;
- there is a death of someone to whom he or she was close; or
- the child is separated from his or her parents without fully understanding the reason for the separation.

It is not difficult to see that all the causes above stem from some failure in the relationships the child has with the people around him or her.

Signs that indicate a child is emotionally upset could include the following:

- The child is aggressive towards parents, other children or siblings. He or she may bully other children.
- The child is withdrawn and finds it difficult to socialise (mix with others).
- The child's behaviour regresses (returns to the behaviour of a younger child) – e.g. he or she starts to wet the bed again.
- The child becomes 'clingy' and seems reluctant to leave the company of a parent.
- An older child may become sullen and argumentative.

Check your knowledge

1 Describe five values that parents should pass on to their children.
2 How do girls' and boys' friendships differ?
3 What is the value of friendships to the child?
4 How does success in school help a child's development?
5 How do unhappy children express their feelings?
6 Describe the behaviour of an emotionally disturbed child.

Relationships in adolescence (11–18 years)

By the time a child has reached adolescence, the number of people he or she comes into contact with will have become much greater. This means he or she will be forming more relationships than previously.

Parents

During the teenage years, the relationship between child and parent is still the most important one in the child's life. The child now relies less on the parent for physical support. The relationship gradually becomes one based more on emotional support, such as affection, trust and approval. However, during this time it can be a very difficult relationship, for both parent and child. Teenagers are experiencing great physical and hormonal changes, and are also learning to develop their own opinions about how they want to live their lives.

Parents have to try to change their attitudes to the child and to recognise that underneath the confident exterior, the teenager is struggling with his feelings about himself and his relationships with other people. The problem for parents is how to negotiate this change without damaging the relationship between parent and child. When the child needs reassurance and help, he should still feel he could approach his parents.

If parents can learn to communicate with their child then, hopefully, the relationship between parent and child can remain basically sound. If this can be done, at times of trouble the child will feel able to turn to his or her parents for help and assistance. A child who does not feel loved will lack self-esteem and self-confidence, which will affect the child's ability to make decisions for him or herself when the child is an adult.

Case study

Mark

Mark is an only child. His father died when he was 5 years old. He has always been close to his mum. Mark is now 15. His friends are keen on heavy metal music and he has bought a second-hand guitar so he can join in the band a few of them want to form. He has bought some new clothes that are similar to the clothes his friends are wearing. His mum thinks both the clothes and the music he makes are dreadful and tells him so regularly.

▶ 1 How is Mark demonstrating his independence from his mother?
2 How is Mark illustrating typical teenage behaviour?

▶ 1 Both Mark and his mum know that the relationship between them is changing. How is the change affecting his mum's behaviour?
2 How is the change likely to affect his mother?
3 How can Mark and his Mum ensure that their relationship remains a close one?
4 What would be the benefits to both of them if they were able to do this successfully?

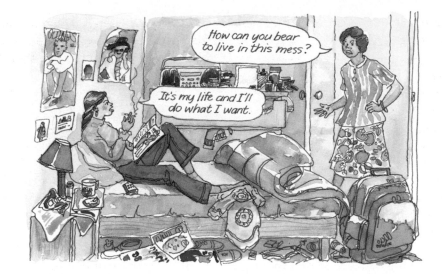

Siblings

Many siblings don't get on with each other when they are teenagers. Arguments, jealousy and unpleasantness between sisters and brothers are unfortunately common.

Siblings can also provide support in times of trouble (e.g. if the parents divorce). The parents' treatment of their children is very important. Comparison between siblings by the parents is not advised. It is likely the less favoured child will take his or her feelings of resentment out on the sibling rather than on the parents, whose approval he or she is still trying to gain. If the parents have shown favouritism, the poor relationship that develops between all family members is likely to continue into adulthood. This can sour relations between siblings for ever. However, relations between siblings generally improve as they become older.

Activity

Divide a piece of paper into two columns, heading one column 'Advantages of having siblings' and the other 'Disadvantages of having siblings'. Fill in both columns, drawing on your experiences. If you have no siblings, try to imagine what it would be like to have them.

Friends

Friends become even more important to teenagers than before. They no longer have solely same-sex friends. As teenagers get older, the sexes will mix more easily until some boys and girls begin to pair off as couples.

Teenagers' relationships with their friends are extremely important to them. Most teenagers want to belong to a group, as belonging helps them to feel more secure. This is shown by the way teenagers often choose similar hairstyles and clothes. These are obvious signals to others of what the group has in common.

When a young person has no friends

Figure 13.3 suggests some reasons why a child might have no friends.

May be different from others (clothes, accent or hairstyle different from peer group)

May have features others laugh at or criticise (e.g. being overweight, having red hair or a slight speech impediment)

Why teenagers have no friends

May have very different values from the peer group or may be much less or much more able than peer group

May lack social skills (e.g. very quiet or over-domineering)

Figure 13.3 Why teenagers might have no friends

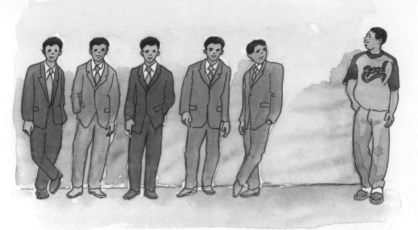

People who differ in appearance from the group may not fit in

Parents may also be concerned that their teenage child is getting involved in drug-taking or other destructive behaviour. In these situations, the child's best defence is her self-confidence and self-esteem, which will help or stand against the pressure of the group and ensure she doesn't get drawn into behaviour she (and the parents) would rather avoid.

Teachers

Learning takes place most successfully if the relationship between teacher and student is a good one. Like all relationships, this only happens if both people try to make it work. The qualities a good teacher should have are shown in Figure 13.4.

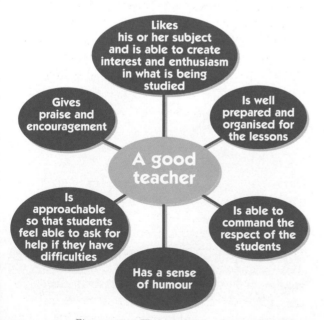

Figure 13.4 The qualities of a good teacher

Text in diagram:

- Likes his or her subject and is able to create interest and enthusiasm in what is being studied
- Gives praise and encouragement
- Is well prepared and organised for the lessons
- **A good teacher**
- Is approachable so that students feel able to ask for help if they have difficulties
- Is able to command the respect of the students
- Has a sense of humour

If both student and teacher have a good relationship, there is a greater chance that the student will both enjoy what he or she is taught and make progress in the subject. This leads to greater success in exams and increased self-confidence in the student.

Sexual relationships

Teenagers start to become involved in sexual relationships in their early teens. Girls may be a little younger and boys a little older as girls mature physically before boys.

Relationships often follow a similar pattern. In the mid-teens they tend to be short lived but, as the teenagers get older, they will last longer and be more intense. By 18 years old, about 50% of girls and 75% of boys will have had sexual intercourse. Longer-term relationships in the late teens prepare the individuals for adult life when, hopefully, they will settle into a *monogamous* relationship (a sexual relationship with one person only).

When relationships go wrong

When relationships go wrong, the effect they have on the individual can be severe. As in young children, the behaviour of an individual often indicates that something is wrong (see Figure 13.5).

Bullying

Bullying goes on at school principally because there are large numbers of children present in one place. There are plenty of victims available for those teenagers who want to bully others.

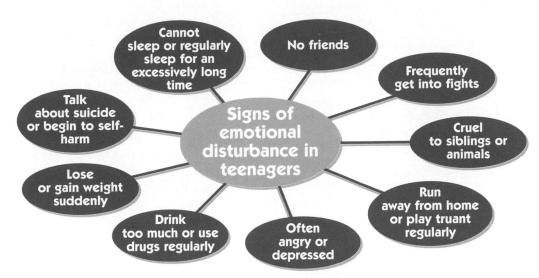

Figure 13.5 *The warning signs of emotional disturbance in teenagers*

Bullying takes many forms, which can include the following:

- Physical violence to the person and his or her property.
- Threats of violence.
- Verbal abuse often based upon someone's appearance.
- Spreading untrue, unpleasant rumours about someone.
- The threat of exclusion from the peer group if all members do not do as one person decides.

Bullying behaviour is thought to stem either from feelings of anger about something or feelings of inadequacy. These feelings generally arise from the bullies' poor relationship with family members. These poor relationships can result in feelings of inadequacy, anger or resentment. Inflicting pain on somebody else helps to make the bully feel better about him or herself.

Delinquency

Teenage delinquency could include behaviour such as regular heavy drinking, a serious drug habit or promiscuity. The term also applies to those teenagers who break the law regularly. Poor self-esteem and lack of confidence are usually a cause of such behaviour. Studies show that delinquents often have parents who show little interest in their child or, in contrast, are unreasonably heavy handed in their punishment of the child. Lack of success in school can also make the existing problems worse.

School refusers

School refusers quite simply refuse to go to school. Attendance at school can result in the teenager suffering intense feelings of anxiety. This makes the situation worse and becomes another reason to not attend school. The child may be unusually frightened of failure in a subject or number of subjects, or be scared of a particular teacher. Alternatively, the teenager may be anxious about some aspect of his or her home life. He or she feels it is necessary to remain at home to ensure that nothing goes wrong in his or her absence.

Due to the long absences from school, the teenager often has few friends. School refusal is uncommon and not easily understood by other pupils, who can be unhelpful in their attitude when the sufferer tries to return. This can make the situation worse.

Suicide and self-harm

Suicide and self-harm are often attempted by those students with some sort of mental disorder, such as depression or acute anxiety. They often occur in children from families with severe problems such as mental illness, long-term unemployment or parents with criminal backgrounds. In these families the child may feel unloved or unwanted. There is not enough time to give the child the attention he or she needs.

The intense unhappiness such young people feel means they may not relate well to others of their own age. The feeling of loneliness becomes even more intense. Students who feel depressed should seek help and support from their teacher, parents, friends or organizations such as The Samaritans.

Check your knowledge

1   Why can there be difficulties in the relationship between parents and teenagers?
2   Describe the benefits of having siblings.
3   Why do some teenagers have no friends?
4   How can teachers work towards a good teacher/student relationship?
5   Describe signs of emotional disturbance in teenagers.
6   What are the causes of school refusal?
7   What are the causes of self-harm in teenagers?

Relationships in adult life

The period of adulthood is a very long one. During this time individuals will go through many different experiences that bring them into contact with a great many different people. Such experiences include:

- going to college or university;

- getting married;
- having children;
- building or changing career;
- the death of parents; and
- moving house or moving to another part of the country.

Except for the death of parents, the list of events above is generally exciting and is under the control of the individual. Many other events that happen to people are out of the person's control and therefore may be much more difficult to deal with. Such events could include:

- divorce or the breakdown of a long-term relationship;
- redundancy or business failure;
- serious illness or injury to the individual;
- serious illness or the death of a child; and
- financial problems.

In all cases, the problem will be lessened if the individual has good relationships with the people he or she is involved with. The support and assistance of people close to a person can be of great help when things are not going well.

Marriage and cohabitation

While the number of people who marry is declining, the number of people *cohabiting* is going up. This shows that most people have a need for a close, intimate relationship with one other person. The number of people cohabiting has increased greatly in the last 25 years. Approximately 30% of people under 35 years old are cohabiting.

Checkpoint

When adults **cohabit** they live in a monogamous sexual relationship similar to marriage but without going through the legal ceremony. They do not have the legal protection of marriage (rights over their children, etc.).

Marriage is good for a person's emotional and physical health. In a happy marriage the partners:

- see each other as their best friend;
- share the same sense of humour;
- care for each other, particularly when one is under stress;

- continue to find the other person interesting to be with; and
- benefit from a successful relationship that gives both people more self-confidence.

For these reasons, many people go on to remarry even though their first marriage has ended in divorce.

When adults become parents

When adults become parents, they will draw on their own experiences of being children as a guide to help them parent their own children. For example, some adults remember that, in their childhood, a sibling was favoured above themselves. These adults are more likely to take care that they do not have favourites among their own children. The child will also have an impact on the parents. By their behaviour, children can influence the way the parent behaves towards them (e.g. by throwing tantrums). This will affect the way parents react.

Becoming a parent is perhaps one of the biggest decisions people ever make. If the parents feel they have done a good job of raising their children, the parents will rightly feel great satisfaction at their achievement as parents and pride in their children.

Friends

We tend to become friends with people with similar attitudes to ourselves. We also become friendly with those people who meet our emotional needs.

Friendships bring many benefits to our lives. Friendships:

- provide emotional support when things go wrong;
- provide an alternative view of the world from our own;
- introduce us to other interests and people;
- increase enjoyment of an activity by taking part in the activity with us; and
- increase our self-confidence and self-esteem.

Children with many friends of their own age often have parents with a stable, long-established circle of friends of their own. The

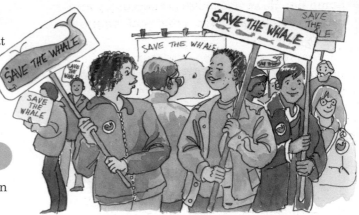

We often become friends with people who have similar attitudes and beliefs to ourselves

benefits of friendship for adults who are also parents can affect positively the chances of children having the same good experiences.

Work colleagues

Increasingly, work is a place where people make friendships that are valuable to them. In Britain, people work longer hours than people in any other country in Europe. As more and more people go out to work, many friendships are made in the workplace.

Like any other relationship, if a person feels valued by his or her colleagues, he or she will feel better about him or herself. If friendships are formed at work there is someone to share gossip with. There is also someone to understand exactly what problems you are having. To have no friendships at work,

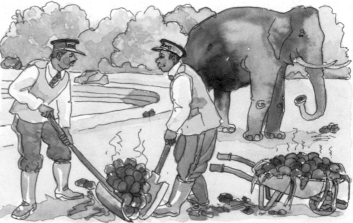

Only colleagues fully understand the problems people encounter at work

when people spend so much time there together, gives a person feelings of isolation and loneliness.

Case study

Ravi

Ravi works in a large restaurant as a chef. He has worked there for four years. He lives in accommodation above the restaurant with three other chefs and the restaurant under-manager. On Monday evenings some of them go out together. This is the only evening when the restaurant is closed. They try not to discuss work, but this can be difficult, especially if the manager has been telling them off! In the summer, if they are free together, Ravi and Jim, another chef, take their motorbikes for a run. They like going into the country where the roads twist and turn and real skill has to be used to keep the bike on the road. At weekends a crowd of the chefs (plus any of the casual weekend staff) often go to a club after the restaurant has shut. Ravi hasn't got a regular girlfriend as it is difficult to keep a relationship going with the hours he works.

1   What particular features of Ravi's job will make his colleagues important to him?
2   What benefits do you think Ravi gets from his friendships with his colleagues?
3   How will Ravi's relationships with his work colleagues help (a) his self-esteem and (b) his self-confidence?

When relationships go wrong

Loneliness

People who are lonely feel that way because of the difficulty they have in making and maintaining deep, satisfying relationships with other people. A small number of people feel loneliness as part of their personality (as opposed to those who feel lonely simply because they have moved to a new town, for instance.) Loneliness in these people often arises from their inability to form any deep relationships with other people. Figure 13.6 suggests some reasons why people might be unable to form relationships.

Loneliness causes people to have unpleasant feelings about themselves. It is a negative emotion to experience. It can contribute to loss of self-esteem and self-confidence. Training programmes concerned with helping people to improve their social skills have proved to be useful to people who feel long-term loneliness.

Check your knowledge

1   What is cohabitation?
2   What are the features of a happy marriage?
3   How does a person's childhood experiences affect his or her behaviour as a parent?
4   What are the benefits of friendships?
5   Why do some people have difficulty forming relationships?
6   Why is loneliness damaging to the individual?

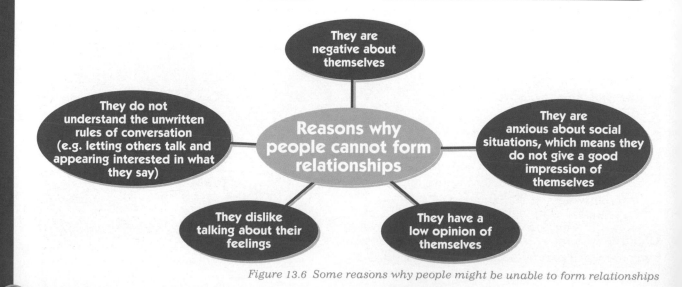

Figure 13.6 Some reasons why people might be unable to form relationships

Relationships in old age

Because of better health care, diet and greater wealth, the number of elderly people in society will continue to rise over the next decades. As a group, they are a significant section of the population to be considered when governments are planning housing, health care and welfare benefits for the future. Sometimes this group is called 'the grey vote'.

Personal and sexual relationships

Everyone, no matter what his or her age, needs the companionship and emotional support that close relationships can bring. Inevitably, many elderly people live alone, due to the death of a long-term partner or because they never married. For those elderly people whose partners are still alive, it may be very important to them to continue to have a sexual relationship. Some elderly people find that their sex lives improve as they get older due to greater familiarity and increased confidence.

If the health of one of the couple declines, it is common for the other person to become the prime carer of the other. This can bring a strain to a marriage as one person has to take over the role of the other within the home, which may cause the person who is ill to feel he or she has lost some control of his or her life. If an elderly person is left on his or her own, there is evidence to suggest that women cope better than men. They have spent more time there on their own so they are more content with their own company.

Relationships with the family

Relationships between family members are at best very supportive and at worst argumentative and destructive to everyone. Family members are usually the first to be called upon for assistance if an elderly person can no longer manage to live a completely independent life. However, due to the changes in families nowadays, elderly people may not have the support to call on they used to have. Changes in family structure include the following:

- Many couples are deciding not to have any children at all.
- Families live longer distances from each other, making regular support impractical.
- Many more women have full-time jobs and are reluctant to give them up to provide care for elderly relatives.
- As the state provides more care, people feel they need to do less. People feel the state should provide support in a way people did not expect it to do years ago.

Caring for elderly people

Problems can occur in families when the roles start to change because of the poor health of an elderly person. Although unwell, the person may resent having to give up his or her independence even though he or she knows he or she needs help. At the same time, the adult 'child' has to accept that he or she can no longer look to a parent for help and support. Caring for an elderly person is not an easy task. If relationships between family members are already not good, they are likely to become worse when one needs the regular care and attention of the other.

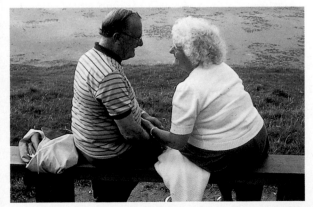

Many elderly people have a very satisfying sex life

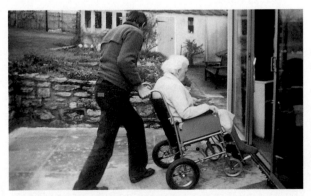

Caring for elderly parents can put a strain on the relationship between parent and child

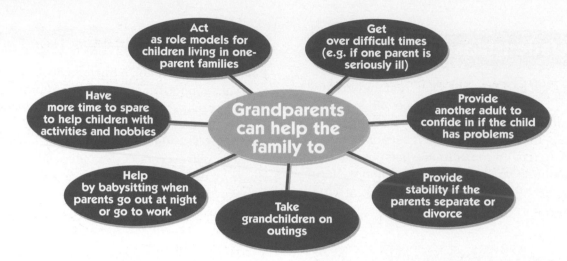

Figure 13.7 Some reasons why parents look forward to becoming grandparents

The role of grandparents

Many parents look forward to the time when they become grandparents. Some of the reasons for this are shown in Figure 13.7. However, if the relationship between the generations becomes distant due to disagreements, all generations of the family will miss out. The grandchildren may not really get to know their grandparents. Both generations lose the opportunity to love and value each other.

Friendships

The companionship of friends can be very important, particularly for many elderly people who live alone. The problems for the elderly in maintaining friendships include the following:

- Like partners, friends die.
- Social contact becomes more limited, so the chances of meeting new people decrease.
- Physical problems (such as poor hearing) can affect self-confidence.

The best way to help elderly people to make more friends is to encourage them to have as wide a list of activities as physically possible. This will bring them into contact with different people so that friendships arise naturally.

When relationships go wrong

The following are some causes of unhappiness in elderly people:

- They may resent their loss of status now they are no longer working.
- They may dislike their children becoming the decision-makers at home and in society.
- They may not approve of their children's choice of partner or way of bringing up the grandchildren.
- They may resent the way illness or old age means they cannot do as much as they used to.

All these reasons can cause a breakdown in the relationship between the generations. This comes at a time when the elderly are probably beginning to need the help and support of their children more than they have ever done before.

Loneliness

Many elderly people live alone and their friends may have died. It is therefore very important that they maintain good relationships with their family. However, if the elderly person makes no effort to maintain the relationship, he may find himself isolated and alone.

If the elderly person does not mix with others, he is likely to become depressed and unhappy. Everybody needs some human contact and, if this becomes very limited, either mental or physical illness begins. If the person has only a poor quality of relationship with his children, he will quickly begin to suffer from extreme isolation.

Figure 13.8 gives a summary of the effects of personal relationships at different stages of a person's life.

Good relationships can produce	Poor relationships can produce
Infancy Secure attachment between the infant and parents A rich learning environment A safe, loving environment which meets a child's emotional needs	A failure to make a secure or safe emotional attachment between parents and the child Neglect or rejection of the child
Early childhood A secure home from which to develop slowly Parents who can cope with the stressful behaviour of young children Friendships with other children	A stressful home situation Neglect or rejection of the child Inconsistent attempts to control a child Parents who become angry or depressed because of the child Isolation from other children
Later childhood Membership of a family or care group Socialisation into a culture Friendships with others at school Increasing independence from parents A feeling of being confident and liked by other people A feeling of being good at things	Stress and change if parents fight each other or separate No clear feelings of belonging with a group or culture Limited friendships Feelings of not being liked by others Feelings of not being good at anything or not as good as others
Adolescence Independence but still with the support of the family A network of friends, a sense of belonging with a group of friends A culture shared by friends A positive environment that has opportunities for the future	Conflict and fighting with parents and family Few friends, feeling depressed and rejected No feeling of belonging with other people No clear sense of who you are The feeling that life is not worth much
Adulthood A network of friends and family who help and support you A secure, loving, sexual relationship Good relationships with work colleagues The ability to balance time pressures among work, partner and other family relationships A feeling of being secure and safe, with other people to help you	Feelings of isolation, loneliness, rejection and no feeling of belonging with friends No support Changing relationships No social protection from stress Low self-esteem
Old age A network of family, friends and partner to provide emotional support Control of own life A sense of purpose	Few friends, no social support No social protection from stress Isolation No sense of purpose

Figure 13.8 *The effects of personal relationships at different stages of a person's life*

Check your knowledge

1 How has family structure changed over the last fifty years?

2 Describe the problems encountered in caring for the elderly.

3 How can grandparents help the family?

4 Why can it be difficult for the elderly to maintain friendships?

5 Describe some causes of unhappiness in the elderly.

Abuse, neglect, lack of support and their effect on personal development

If relationships become very poor, they may become *abusive* (i.e. harmful to the people involved). Abusive relationships occur when one person has power over another. He or she uses this power in a way that is unreasonable, unkind and without thought for the harmful effect on the other person. Abuse most commonly occurs between parent and child, husband and wife (or male and female partner) and carer and elderly person.

Child abuse

Child abuse can be divided into three types:

1   Physical abuse.
2   Sexual abuse.
3   Emotional abuse or neglect.

Someone in the child's family is usually the perpetrator of abuse.

Who carries out child abuse?

A recent survey by the charity Banardo's found that men abused 95% of girls and 80% of boys. Women abused the rest. The abuse took place either in the home of the child or the abuser. The child may suffer from more than one type of abuse at the same time.

What causes child abuse?

Abused children are likely to come from a home where there is one or more of the following problems:

- There are arguments between the child's parents or the child may live in a lone-parent or reconstituted family.
- There may be too many children in the family so the parents do not cope well.
- There may be a poor attachment between parent and child.
- The family is under stress because they live in poor housing, have money troubles, are unemployed or feel socially isolated.
- The child may be disabled, unwanted, difficult to discipline or disliked.

It should be understood that many children are brought up in homes that suffer from one or more of these problems but they are not abused. However, if these factors exist, there is an increased chance of the child being abused.

Physical abuse

This is defined as a child who is suffering from non-accidental injury (e.g. bruising, cuts, broken bones, etc.). This can happen as a result of too harsh discipline or because of shaking or rough handling. Physically abused children may:

- be aggressive to others – they may bully other children;
- lie, steal or truant from school;
- be reluctant to remove their clothes for PE lessons to reveal bruising;
- have difficulty in making friends; or
- underachieve at school.

Sexual abuse

A child who is sexually abused has been involved in sexual activities he or she does not understand. Examples of such behaviour include inappropriate touching, looking at pornography, being encouraged to watch the sexual behaviour of others or involvement in sexual intercourse. Abused children are often encouraged by their abuser to believe they are responsible so they don't tell anybody in case they are blamed for the behaviour. Sexually abused children may:

- show signs of sexual behaviour at a young age;
- be very tired as abuse often occurs at night so their sleep is disturbed;
- be withdrawn and unwilling to talk and mix socially;
- start to wet themselves having previously been dry;
- be badly behaved and underachieve at school; or
- if they are older, run away, drink too much or take drugs.

Emotional abuse or neglect

Parents should provide children with a loving environment where the child feels valued. Their needs should be considered and they should be able to make an attachment with one or more adults. An emotionally abused child does not have care of this type. They may be physically well cared for but their parents may not understand or care if the child's emotional needs for love, security, comfort and encouragement are not met. Emotionally abused children may:

- be slow to speak and walk;
- grow more slowly than they should;
- show little emotion with people;
- have difficulty forming relationships with their peer group; or
- underachieve at school.

Unless stopped by a person close to the child, abuse may go on over a very long period of time. The effects on the victim are therefore very serious. The long-term effects of all types of child abuse include the following:

- Intellectual development is slow and progress in school is affected.
- Abuse can lead to poor concentration and aggression, which also affects progress in school.
- The child may be self-destructive or may destroy his or her toys, or those of other children.
- The child will have poor self-esteem and lack confidence.
- The child will not mix well with other children, increasing feelings of isolation.

Domestic violence

Domestic violence can include the following types of behaviour:

- Pushing, hitting, intimidating or battering a person.
- Rape or attempted rape of a person.
- Verbal abuse (e.g. insulting and/or continually criticising a person).
- Keeping a person isolated either by imprisonment in the home or by preventing a person having enough money to enable him or her to go out.
- Threatening a person with any of the behaviours listed above.

Domestic violence most commonly occurs between couples who cohabit. At greatest risk are people under 25 years old and those with financial troubles. Domestic violence is more likely to occur in working-class families and in homes where the man is unemployed. Men are responsible for most domestic violence. However, it should be remembered that a small number of women are violent towards their partner.

The long-term effects of domestic violence

The physical and mental damage can be very severe. Long-term effects on the victim will include low self-esteem, feelings of guilt, shame and depression. The abused partner may suffer from long-term physical damage. Even if the children of the couple are not physically harmed, they will have a unhealthy view of adult relationships because they have witnessed violence in their home regularly.

Case study

The Hardy family

Susan Hardy has three teenage sons. She has been divorced from her husband for three years. Her ex-husband had a vile temper and used to humiliate Susan verbally in front of the their friends and the boys. Since the divorce, he has not paid maintenance for his sons, as he should do. As a result Susan is often short of money.

Susan's middle son, Christopher, often demands money from her although he knows the family is not well off. He has recently started hitting his mother if she does not do as he demands. As Christopher is now bigger than her, Susan is frightened of him and is totally unable to discipline him.

1. Describe the feelings Susan will have about herself.
2. Describe the feelings she will have about Christopher.
3. What kind of role model has Mr Hardy been to his sons?
4. Why do you think Christopher is behaving in this way?
5. What effect will Christopher's behaviour have on his brothers?

1. Children learn how to behave by modelling (copying adults). How is Christopher likely to behave as an adult when he marries or cohabits? Give reasons for your answer.
2. The relationship between Christopher and Susan is a negative one. What effect will this have on the self-esteem of (a) Christopher and (b) Susan?

Abuse of elderly people

The problem of the abuse of elderly people has only recently been recognised. It was first identified in the 1970s. The following types of abuse of the elderly have been recorded:

- Physical abuse (e.g. pushing, assault, burns, fractures).
- The quality of care is so poor it leads to medical problems (e.g. malnutrition, dehydration, pressure sores).
- Psychological abuse (e.g. threats, verbal abuse).
- Violation of basic rights (e.g. opening the elderly person's post, not allowing him or her to vote, not allowing him or her to practise his or her religion).
- Financial abuse (e.g. taking the person's money).

Who carries out the abuse?

A person who cares for the elderly person usually carries out the abuse. There has possibly been an increase in abuse due to the larger numbers of frail, elderly people who need greater care from someone else. The reasons for such abuse include the following:

- Stress due to isolation and lack of sleep.
- Physical exhaustion due to meeting the person's needs, possibly through the night as well as during the day.
- Frustration due to the severity of the person's condition.
- Personality clashes between family members that always existed but were not a problem while the two people were not spending so much time together.
- Arguments between family members about the elderly person that result in violence against the person.

Long-term effects of abuse

The long-term effects of abuse on the elderly person will be to make his or her life very unpleasant. They will have feelings of fear, shame and embarrassment that they are not able to prevent this awful experience happening to them. It is possible the carers will feel ashamed of themselves, as they are likely to know that their behaviour is wrong, but are unable to stop because of the problems and frustrations they feel in caring for the elderly person.

Lack of support

Most people will encounter difficult times during their lives. You looked earlier at some of the problems adults have to face and resolve (see page 210). Few adults are fortunate not to experience at least one of the problems mentioned here. Those people who have no one to turn to at times of difficulty will suffer from stress. Having someone to turn to helps to make the problem seem less difficult. They may also suffer from feelings of isolation and loneliness as they are forced to recognise there is nobody they can go to to ask for help. This will be another factor that could contribute to low self-esteem. You will learn more about the types of support available to people in Chapter 15.

> ### Check your knowledge
> 1 What factors increase the possibility of domestic violence?
> 2 What are the long-term effects of domestic violence for the victim?
> 3 Describe the types of abuse suffered by the elderly.
> 4 Who abuses the elderly?
> 5 What are the reasons for the abuse of the elderly?

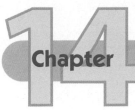

Chapter 14 Self-concept

What factors influence the development of a person's self-concept?

Everyone has a view of him or herself and this is known as his or her self-concept. This is based on the beliefs people have about themselves as a person and also on what they believe others think about them. In this chapter you will learn how a person's self-concept is affected by such factors as his or her:

- age
- appearance
- gender
- culture
- emotional development
- education
- relationships with others
- sexual orientation
- life experiences.

What is self-concept?

Our self-concept describes the sum total of the ways in which we think about ourselves. There are two aspects to our self-concept. The first is our *self-esteem*, which means how highly we think about our abilities and our self. The second aspect is our *self-image*, which we gain from people's reaction to us. Self-esteem and self-image add together to form the self-concept.

Children gain self-esteem from the way they are treated by their parents or carer when they are very small. A child who is loved and valued when young will have good self-esteem. If other people regularly praise you, your self-image will improve. This is why praise is important to people (see Figure 14.1).

Some people may view themselves positively in all areas of their lives, which might mean they have a very positive self-concept. Other people may not rate themselves highly in

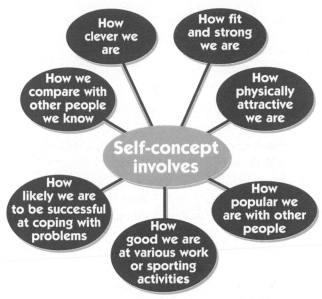

Figure 14.1 Self-concept

any aspect of their lives, which might mean they have a poor or negative view of themselves. Many people may have a mix of good and less good comments. Each person develops his or her own special view of him or herself. This is because of the experiences people have had as they have grown and developed.

Activity

▶ Use the spider diagram shown in Figure 14.1 to begin to describe your own self-concept. Use each 'leg' of the spider and comment on how you see yourself. Try to be honest; it can be easier to say you are not good at something than to state you are talented in a particular area!

▶ Look at the statements you have made. Do you have an area in which you feel your self-concept is particularly good? For example, if you are good at sports and try to keep fit, you might find your physical self is very positive. Is there an area you think is rather weaker? In your notes, use the diagram to describe yourself honestly.

Positive self-concept	Negative self-concept
You are motivated to do something because you have often been successful	You lack motivation because, when you have tried new things before, you often did not do very well
You are confident in social situations because you usually get on well with people	You lack confidence , especially when meeting new people; new people make you feel anxious as you fear you will have nothing to say
You are generally happy with your life	You are unhappy a lot of the time
You have enough self-confidence to cope with new challenges and to view them positively	You often find life difficult and do not enjoy new challenges, as you are afraid of failure

Figure 14.2 How our self-concept affects us

Why is self-concept important?

Our view of ourselves is important because it can affect us in the ways shown in Figure 14.2. Note that people with a good self-concept will not find everything in life easy. They will not be successful all the time. However, they will be more positive about life and more willing to 'have a go' at new experiences. As they have a positive attitude they are more likely to experience success (see Figure 14.3).

If we think we are good at school or work we will probably enjoy going there. Our concept of ourselves will make us want to be there. If we think we are not good at a new subject or task, we will be less keen to get involved. The way we think about ourselves influences what we do and how we feel.

Self-concept development

Our self-concept develops and changes because of the experiences we have. Therefore we should perhaps seek out new life experiences that might help us to change our self-concept.

How does self-concept develop? When we are born we do not understand anything about the world we are born into – we do not know we are an individual person. The beginnings of self-awareness may start when an infant can recognise his or her own face in a mirror. This happens somewhere between 1½–2 years of age, when an infant begins to demonstrate he or she is different from other people.

From this point on, children begin to form ideas about themselves. Children are influenced by the environment and culture they grow up in; they are also influenced by the relationships they have with their family and friends. As

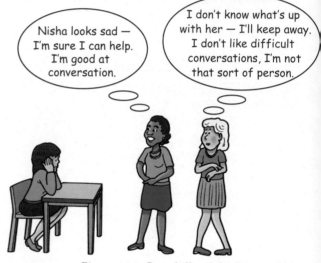

Figure 14.3 Our skills at dealing with the problems of others vary

children's ability to use language develops this will also affect how they can talk and how they can explain things about themselves.

The self-concept we have when we are very young is influenced by our family or carers. Hence primary-school age children are influenced by the adults around them but as we grow older our friends gradually take their place. As adolescents, we often compare ourselves with others and choose a particular set of friends accordingly.

Our self-concept doesn't usually settle down until we are ready to go out to work full time, or until we plan to leave home and live with a sexual partner. Until this time of life it may be that we experiment with ideas of what we may be like and what we may be good at. Adult commitments perhaps force us into making decisions about ourselves. It could be for this reason that some people may not be able to explain their self-concept clearly until they are in their early 20s (see Figure 14.4).

Age	Stage of development
1½–2 years	Self-awareness develops – children may start to recognise themselves in a mirror
2½ years	Children can say whether they are a boy or a girl
3–5 years	When asked to say what they are like, children can describe themselves in terms of categories, such as big or small, tall or short, light or heavy
5–8 years	If you ask children who they are, they can often describe themselves in detail. Children will tell you their hair colour, eye colour, about their families and to which schools they belong
8–10 years	Children start to show a general sense of 'self-worth', such as describing how happy they are in general, how good life is for them, what is good about their family life, school and friends
10–12 years	Children start to analyse how they compare with others. When asked about their life, children may explain without prompting how they compare with others. For example: 'I'm not as good as Zoe at running, but I'm better than Ali'.
12–16 years	Adolescents may develop a sense of self in terms of beliefs and belonging to groups – being a vegetarian, believing in God, believing certain things are right or wrong
16–25 years	People may develop an adult self-concept that helps them to feel confident in a work role and in social and sexual relationships
25 onwards	People's sense of self will be influenced by the things that happen in their lives. Some people may change their self-concept a great deal as they grow older
65 onwards	In later life it is important to be able to keep a clear sense of self. People may become withdrawn and depressed, without a clear self-concept

Figure 14.4 The development of self-concept

Check your knowledge

1 What do we mean by 'self-concept'?
2 Why is your self-concept important?
3 How does a positive self-concept help you?
4 Describe how a child's understanding of self-concept changes as he or she gets older.
5 How does adulthood affect self-concept?

Influences on self-concept

Age

Age makes a big difference to the way children describe themselves and to the way adults think about their lives. Our self-concept grows and changes as we get older. Some general differences in self-concept between various age groups and the way our self-concept develops are shown in Figures 14.5 and 14.6.

Age	Expression of self-concept
Young children	Self-concept limited to a few descriptions, for example, boy or girl, size, some skills
Older children	Self-concept can be described in a range of 'factual categories', such as hair colour, name, details or address, etc
Adolescents	Self-concept starts to be explained in terms of chosen beliefs, likes, dislikes, relationships with others
Adults	Many adults may be able to explain the quality of their lives and their personality in greater depth and detail than when they were adolescents
Older adults	Some older adults may have more self-knowledge than during early adult life. Some people may show 'wisdom' in the way they explain their self-concept

Figure 14.5 The differences in self-concept between various age groups

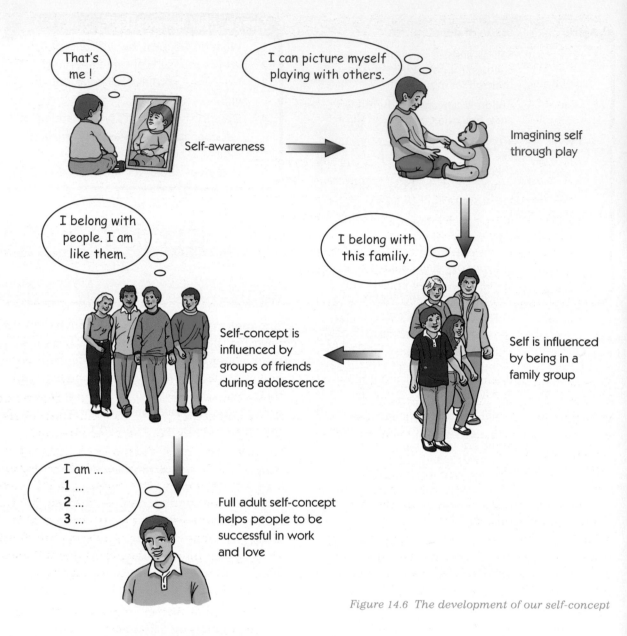

Figure 14.6 *The development of our self-concept*

Appearance

Somewhere between 10 and 12 years of age, children start to analyse the ways in which they are like or not like others. The physical shape of our body, our height, weight, hair, eyes and skin colour all influence how we see and think about ourselves. Many people think there is an 'ideal' look that they should resemble. If we think we look good then we have a positive self-image. If we think we do not look good we may have a negative self-image. A negative self-image may contribute to a low self-concept.

Clothes, hairstyle, make-up and body shape are seen differently by different people. No one looks attractive to everyone. What you see as attractive may be so because of your own age, culture and lifestyle. The important issue is to feel positive about the way you look. We can easily develop a negative self-image if we do not understand the way other cultures or personal beliefs influence other people's opinions of our appearance. A poor self-image may cause us to lack confidence or to feel depressed about our relationships with other people.

▶ Use fashion magazines to collect pictures of male and female models. Describe what type of body and facial features are needed to make a successful model. Do you know many people with those types of features? Do these pictures influence you? Put your thoughts in your file.

▶ Now think of the people you know, of your age and older. How similar are these people to the appearance of the models opposite? How do you think images in magazines affect our view of what is a desirable body? Use your opinions to write a newspaper article, explaining why photographs of the 'perfect' body should not heavily influence people. You can use Microsoft Publisher to produce the article in a newspaper format.

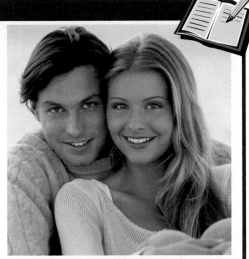

Many people think these models have a desirable appearance

Gender

Very early in life children seem to be able to classify themselves in terms of gender – children know if they are a boy or girl. Gender is a major social influence that affects how we understand ourselves. There tend to be different social expectations of men and women.

Nowadays the differences between the sexes are not as marked as they used to be. At school, students are very aware of instances of sexism. They are quick to point out when one sex is being treated less well than the other. Boys and girls expect to have exactly the same opportunities.

Despite all the changes, some gender differences still exist. You will have looked at some of these differences in Chapter 12, when you saw how gender affects level of education and type of employment.

It would appear that, despite their educational success, women do view themselves differently from men. Women tend to choose different types of jobs. They are more likely to interrupt their career to look after children. They appear still to put the needs of family before their career so that their progress in the workplace is held back. In this way, a woman's self-concept as the carer of the family affects the decisions she makes about the kind of life she wants to lead.

Culture

Different people have different customs and ways of thinking. Your family or the community where you grew up may have different beliefs and expectations from other families and communities. These differences influence the way we think. We call this range of influences 'cultural influences'. Our culture can influence how we understand ourselves because different cultures create different ideas about what is normal or what is right. Sociologists call these ideas *norms*. Some of the norms that influence what we think of as right or wrong are described below:

- Most white British people will not eat frog's legs, snails or horse meat.
- Parents in professional jobs generally value education. They expect their child to do well at school.
- Parents who do not smoke will discourage their children from starting to smoke.
- People from some ethnic minority groups are more likely to live in an extended family.
- People with a strong religious belief may teach their children that sex before marriage is wrong.

What you think of as important, or right or wrong, will be influenced by the norms of the people around you. Your self-esteem (how you feel about yourself) will be influenced by cultural beliefs about what is right or wrong.

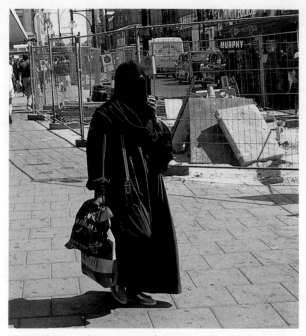

According to the culture of their country, women may have to wear certain clothing. How do you think this will affect their self-concept?

his or her likes and dislikes and aspects of his or her life, such as his or her home and school. However, they may not be emotionally mature enough to compare themselves with another person.

By late adolescence, people are emotionally mature enough to draw comparisons with their peer group. A teenager may say 'I am not as good at meeting new people as my friends are'. The peer group is particularly important to this age group so these comparisons with others will help the person form a view of his or her self-concept. Adolescents will begin to have views on issues such as animal rights or the protection of the environment. These are more abstract ideas, and the person needs emotional maturity to be able to form clear opinions on such issues.

By the time a person is an adult, he or she is emotionally mature enough to have personal insight. He or she will also have the necessary language to describe his or her self-concept in detail.

Check your knowledge

1 Imagine you are 8 years old again. Use the information in Figure 14.5 to help you describe your self-concept at that age.
2 How does appearance affect self-concept?
3 How do ideas about gender affect women's careers?
4 What are 'cultural influences'?
5 What are 'norms'?
6 Suggest two norms of British society.

Emotional maturity

A person's understanding of his or her own self-concept is dependent on his or her own emotional and intellectual maturity. A person needs complex language to describe his or her self-concept accurately so language development must come first. For this reason alone, small children cannot describe their self-concept.

At the age of 2 years, a child can say if he or she is a boy or girl. He or she may know his or her age but will not be able to describe him or herself in any more detail. This is, however, the first stage in having a self-concept. By 10 years old, a child can describe his or her appearance,

Activity

▶ You are now old enough and mature enough to be able to describe your self-concept. Try to describe yourself, beginning with your physical appearance. Then try to describe your personality, including what you see to be your strengths and weaknesses.

▶ Now swap your description with that of your friend's. From what you know of your friend, do you think your friend has described him or herself accurately? How accurate does he or she think you have been about yourself? You may find a difference between your view of yourself and other people's view of you. Put your comments in your file.

Education

Our idea of who we are is strongly influenced by our experiences at school. Young people spend more than half the time they are awake at school, doing homework or meeting with friends from school. Later experiences at college or university can also confirm or change what we think about ourselves (see Figure 14.7).

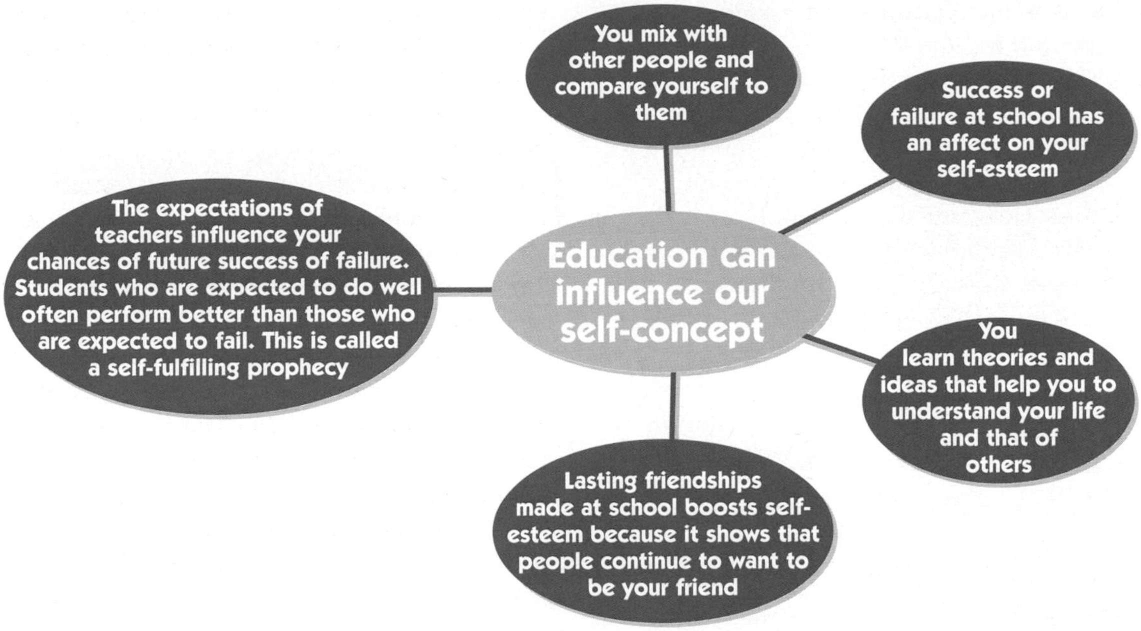

The expectations of teachers influence your chances of future success of failure. Students who are expected to do well often perform better than those who are expected to fail. This is called a self-fulfilling prophecy

You mix with other people and compare yourself to them

Success or failure at school has an affect on your self-esteem

Education can influence our self-concept

You learn theories and ideas that help you to understand your life and that of others

Lasting friendships made at school boosts self-esteem because it shows that people continue to want to be your friend

Figure 14.7 How education influences self-concept

Activity

So far in your life you will have formed a relationship with some (if not all) of the following people:

- mother, father or an adult who cared for you when you were a small child
- brother(s) and sister(s)
- other family relatives (e.g. aunts, uncles, grandparents)
- school friends
- teachers
- family friends and neighbours.

▶ For each of the people with whom you have formed a relationship, try to suggest at least one way he or she has affected you or taught you something. This is the way these people have contributed to your self-concept.

▶ Now analyse the list of people you have named and the comments you have written. Decide which of them had the most effect on you and which had the least. You are now identifying the relationships that had the most significant effect on the development of your self-concept.

Relationships with others

The relationships we form are crucial to our development into happy, emotionally secure adults. Our relationships will affect our self-concept.

Our first relationships are with our parents (or another adult who acts as the main carer). As you have seen in Chapter 12, parents give the child self-esteem by the way they love and interact with the child. The child will come into contact with other people – for example, members of the extended family such as aunts and uncles. These are adults who, hopefully, will value the child and give the child the feeling of being liked and thought of as important. This will help foster a good self-image in the child. This contributes to the development of a positive self-concept.

As the child grows towards adulthood, he or she will form relationships with many other people. Some of these relationships will be less successful than others but most of us gradually realise we cannot get on well with everyone. So long as some of the relationships are satisfactory and fulfil our emotional needs for closeness and being valued, our self-concept will develop in a positive way.

Adults come into contact with a wide variety of people when they begin work. People also start to have sexual relationships. Some of these people will have less effect on us than others, depending on the amount of time we spend with them and the value we place on their opinions. However, all the people with whom we form a relationship will affect us to a greater or lesser degree. These relationships will influence our self-concept and its development.

Sexual orientation

Sexual orientation refers to our sexual behaviour and choice of partner. Most people are heterosexual (i.e. sexually attracted to the opposite sex). A minority are homosexual (i.e. attracted to the same sex). An even smaller number are bisexual (i.e. attracted to both sexes).

A person's sexual orientation is certain to form part of his or her self-concept. It will be particularly significant to those who are homosexual. This is because to admit to being homosexual can still be a very traumatic thing to do. A young person who is homosexual may encounter the following problems:

- His or her parents may express sadness and disappointment when they realise their child will not marry and form a 'conventional' couple.
- Acquaintances may express *homophobic* attitudes.
- He or she may suffer prejudice at work.
- Some people believe that homosexuals should not have jobs that involve them coming into contact with children. This can cause problems for homosexual teachers, youth workers, etc.
- Pension regulations and housing laws do not allow the same privileges for homosexual partners as they do for heterosexual couples.
- There is considerable public opposition to homosexual couples being allowed to

foster or adopt children. (There is less opposition to lesbian couples who wish to foster and adopt.)

Checkpoint

Homophobia is the intense dislike of homosexual people.

Due to the problems homosexuals face in society, some young people feel confused and even fearful as they accept they are homosexual. The prejudice that still exists in society can have a harmful effect on individuals' view of themselves. It can be difficult to be positive about yourself if you are receiving negative signals about a significant aspect of yourself. Self-concept will therefore be affected greatly by sexual orientation.

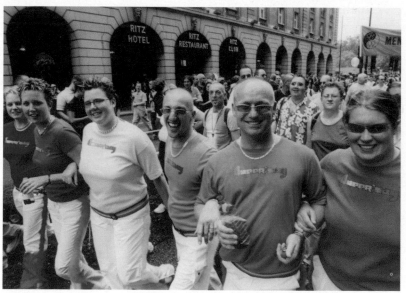

Sexual orientation can have a significant effect on self-concept

Life experiences

As a person gets older, he or she will inevitably have different life experiences. By getting through each experience and learning to cope with the situation, a person learns something about him or herself. Figure 14.8 shows some common life experiences and the things a person may discover about him or herself as he or she goes through them. Through each life experience, therefore, the person learns something about him or herself.

Life experience	What I can learn about myself
Starting school	Do I like being told what to do? Do I like learning new information and skills?
Getting a job	How do I deal with money? Do I dislike someone bossing me about?
Getting married	Do I find it easy to be faithful to one person? Does domesticity bore me? Is my home important to me?
Having children	Do I like having the responsibility of a baby? Do I like caring for a child? Do I resent the loss of my freedom now I have a baby to consider?

Figure 14.8 How life experiences help us understand ourselves

Case study

David

David is a black 4-year-old who is starting nursery school. Until now he has always been at home with this mother. He has played with other children many times in his home and also when his mother visited friends. David is an only child. He has a close, loving relationship with his mother.

David's first reaction to school was one of shock – there were so many other children and it was noisy. He had always looked to his mother for guidance, but she was not there and he was on his own. David had been told all about school, but he could not really understand or imagine what it would be like. Another adult who looked very different from his mother was trying to get him to join in a game. David felt frightened and lost. David cried for his mother and told staff he wanted her. A kind teacher who looked a little like his aunt spent time with him and he felt better.

Later in the day, David enjoyed some food and joined in making music with the other children. When his mother came to collect him he was relieved. He did not really feel safe until

she appeared. Now he felt tired, but important. He had been to school, had learned about music and his mother made him feel everything was all right and safe again. This was a real adventure!

1 How was David affected physically on his first day at school?
2 What intellectual activity did David take part in on his first day?
3 How was David affected emotionally by his first day at school?
4 How did David's mother prepare him socially for his first day at school?
5 How did adults at school help David cope with the change he experienced?

1 Describe your first day at school.
2 Did you feel a sense of uncertainty, tiredness, excitement or fear when you went through this change?
3 Were your experiences positive or negative?

Life experiences also help to form our self-concept. By experiencing as many different things as possible, a person discovers his or her ability to cope, enjoy and learn from the experience. Sometimes, people are placed in unpleasant situations where they learn about their ability to cope in extreme conditions most people are not exposed to. Their self-concept is altered as a result.

Most people do not go through ordeals like the ones just described. However, if we think about it carefully, the experiences we all go through help both to form self-concept and to help us to learn about our own self-concept (see Figure 14.9).

List the life experiences you have had so far. The list could include starting primary school and the birth of a younger sister or brother. Think about each event in turn. What did you learn about yourself through each event? Be as honest as you can. Do you see how your life experiences so far have helped you to understand your self-concept?

Think about the life experiences you hope to have as you get older (e.g. going to college, getting married, etc.). Use Figure 14.9 to help you forecast what you will learn from each.

	Physical	Intellectual	Emotional/social
Babies	A good home with a healthy diet, ensures good physical health	Toys to play with and the attention of adults ensure a good basis for intellectual development. At this age the baby has no understanding of self-concept	Good carers and attention of other adults ensure a satisfactory attachment relationship, forming the basis of the baby's ability to make sound, lasting personal relationships when he or she is older
Young child	Good health and growing confidence in physical skills (for example, being on the football team) ensures increasing self-confidence	If the child achieves well at school, he or she begins to gain self-confidence in his or her intellectual abilities. The individual still has little clear understanding of self-concept	The child begins to make friends with other members of the peer group. Parents should ensure that the child begins to understand the 'norms' of his or her culture so the child feels secure among the people with whom he or she mixes
Adolescent	The individual starts to have an interest in his or her personal appearance. If the child is happy with his or her appearance, this will contribute to the satisfactory formation of self-concept. Individuals who enter puberty early may gain self-confidence as other members of the peer group hold them in high esteem.	Success in exams and good educational achievement in school help to increase self-confidence. The individual is now old enough to have some understanding of his or her own self-concept	Good relationships with friends and the first sexual relationships will affect self-concept. Excellent or poor self-confidence in gender role will also have an effect
Adult	A pleasant home ensures physical good health. Illness or physical damage to the body can have an effect on self-concept	Adults have a greater under-standing of their self-concept. Success at work (which can be partly linked to their level of educational success) will help to increase self-confidence and self-esteem	A satisfactory sexual relationship will increase self-esteem. Lasting personal relationships will also be of positive benefit to the individual. Feeling confident within your culture increases self-confidence, as does an ability to cope with life experiences capably
Later adulthood	Poor health and the change in a person's appearance due to the ageing process may affect self-concept adversely	Retirement may cause individuals to lack the self-esteem that comes from achievement at work. Self-concept may be badly affected by no longer working	Old friends can help provide emotional support after the death of a partner. Different life experiences will affect self-concept depending on whether the individual coped well with each experience

Figure 14.9 Factors that affect self-concept at different life stages

Check your knowledge

1 What is needed before people can describe their own self-concept?
2 How does self-concept develop in adolescents?
3 How do educational experiences affect self-concept?
4 How does the extended family affect the child's self-concept?
5 Use Figure 14.10 to identify which people appear to have the greatest effect on self-concept. Try explaining why some people are more influential than others.
6 What is meant by sexual orientation?
7 What problems can homosexuals face in society?
8 How do our life experiences affect self-concept?
9 How do life experiences help you to know yourself better?

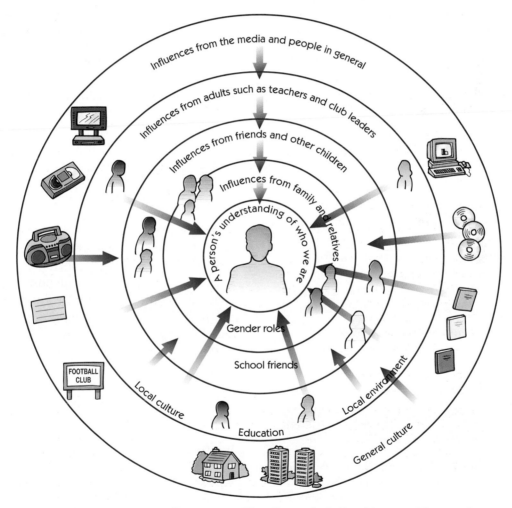

Figure 14.10 The effects of relationships on self-concept

Chapter 15: The effects of life events on personal development

Key issue

How can life events affect an individual's personal development?

Life events are expected or unexpected experiences that can have a major impact on an individual's personal development. These may include events that result in the following:

- Relationship changes (marriage, divorce, living with a partner, birth of a sibling or own child, death of a friend or relative).
- Physical changes (e.g. puberty, accident or injury, menopause).
- Changes in life circumstances (e.g. moving house, starting school, college or a job, retirement, redundancy or unemployment).

By the end of this chapter you will be able to identify and describe the effects such examples of expected and unexpected life events can have on an individual's personal development. You will learn how individuals adapt and use sources of support to cope with the effects of life events. Sources of support may include:

- partners, family and friends;
- professional carers and services; and
- voluntary and faith-based services.

Life events

As people go through life, they will have to cope with various different life events. All major life events will involve change of some sort. For example, when a child starts school, he or she has to get used to spending time without his or her parents or a familiar adult.

Some of the events that happen during life are to be expected. We know these events will occur and we choose to experience them. Examples of these types of events are:

- starting a new school;
- going through puberty;
- starting work;
- getting married; and
- retirement.

Other life events are unplanned. Some of these may be unpleasant or difficult to cope with (but not all!). For example:

- the birth of a brother or sister;
- physical injury or illness;
- divorce or the breakdown of a serious relationship;
- redundancy or business failure;
- the death of a friend or relative;
- winning the lottery.

Positive and negative effects of life events

Change usually involves some level of stress. When people choose to change (e.g. start a new job), the stress may be experienced as excitement. People may feel 'butterflies in the stomach' on their first day at work, but they may also look forward to meeting new people and learning new things. Some changes, such as the death of a friend, are experienced as being negative and these will usually cause people to become very stressed.

Life events involve some stress because change can cause:

- a sense of loss for the way things used to be;
- a feeling of uncertainty about what the future will be like;
- a need to spend time and/or money and/or emotional energy sorting things out; and
- a need to learn new things.

Changes in relationships

Throughout life, emotional relationships are of central importance to human health and happiness. Research suggests that people who

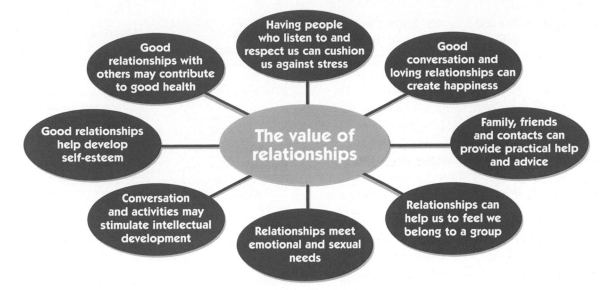

Figure 15.1 *The value of relationships*

have strong, loving relationships are happier than those without.

Talking with friends and family and colleagues may protect us from the stresses we may otherwise face in life. Parents protect us when we are young, while adult relationships with partners and friends help us cope with life events in adult life. The benefits of good relationships are summarised in Figure 15.1.

Marriage

Checkpoint

In Britain, **marriage** is the legal union of one man to one woman. Gay and lesbian couples cannot at the moment be registered as married.

Marriage involves a commitment to live with a partner permanently. It ties the financial resources and networks of family relationships together. Marriage is a big change in life and it usually involves moving house and leaving your family. This may cause a sense of loss. Many people feel some anxiety about getting married because of the adjustments that will have to be made if the marriage is to last.

As you have seen previously, marriage is generally thought to be good for a person. Married people live longer and are ill less often than divorced people. If the marriage is a happy one, although the initial change may be difficult, the couple will feel the benefit of the support of the partner.

Divorce

At present, one in three marriages are likely to end in divorce. In the past it was often difficult to get a divorce. Divorce is much more common nowadays and many people who divorce go on to remarry. Each year, over a third of marriages are likely to be remarriages.

Although many people experience divorce negatively, it may be better than living in a stressful situation. However, even if the couple involved know they will be happier if they separate, they are both likely to feel a sense of failure. This is because people get married believing they have chosen a partner for life. Marriage is a public statement of their intentions to live happily with the person each has chosen. It is therefore very disappointing for the couple involved to realise they made such a big mistake.

Divorce is an example of an unexpected, unpleasant life event. People may be affected emotionally for some time, especially if they didn't want the marriage to end. At the end of this chapter you will learn about services that can help people cope with traumatic events like divorce.

Living with a partner

These days many couples live together before getting married. In 1999, 39% of men and women aged between 30 and 34 years of age were living with someone outside marriage. Some people may choose not to marry because they have been married before and do not want the risk of being divorced for second time. Whatever the reasons for not marrying, the decision to live with someone is not one to be taken lightly. The same sorts of practical arrangements concerning money, friends and family have to be made as if the couple were married.

However, many cohabiting relationships do not last as long as marriages. Government statistics show that, between 1986 and 1999, the average cohabitation for single men lasted only three years. If the relationship ends, the couple are likely to have the same feelings of loss and disappointment as couples who are divorcing. There will be the same practical problems to resolve concerning where they will live and what happens to the children.

Birth of a sibling

Gaining a new brother or sister changes our relationships with our parents and other family members. Children may have mixed emotions about the new arrival. Some of the feelings that may be experienced by a child are described in Figure 15.2.

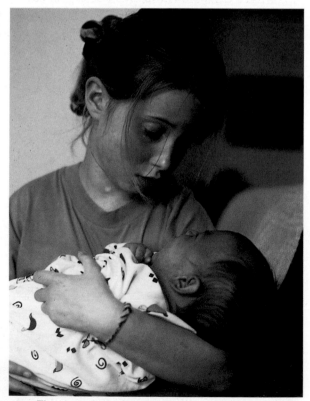

The arrival of a baby brother or sister has a great effect on the whole family

Positive	Negative
Feeling important because you can care for the new infant	Feeling rejected because your parents seem to spend more time with the infant
Feeling pleased because there are more people in your family group	Feeling you have been replaced in the family and are not important
Feeling valued because you are the older child	Feeling your attachment to the family and parents is threatened
Making a relationship or attachment with your new brother of sister	Feeling you are in competition with your brother or sister

Figure 15.2 The positive and negative feelings associated with gaining a new brother or sister

The birth of your own child

Becoming a parent involves a major change in life. Many parents experience their relationships with their child as an intense, emotional experience. However, parenthood brings many problems:

- Parents lose sleep when the baby needs attention in the night.
- The parents' social life has to change as babysitters are needed if the parents are to go out.
- There may be a loss of income if a parent decides to give up work to look after the child.
- Parents can lose out on career opportunities if they take a 'career break'.
- If both parents decide to work, child care can be expensive and occasionally unreliable.
- Children need toys, clothes and special equipment, such as pushchairs, cots, etc. These can be expensive to provide.
- Children need a lot of attention and care.

Activity

▶ Read the account on this page describing how parenthood affects the lives of adults when they become parents. Consider all the changes mentioned. Analyse the list in terms of the PIES (e.g. loss of sleep affects people physically and possibly intellectually if they are unfit for work the next day).

▶ Use the list above and an ICT program such as Microsoft Publisher to produce a leaflet to be given to new parents informing them of the changes to their lives that will occur when they become parents.

Death of a friend or relative

Bereavement means losing someone you have loved. It causes a major change in people's lives. There is a very strong sense of loss – you may lose the main person you talked to, the person who helped you, your sexual partner and a person who made you feel good. Bereavement can mean you have to live a new life as a single person again.

People who try to cope with a major loss often experience feelings of:

- disbelief the person is dead;
- sadness and depression;
- anger or guilt; or
- stress because they have to cope with a new lifestyle.

Case study

Alice

Alice is 86 years old. Her husband has recently died. Although he was elderly, his death was a shock to Alice, as his health had seemed much better than hers. The couple were married for 53 years. Alice suffers from a heart complaint and had become very dependent on her husband in the years leading up to his death. Alice now lives alone. She has a son and a daughter who visit her each week. Her children have organised for someone to come to her house each morning and evening to see that Alice is all right.

▶ 1 Describe how Alice will be feeling as she comes to terms with her husband's death.
   2 Describe the practical problems Alice will be having now she is living on her own.

▶ 1 How will Alice's physical, emotional and social health and well-being be affected by her husband's death?
   2 How will the death of her husband affect Alice's (a) self-confidence and (b) her self-esteem?

Check your knowledge

1 Give four examples of expected life events.
2 Give three examples of unexpected life events.
3 Why do life events cause stress?
4 Explain why divorce can be a very unpleasant life event.
5 Why should cohabitation be seen as a major life event?
6 How does the arrival of a baby affect other children in the family?
7 How does the arrival of the first child affect the new parents?
8 Why can the death of a friend or relative be a traumatic event?

Physical changes

Puberty

Puberty is the time when adolescents have developed physically so they are able either to father a child or to become pregnant. At this time there is great development of the sexual characteristics (see Chapter 11). Puberty can be a difficult time for both boys and girls. Both sexes may be embarrassed at the way their bodies are changing. The actual physical changes can be difficult to deal with. Boys' voices break, which can be a source of amusement to others. Girls have to cope with menstruation.

Puberty can be particularly difficult for those individuals who begin earlier or later than average. There is some evidence to say that those who enter puberty are 'looked up to' because they are obviously more advanced than others. Teenagers who do not start puberty until later than average may feel isolated. A child who has not begun puberty may feel left out. The problem is particularly significant in boys.

Accident or injury

Accidents or injuries can strike any person at any time in his or her life. They can vary greatly in seriousness. Some accidents can be very serious but, in time, the person will make a full recovery. In other cases, the damage that results from the accident can result in permanent changes to the body.

Changes such as injury and illness can be unexpected and very negative in their effects. A sudden disability, such as the loss of sight or the loss of a limb, can cause a person to react in a similar way to the death of a friend or relative. Injury can also cause problems with self-esteem and self-image, as people have to adjust to their changed appearance and ability. When dealing with this type of life event, the support of family, friends and health care professionals is invaluable.

Activity

▶ Imagine a new student is going to join your school. Carry out an inspection of your school to see how suitable it would be for a student in a wheelchair. How many areas of the school could he or she gain access to? Which subjects would it be very difficult or impossible for him or her to take part in? Could the student have access to the dining hall or the toilets? Put your conclusions in your file.

▶ Now make recommendations for changes to be made to the building to improve its suitability for those students in a wheelchair. The report is to be given to the school governors so, to improve the appearance of the report, you could use a suitable word processing package and include an image or chart.

Menopause

This is the time in women's lives when menstruation stops. This usually happens between the ages of 45 and 55 years. A woman's feelings about this event may be mixed because the menopause occurs at a time in a woman's life when other changes are also occurring. For example, children may be leaving home or she may be considering retirement (see Figure 15.3).

There is now considerable medical help available for women who find the menopause an unpleasant physical and psychological experience. *Hormone replacement therapy*

Positive feelings about the menopause	Negative feelings about the menopause
Problems associated with periods end	No longer able to have children
No longer any need to use contraception, leading to increased enjoyment of sex	A feeling she has no 'role' now children have grown up
Increased confidence	Sadness at signs of physical ageing such as wrinkles and weight gain
Increased time available as children no longer demand as much attention	Symptoms of the menopause include hot sweats, insomnia and mood swings, which can be unpleasant to cope with

Figure 15.3 Feelings about the menopause

(HRT) can lessen the worst symptoms and make the experience more bearable for those women who are having severe symptoms.

Check your knowledge

1 What is puberty?
2 Why can teenagers find puberty difficult?
3 What is the effect of early puberty on the individual?
4 Explain why illness and injury are negative life events.
5 What is the menopause?
6 Why do some women find the menopause an unpleasant life event?
7 What help is available to women going through the menopause?

Changes in life circumstances

Moving house

Moving house is very stressful for a wide variety of reasons:

- People are often emotionally tied to their homes because important events have happened while they lived there.
- Moving house is physically hard work. Packing and unpacking can be a very big job.

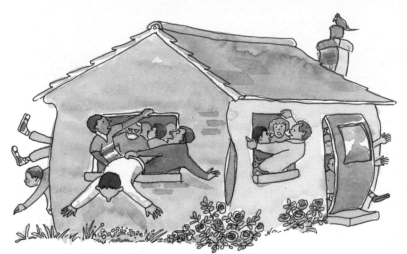

Many people have to move when the house becomes too small for the family

children feel a little afraid at leaving their parents and being with different people. A family might help their child in the following ways:

- Ensuring the child goes to playgroup so he or she is used to some separation from his or her parents.
- Encouraging independence in the child.
- Making sure the child knows and understands what is going to happen when he or she first goes to school.

- People become friends with the neighbours. Children may have good friends who live nearby. It can be difficult to leave them.
- Children may need to go to a new school as a result of the move. They are likely to be concerned about this.
- The process of buying and selling a house can take months. People can agree to buy your house and then change their minds. This can be very frustrating for the house sellers.
- Moving house is very expensive. Money is needed for estate agents, legal bills, the removal firm and furnishings in the new house.

Starting school

When starting at school, a child's family can help by understanding what is involved. Most

Professional carers, teachers and classroom assistants might help by understanding the change children face. They should all help to reassure the child when he or she first arrives at school.

Starting college

Starting college is usually an expected, enjoyable life event. Colleges usually treat the students in a more adult way. For example, students do not wear uniform and are allowed to leave the college when they don't have lectures. Although college is usually an enjoyable experience, some students may have difficulty in adjusting to the different system when they first start (see Figure 15.4).

However, most students enjoy their time at college and, once they are used to the system, find it a useful and memorable experience.

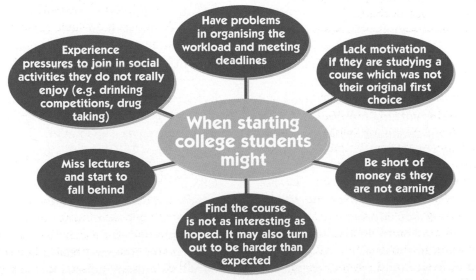

Figure 15.4 The problems students might encounter when starting college

Case study

John

John has been at college for two terms. His parents wanted him to stay at school to do his AS levels but he was adamant he wanted to go to the local FE college. He was looking forward to the more relaxed routine at college and not having to wear a school uniform any more. However, he is now beginning to think that he should have stayed at school. He doesn't like the college lecturers as much as his schoolteachers. He is also finding it hard to organise his time and work routine. He hated it at school when teachers nagged for coursework but now no one is pushing him he is finding he is falling behind.

▶ 1 What was the attraction for John of attending college to do AS levels?
2 Why is John finding college more difficult than he expected?
3 What could John do to resolve the problem?
4 What could happen if the problem is not resolved?

▶ How could failure at college affect John's:
1 Self-esteem?
2 Level of educational attainment?
3 Employment prospects?

Starting work

As when starting at college, most people are both excited and anxious when starting a new job. A person will be anxious because he or she will be meeting new people and he or she will want to get on well with them. The person also hopes to be able to cope with the demands of the job. He or she will be excited because having a job is a sign of adulthood. The job will mean this person is earning money so he or she can be truly independent for the first time in his or her life.

Retirement

The nature of work is changing rapidly. More people look forward to retirement at an earlier age than workers did 50 years ago. Retirement can represent a major change for people who have worked in a demanding full-time job for many years. The following problems can occur:

- There may be a feeling of loss as people no longer have the status associated with work.
- Self-concept can be affected as the person is now seen as an 'OAP'.
- There can be loss in social contact as people no longer see work colleagues on a daily basis.
- There may be a considerable drop in income.
- People feel they are no longer contributing to society.

On the positive side, many people enjoy the chance to take up hobbies they have had little time for before. They also enjoy the company of old friends and family. Retirement offers freedom from the daily routine and commitment of work.

Redundancy or unemployment

Redundancy means you are no longer needed to do the job you have been doing. As a result, you no longer have a job. Older workers may choose to give up their job when cutbacks in a workforce are needed. This is called voluntary redundancy.

If a person has been working for a company for longer than two years, he or she may get redundancy pay. Sometimes the workers are aware the company has been having a difficult time financially. The workers may therefore not find redundancy too much of a shock. On the other hand, sometimes workers have no warning at all. They are told they are no longer needed and have to leave the building immediately, without even having the chance to say goodbye to their colleagues. This can be very distressing for people.

Unemployment can be a very unpleasant experience. Men tend to find it more difficult to cope with than women because, even now, there is greater expectation that men should earn money. The person is likely to suffer from a loss of status and possibly self-respect (see Chapter 12). Unemployed people may feel depressed because they have less money than they used to. They may not know how to fill their time because they are so used to having a job to go to. They may therefore feel very bored. At a time like this, the support of family is very important.

Sometimes, being made redundant can turn out to be a good thing for a person. Because he or she no longer has a job, the person can take the opportunity to learn a new skill. He or she may decide to start his or her own business or try to make some money out of something that was previously only a hobby (e.g. selling his or her own paintings or becoming a full time gardener).

Check your knowledge

1. Explain why moving house can be a stressful life event.
2. How can the family help a child adjust to starting school?
3. How do teachers and classroom assistants help small children adjust to starting school?
4. What problems might students have at college?
5. Why are people nervous when they first start work?
6. Why do some people have difficulty adjusting to retirement?
7. What are the benefits of retirement?
8. What is redundancy?
9. How can redundancy sometimes be a positive life event?

Sources of support

Coping with life events is easier if you have other people to help you. Different types of support are available to people.

Partners, family and friends

Most people have family and friends to help them cope with life events. Family and friends can offer help and support to meet different types of needs.

Physical needs

Family and friends can provide practical help and support to meet the physical needs of someone coping with a major life event. Such support could include:

- Helping move furniture when a person moves house.
- Providing transport for a person who is disabled.

Intellectual needs

Family and friends can help people to understand the changes life events can bring. Sometimes they can offer useful advice or information to help with the change. Examples of advice and information include:

- Advice about managing money when a person moves house.
- Sharing your own experiences of grief and loss.

Emotional needs

Family and friends often give us an emotional 'safe place' to get away from stress and pressure. Friends can help us through periods of stressful change by helping us to feel we matter. Examples of emotional support include:

- Listening to one another.
- Using conversation to show we understand how other people feel.

Social needs

Friends and family create groups of people we belong to. Mixing with other people who like us is very important when we have to cope with changes in our lives. Change is easier if we can talk to and be with other people. Examples of social support include:

- Visiting friends or relatives in hospitals.
- Being able to talk to your parents about marriage, childbirth or divorce.

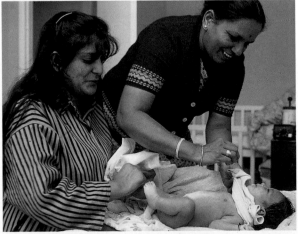

The family often provides help and support when people are in difficulties

Professional carers and services

Some people do not have close friends and family who can provide the help that is needed in the event of a change in the person's circumstances. On other occasions, the help needed is more specialist than can be provided by family and friends. For example, an elderly person with no family nearby may be widowed. As a result of his or her bereavement, the person may need help every day with meals and shopping. He or she may also need emotional support. In this case, specialist help would be needed. There are many types of help available to people who need it (see Figure 15.5). This list gives some examples of the types of help that are available: there are many other types of support available to people who need assistance.

The *local authority* is the organisation that administers help at a local level. It investigates the needs of the area and tries to provide help to meet them. The *area health authority* administers medical support services locally. The *Department for Work and Pensions*, through local offices, administers benefits such as the Job Seeker's Allowance or Working Families Tax Credit. As it can be difficult knowing where to start to ask for help, most towns have a *Citizens Advice Bureau (CAB)*. The staff will know which office or department an individual should approach for help. Alternatively, the public library usually has information to point people in the right direction to find help.

As well as providing specialised support, professional carers also help people to cope with life events by:

*   using their understanding of people and change;
*   using good listening and communication skills (see Chapter 4); and
*   working with values that respect the diversity, rights and confidentiality of the person seeking help (see Chapter 5).

Voluntary and faith-based services

Voluntary services are organised by people who often give their services for nothing. They do not make profits. Some are registered as charities (e.g. Banardo's). They may be funded by the government or by the local authority because there are always expenses such as telephone bills, heating and lighting of an office, etc. The people who use the service may be asked to pay towards the service they receive. If the person has little money, he or she may receive the help for free. Examples of voluntary services include the following:

*   Relate, which helps couples and young people who are having relationship problems.
*   MENCAP, which helps people with learning disabilities and their carers.

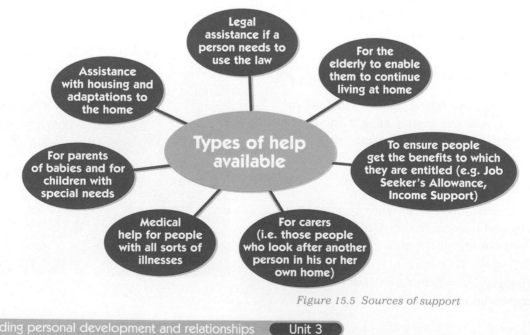

Figure 15.5 Sources of support

- Gingerbread, which helps lone-parent families with all aspects of caring for children.
- Victim Support, which visits and counsels people who have been the victims of crime.
- Help the Aged, which deals with all aspects of life for elderly people and their carers.
- The Leukaemia Care Society, which gives help and practical support for people with leukaemia and their families.

There are many other voluntary groups offering support to people in difficult situations. Many of these voluntary groups operate all over the country, with local offices where people can go to get help.

Checkpoint

A **chronic** illness is one that is not usually life threatening but for which there is no cure (e.g. diabetes or eczema).

There are support groups for most serious or chronic illnesses. These groups are particularly helpful as the people who run them often have the same medical problem themselves so they understand fully the problems other sufferers are having.

Faith-based support groups may also be run nationally or on a local basis only. They support those people of their faith who need the help they are offering. An example is the Catholic Children's Rescue Society, which provides housing help for young Catholic women who are pregnant or who have a small child. Local churches may organise befriending services for people who have recently been bereaved or for the elderly who live alone without family nearby. If the area has an ethnic community, often members will organise and run support groups for anyone in the community who needs help.

Check your knowledge

1   How do family and friends provide physical help and support to an individual?
2   How do family and friends provide emotional help and support to an individual?
3   Why do people sometimes have to seek specialist help and support?
4   Give five examples of specialist support that are available to people.
5   What type of help is provided by the Department for Work and Pensions?
6   How does the Citizen's Advice Bureau help people?
7   Give five examples of voluntary services that provide support to an individual.
8   How do faith-based support groups help people?

Assessment

Unlike Units 1 and 2, Unit 3 is assessed by a test. This section is designed to help you prepare for the test. It explains how to give answers with enough detail and knowledge to ensure you get a good mark.

In the assessment you will be asked to link all the information you have learnt about in Chapters 11–15. This will allow you to demonstrate your ability to use ideas from the five areas of the unit to comment on the personal development of the individual. You should already have had practice at doing this through the use of case studies in class.

An example of a case study is provided here. Following the case study are the kinds of questions you will be asked in the test. You should read the case study carefully. Then try to answer the questions as fully as you can and include plenty of detail.

When answering the questions always remember the following points:

- You should always try to refer to personal development in terms of PIES (physical, intellectual, emotional and social development).
- Always look to see how many marks are awarded for each question. If there is only one mark, the examiner is only looking for one idea. However, if there are three marks you will be expected to make three separate points in your answer.
- The number of lines you are given on the paper for your answer also provides guidance as to how much information is required.
- If you are asked to use ideas from the case study to support your answer, make sure you do. The case study will have been written with ideas included to enable you to do this.

When you have answered the questions as fully as you can, use the mark scheme that follows to mark your own work. Remember that in questions 2 and 5 the answers given are only a selection of possible answers. Be sure to read the analysis of answers section carefully as this will give you more information to ensure you do well in the test.

Case study

Anna

Anna is 38. She is happily married to Stephen and has two children. Her younger child has asthma.

The family has recently moved to a new area of the country due to Stephen's promotion at work.

Anna has managed to find work in a local solicitor's office. The rest of the staff have worked there for a long time but Anna is beginning to feel as though she fits in.

Eventually, she wants to have a better job, so she is doing an Open University degree in her spare time.

Now answer the following questions.

1   Identify Anna's **life stage**.   (1 mark)

2   Identify the types of **relationships** Anna has with the following people. Describe the possible **positive** and **negative** effects these relationships could have on Anna's development:
   (a) Anna's relationship with Stephen.   (5 marks)
   (b) Anna's relationship with the people at the office   (5 marks)

3   Complete the sentences below to show whether the life change is **expected** or **unexpected**:
   (a) Moving house is an example of
        an ————————————— life change   (1 mark)
   (b) Getting married is an example of
        an ————————————— life change   (1 mark)

4   Anna and Stephen have to cope with their child's asthma. Describe the types of **formal** and **informal** support Anna and Stephen can receive to help them cope.   (5 marks)

5   The **self-concept** is affected by various different factors. Describe the physical, intellectual, emotional and social factors that will affect an adult like Anna.   (12 marks)

Total: 30 marks

Mark scheme and analysis of answers

Question number	Marks	Correct answers	Analysis of answers
1	1 mark	Adulthood	Always use the correct terms to describe the life stages e.g. a person aged 11 – 18 is an adolescent not a teenager.
2(a)	1 mark to identify the relationship. 4 marks for any of the factors you have correctly identified = 5 marks	Intimate/sexual Source of support Raised confidence/self-esteem Security from their shared history Someone to share good and bad times with Able to reveal her true self Someone to share problems with May find a monogamous relationship very restricting	Again, when asked to identify a relationship, the answer will be one of the four types of relationships that you leant about in Chapter 13. If the question asks you to give positive and negative responses in your answers, you must do so or you will lose marks. When answering questions like this one, you should realise that a wide range of answers is acceptable so don't be afraid to use your imagination. The answers given are suggestions of correct answers, but other ideas could be acceptable.
2(b)	2 marks to identify the relationship 3 marks for any of the factors you have correctly identified = 5 marks	Working/friendship Source of support Source of information about the new area in which she lives Raised self-confidence as Anna makes new friends Negotiating the consequences and possible conflicts of having friends as colleagues	
3(a)	1 mark	Unexpected	
3(b)	1 mark	Expected	
4	5 marks. Answers must include at least one example of one type of support	Formal – GP/health centre Asthma sufferers support group Hospital department Pharmacy Informal – family/friends Neighbours Work colleagues	If the answer asks you for two types of support, you must include both types to get full marks for your answer.

Question number	Marks	Correct answers	Analysis of answers
5	12 marks. Must include at least one physical, intellectual, emotional and social factor for full marks. Each of the four factors named and then described earns a maximum of 3 marks	**Factors** Appearance (physical) – looking good makes you feel better about yourself Emotional development – maturity means you understand yourself better. Education (intellectual) – a good education gives self-confidence Relationships with others (social or emotional) – good relationships with colleagues help increase self-esteem. A happy marriage provides self-confidence Life experiences (social or emotional) – wider experience of life and successfully dealing with life's problems increases self-confidence. Gender (social) – what is expected of them in society. People who feel esteemed by others, have increased self-confidence Sexual orientation (social or emotional) – is the individual happy about his or her sexual orientation? Cultural (intellectual or social) – the individual should feel that his or her culture allows him or her to fit in with the society in which he or she lives	As in question 2, the answers for this question can be very varied. However, you should confine your ideas to those based broadly on the factors that affect the self-concept that you studied in Chapter 14. The answers given in the previous column are examples of correct answers. There are many other variations on these that would also be acceptable.

Index